PSYCHIATRIC NURSING

Candace De Vieira

ALLIED
HEALTH
PRESS

Psychiatric Nursing

Author: **Candace De Vieira**

Allied Health Press
4164 Lakeshore Road
Burlington ON L7L 1A4
Canada
www.alliedhealthpress.com
Email: orders@arclereducation.com

ISBN: 978-1-77956-246-3

ABOUT THE AUTHOR

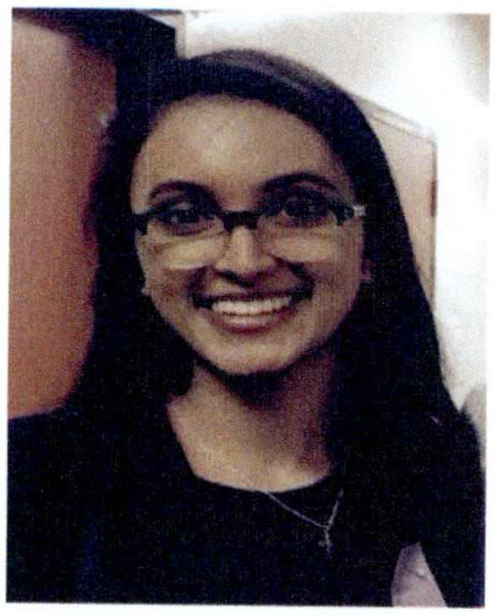

Candace De Vieira is a Board Certified Psychiatric Mental Health Nurse Practitioner who currently practices in the heart of New York City. Working diligently throughout the pandemic, she practiced as a mental health nurse while completing her graduate studies at Adelphi University to earn a master's degree in nursing. Specializing in child and adolescent psychiatry, she has worked her way up the ranks from a new graduate nurse to a nurse educator, culminating in her promotion to a Psychiatric Nurse Practitioner. Her passion has always been to work with children. Along with working in the mental health field, Candace has also practiced as a pediatric registered nurse in long term care, as well as an elementary school nurse. As a Psychiatric Nurse Practitioner, she particularly enjoys working with younger children in the diagnosis and treatment of such illnesses as DMDD and ADHD. Her desire for others to have a better understanding of mental health, and to reduce the stigma associated with mental health, have prompted her to pursue her Doctorate degree in Nursing, in order to function in both leadership and nursing research. In her free time, Candace has a strong love for singing and music, doing both while volunteering at her local church.

Word Roots, Prefixes, and Suffixes by Chapter

Chapter 1 Overview of Psychiatric–Mental Health Nursing

neur/ o/ tic having a neurosis

neur/ o/ path/ ic having a nervous disease

cata- down

dys- difficult

-kinesia movement

Chapter 2 Psychosocial Theories and Therapy

schiz/o split

Psycho- the study of the mind and behavior

Neuro- a mild mental disorder related to stress or anxiety

-phobia fear of open or public spaces

-philia love of books

Chapter 3 Therapeutic Relationships and Communication

somat/o body

Inter- occurring between people, especially in a therapeutic context

Trans- redirection of a patient's feelings for one person to the therapist

Chapter 4 Anger, Hostility, Aggression, and Violence

Bell- Belligerent (hostile, aggressive)

Mal- Malice (the intention to cause harm)

Aggress- Aggression (hostile or violent behavior)

Viol- Violence (physical force intended to hurt or damage)

Pugn- Pugnacious (eager to fight)

Chapter 5 Trauma, Anxiety, and Stressor-Related Psychiatric Disorders

Anx Refers to feelings of fear or uneasiness

psych/ o/ drama the improvised acting out of situations related to mental problems

neur/ asthenia loss of nervous strength

Chapter 6 Symptoms of Mental Illness or Emotional Problems

iatr/o treatment

ment/o mind

para- beside, beyond, separate from

Gastr- Stomach

Hist/o-, Histio- Tissue

Chapter 7 Obsessive – Compulsive, Related Disorders, and Personality Disorders

Obsess- persistent idea

Compuls- drive, urge

Ego- self

Anx- anxiety

Bio- life

-ive relating to

Chapter 8 Schizophrenia Spectrum and Other Psychotic Disorders

Catatonia tension (catatonic)

Halluc- wander in mind (hallucination)

Para- beside, abnormal (paranoia)

Affect- emotion (affective)

Cogn- know (cognitive)

-phrenia mind (schizophrenia)

Chapter 9 Mood Disorders

Cyclo- circle or cycle

Pharmaco- drug

Endo- within

Exo- outside

-algia pain

-tonia tension or tone

Table of Contents

LIST OF FIGURES

LIST OF TABLES

PREFACE

The modern healthcare system often segregates somatic and psychiatric care, leading to fragmented services for individuals with complex needs. This fragmentation can result in isolated treatments for different symptoms, overlooking the holistic nature of health, which encompasses an individual's entire life situation. Many European countries define mental health in terms of the absence of symptoms, rather than as the ability to live a fulfilling life despite symptoms, highlighting a narrow perspective on health.

This narrow view of health neglects its holistic and indivisible nature, particularly affecting those with severe mental illness (SMI). Individuals with SMI experience significant disparities in physical health, leading to increased mortality rates and a shorter life expectancy compared to the general population, often due to stigmatization and inadequate support.

While nursing science has embraced a more holistic perspective on health, nursing practice and research often overlook the positive aspects of health, such as physical, social, and mental strengths. The shift from institutional to community-based mental health services has been inconsistent across countries, leading to ongoing human rights issues for people with mental health problems.

The field of psychiatric nursing has undergone significant changes in recent years, driven by advancements in understanding mental illness, treatment innovations, societal changes, economic factors, and more informed patients and families. This evolution has also impacted the legal aspects of psychiatric nursing practice, with nurses expected to adhere to current laws and standards.

This book examines the key legal issues that influence psychiatric nursing practice in the present day, reflecting the evolving nature of mental healthcare.

The textbook "Psychiatric Nursing" provides comprehensive and up-to-date information on the principles and practices of psychiatric nursing. It covers a wide range of topics including the theoretical foundations of psychiatric nursing, assessment and diagnosis of mental health disorders, therapeutic communication, pharmacology, and evidence-based interventions. The book also addresses legal and ethical issues in psychiatric nursing, cultural considerations, and the role of the psychiatric nurse in interdisciplinary care teams.

Through a combination of theoretical knowledge and practical application, the textbook aims to enhance the reader's understanding of psychiatric nursing concepts and promote the delivery of high-quality care to individuals with mental health disorders. The book aims to serve as a valuable resource for nursing students, practicing nurses, and other healthcare professionals interested in psychiatric care. Therefore, the textbook aims to empower nurses to provide compassionate and effective care to individuals experiencing mental health challenges.

Chapter

1

OVERVIEW OF PSYCHIATRIC–MENTAL HEALTH NURSING

Contents

Introduction

Psychiatric-Mental Health Nursing (PMHN) is a specialized field within nursing that focuses on promoting mental health, preventing mental illness, and providing care and support for individuals experiencing psychiatric disorders or mental health challenges. With a rich history rooted in compassion and advocacy, PMHN encompasses a broad spectrum of roles and responsibilities aimed at addressing the complex needs of individuals across the lifespan.

At its core, PMHN emphasizes the holistic care of individuals, recognizing the intricate interplay between biological, psychological, social, and environmental factors in influencing mental health and well-being. PMHN practitioners strive to foster therapeutic relationships built on trust, empathy, and respect, empowering individuals to navigate their mental health journeys with dignity and autonomy.

The scope of PMHN practice is diverse, encompassing assessment, diagnosis, treatment planning, psychotherapy, medication management, crisis intervention, and community outreach. PMHN practitioners work in a variety of settings, including hospitals, community mental health centers, schools, correctional facilities, and private practices, collaborating with interdisciplinary teams to provide comprehensive care tailored to the unique needs of each individual.

Key components of PMHN practice include mental health promotion and prevention, early intervention, and recovery-oriented care. PMHN practitioners are skilled in assessing risk factors for mental illness, implementing evidence-based interventions to promote resilience and well-being, and supporting individuals in achieving their goals for recovery and recovery.

Furthermore, PMHN practice is guided by principles of cultural competence, trauma-informed care, and advocacy for social justice and equity. PMHN practitioners recognize the diverse backgrounds and experiences of individuals and strive to provide care that is inclusive, responsive, and affirming of individual identities and perspectives.

Psychiatric-Mental Health Nursing is a dynamic and evolving field dedicated to promoting mental health, preventing mental illness, and providing compassionate care and support for individuals experiencing psychiatric disorders or mental health challenges. With a strong emphasis on holistic, person-centered care, PMHN practitioners play a vital role in advancing the well-being and recovery of individuals, families, and communities.

Orientation and Directional Terms

Term	Definition	Illustration
Psychiatric-mental health nursing	Psychiatric-mental health nursing Psychosocial, and neurobiological expertise. PMH nurses promote well-being through prevention and education, in addition to the assessment, diagnosis, care, and treatment of mental health and substance use disorders.	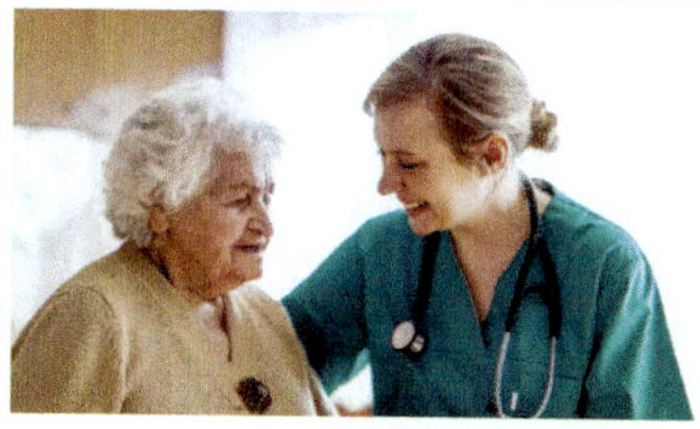
Mental health	Mental health includes our emotional, psychological, and social well-being. It affects how we think, feel, and act. It also helps determine how we handle stress, relate to others, and make healthy choices. Mental health is important at every stage of life, from childhood and adolescence through adulthood.	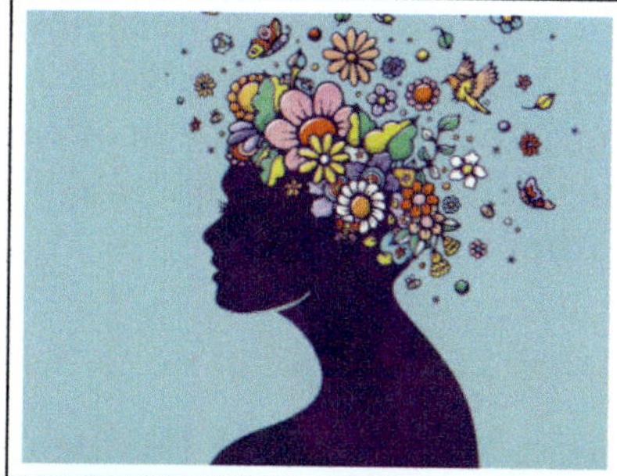
Emergency department	Emergency department, also known as an accident and emergency department, emergency room, emergency ward or casualty department, is a medical treatment facility specializing in emergency medicine, the acute care of patients who present without prior appointment; either by their own means or by that of an ambulance.	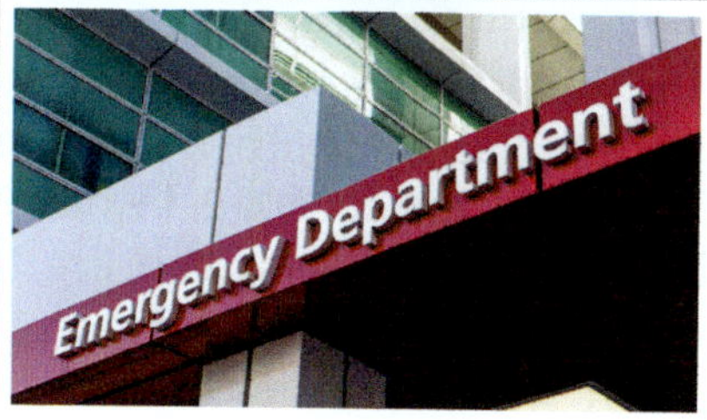
Central nervous system (CNS)	Central nervous system (CNS) is made up of the brain and spinal cord. It is part of the nervous system. The other part is the peripheral nervous system, which is made up of nerves that connect the brain and spinal cord to the rest of the body.	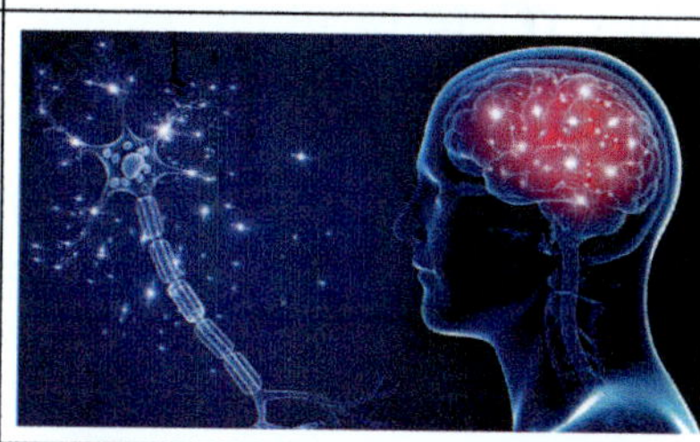
Attention-deficit/ hyperactivity disorder (ADHD)	Attention-deficit/hyperactivity disorder (ADHD) is one of the most common childhood neurodevelopmental disorders. Children with ADHD often have difficulty with inattention, hyperactivity and impulsivity. Kids usually receive a diagnosis during childhood, and the condition often lasts into adulthood. However, effective treatment is available.	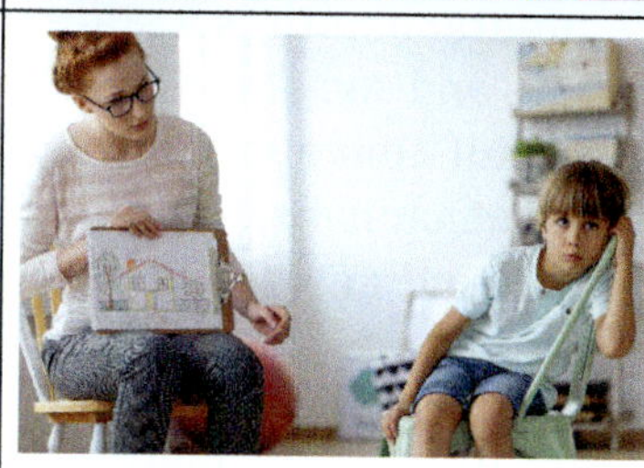

1.1. Mental Health and Mental Illness

It can be challenging to define mental health and mental illness precisely. People are seen as healthy when they can fulfill their social obligations and exhibit appropriate, adaptable behavior. On the other hand, people who act inappropriately or who are unable to perform their duties and responsibilities are seen as sick. Any society's values and beliefs are shaped by its culture, and this in turn shapes how that society views health and illness. What is considered appropriate and acceptable in one society might be considered maladaptive and inappropriate in another.

1.1.1. Mental Health

According to the World Health Organization, being healthy is more than just not being sick or disabled' it also involves total physical, mental, and social wellbeing. According to this definition, being in good health is a state of well-being. Individuals who are in a state of emotional, physical, and social well-being carry out their duties, go about their daily lives with efficiency, and are happy with who they are and how they relate to other people. There isn't one overarching definition of mental health. In general, a person's actions can reveal information about their mental state. Determining a person's mental health can be challenging because every individual can interpret behavior differently based on their values and beliefs. Generally speaking, mental health is a state of emotional, psychological, and social wellness demonstrated by positive self-concept, productive behavior and coping mechanisms, fulfilling interpersonal relationships, and emotional stability.

There are numerous components to mental health, and numerous factors impact it. A person's mental health is a dynamic, or always-changing, state as a result of these interactions. An individual's mental health is influenced by a variety of individual, interpersonal, and social/cultural factors. A person's biological make-up, autonomy and independence, self-esteem, growth potential, vitality, ability to find purpose in life, emotional toughness or resilience, sense of belonging, reality orientation, coping mechanisms, and stress management skills are examples of individual, or personal, factors. Effective communication, the capacity to assist others, intimacy, and a harmonious balance between separateness and connectedness are examples of interpersonal, or relationship, factors. A sense of belonging, the ability to obtain sufficient resources, an intolerance for violence, acceptance of individual differences, environmental mastery, and an optimistic yet grounded perspective on the world are examples of social/cultural, or environmental, factors.

1.1.2. Mental Illness

Disorders affecting mood, behavior, and thought processes, such as addiction disorders, schizophrenia, depression, and anxiety disorders, are all considered forms of mental illness. Mental illnesses frequently result in severe distress, decreased functioning, or both. People feel unhappy with themselves, their relationships, and their inadequate coping mechanisms. Everyday existence can feel oppressive or overwhelming. People could feel as though there is no hope left. It is also possible to examine mental health-related factors from an individual, interpersonal, and social/cultural perspective. Individual factors include one's biological make-up, inability to discriminate between reality and fantasy, unbearable or unrealistic worries or fears, intolerance of life's uncertainties, sense of disharmony in life, and loss of purpose in life. Ineffective communication, an overwhelming reliance on others or a retreat from relationships, a lack of a sense of community, insufficient social support, and a loss of emotional control are examples of interpersonal factors. Lack of resources, violence, homelessness, poverty, an unjustified pessimistic worldview, and discrimination—including stigma, racism, classism, ageism, and sexism—are examples of social and cultural factors. It is crucial to remember that a few of these social and cultural elements can lead to criminal, violent, or maladaptive behavior in addition to feelings of alienation and isolation. This may corroborate a personality disorder diagnosis, but it does not always indicate a mental illness whose symptoms can be managed with medicine. Healthcare professionals are always debating whether this is more likely to be caused by illness or by bad behavior, and the answers are not always obvious.

1.2. Diagnostic and Statistical Manual of Mental Disorders

The American Psychiatric Association publishes the fifth edition of the Diagnostic and Statistical Manual of Mental Disorders (DSM-5), a taxonomy that is updated as needed. Released in 2013, the current edition underwent several significant revisions. All mental disorders are covered by the DSM-5, which also provides detailed diagnostic standards based on research and clinical experience for each. This diagnostic taxonomy is used by all mental health practitioners to diagnose psychiatric disorders.

The DSM-5 has three purposes:

- To provide a standardized nomenclature and language for all mental health professionals;
- To present defining characteristics or symptoms that differentiate specific diagnoses;
- To assist in identifying the underlying causes of disorders.

The classification system allows the practitioner to identify all the factors that relate to a person's condition:

- All major psychiatric disorders such as depression, schizophrenia, anxiety, and substance-related disorders;
- Medical conditions that are potentially relevant to understanding or managing the person's mental disorder as well as medical conditions that might contribute to understanding the person;
- Psychosocial and environmental problems that may affect the diagnosis, treatment, and prognosis of mental disorders. Included are problems with the primary support group, the social environment, education, occupation, housing, economics, access to health care, and the legal system.

Although student nurses do not use the DSM-5 to diagnose clients, they will find it a helpful resource to understand the reason for the admission and to begin building knowledge about the nature of psychiatric illnesses.

1.3. Historical Perspectives of the Treatment of Mental Illness

1.3.1. Ancient Times

In the past, people thought that illness was a sign of the gods' disapproval and actually a punishment for transgressions and sins. Depending on their behavior, people with mental illnesses were perceived as either divine or demonic. People who were viewed as divine were revered and worshipped, while those who were viewed as demonic were shunned, punished, and occasionally set ablaze. Later, Aristotle (382–322 BC) developed his theory that the body's quantities of blood, water, and yellow and black bile regulated emotions to link mental illnesses to physical ailments. These four elements—also known as humors—were associated with joy, serenity, rage, and melancholy. Mental disorders were thought to be caused by imbalances in the four humors, so bloodletting, starvation, and purging were used as therapeutic methods to bring the humors back into balance. These "treatments" continued well into the 1800s (Baly, 1982). There were many strong superstitions and archaic beliefs in the early Christian era (1–1000 AD). Once more, mental health patients were seen as possessed, and all illnesses were attributed to demons. Exorcisms were performed by priests to purge patients of evil spirits. When that didn't work, they resorted to harsher tactics like starvation, flogging, and dungeon confinement.

During the English Renaissance (1300–1600), criminals and those suffering from mental illness were separated. The more "dangerous lunatics" were imprisoned, chained, and starved, while those deemed harmless were permitted to roam the countryside or reside in rural communities (Rosenblatt, 1984). 1547 saw the opening of St. The first-ever hospital for the insane was formally established at Mary of Bethlehem. By 1775, entry to the facility required payment to observe and make fun of the prisoners, who were regarded as less than human animals (McMillan, 1997). The mentally ill were punished during this time because they were seen as evil or possessed in the colonies, which would later become the United States. Offenders were burned at the stake during witch hunts.

1.3.2. Period of Enlightenment and Creation of Mental Institutions

A period of enlightenment about people with mental illness started in the 1790s. The idea of asylum was developed by William Tuke in England and Philippe Pinel in France. It refers to safe havens or refuges where individuals who were mentally ill were not starved, beaten, or whipped (Gollaher, 1995). The ethical treatment of mentally ill people started with this movement. Following a visit to Tuke's institution in England, Dorothea Dix (1802–1887) launched a campaign to reform mental health treatment in the United States. She played a key role in the establishment of 32 state hospitals that provided asylum to the afflicted. Dix promoted appropriate housing, wholesome food, and warm clothing because she felt that society had a duty to care for people who were mentally ill (Gollaher, 1995). The Age of Enlightenment was not long in coming. State hospitals faced difficulties just a century after the first asylum was established. The phrase "insane asylum" gained negative connotation, hospital locations in rural areas were perceived as isolating patients from their families and homes, and attendants were accused of abusing the patients.

1.3.3. Sigmund Freud and Treatment of Mental Disorders

Beginning with Sigmund Freud (1856–1939) and others like Emil Kraepelin (1856–1926) and Eugen Bleuler (1857–1939), the scientific study and treatment of mental disorders began. These men marked the beginning of the discipline of psychiatry as well as the diagnosis and treatment of mental illness. Freud urged society to adopt an impartial perspective on people. In a way never seen before, he studied the mind, its disorders, and how to treat them. Many other theorists expanded on Freud's groundbreaking research by having Kraepelin categorize mental illnesses based on their symptoms, and Bleuler was the one who first used the term schizophrenia.

1.3.4. Development of Psychopharmacology

The discovery of psychotropic medications, or medications used to treat mental illness, around 1950 marked the beginning of a significant advancement in the treatment of mental illness. The first medications to be created were lithium, an antimanic, and chlorpromazine (Thorazine), an antipsychotic. In the ensuing ten years, tricyclic antidepressants, antipsychotics such as haloperidol (Haldol), antianxiety drugs known as benzodiazepines, and monoamine oxidase inhibitor antidepressants were all introduced. For the first time, medication genuinely lessened depression, agitation, and psychotic thoughts. Shorter hospital stays resulted in many patients feeling well enough to return home. In the hospital setting, there was a significant decrease in the amount of chaos, violence, and noise.

1.3.5. Move Toward Community Mental Health

The Community Mental Health Centers Construction Act, passed in 1963, gave rise to a movement that favored treating mentally ill people in less restrictive settings. Deinstitutionalization, the planned transition of care from state hospitals to community settings, started. Community mental health centers offered less restrictive treatment in smaller geographic catchment areas that were closer to the homes, families, and friends of their clients. These facilities offered screening services, education, emergency care, inpatient care, outpatient care, and partial hospitalization. Deinstitutionalization therefore resulted in the discharge of people from lengthy stays in public facilities, a decline in hospital admissions, and the growth of community-based services as an alternative to medical care in hospitals.

Federal legislation was passed to give disabled people an income in addition to deinstitutionalization: Social Security disability income (SSDI) and supplemental security income (SSI). This made it possible for those suffering from severe and chronic mental illness to become more financially independent and to live independently of their families. Because this program was federally funded, states were able to spend less on the care of the mentally ill than they had when these people were in state hospitals. Additionally, in the early 1970s, laws about commitments were modified, making it more difficult to commit patients against their will for mental health treatment. This further reduced the number of patients in state hospitals and, as a result, the amount of money that states had to spend on them.

1.4. Mental Illness in the 21st Century

The National Institutes of Health (2018) estimates that 44.7 million Americans suffer from a mental illness, but only 19.2 million of them have received treatment in the previous year. The age range of 18 to 25 exhibited the highest frequency of mental illness and the lowest percentage of individuals undergoing treatment. Additionally, an estimated 4 million children and adolescents and 15 million adults experience significant emotional disturbances or mental illness that interfere with their day-to-day functioning. For instance, 3–5% of children in school age have attention-deficit/hyperactivity disorder. More than 10 million children under the age of seven live in households where at least one parent abuses drugs or has a serious mental illness, which makes it difficult for these kids to be ready for school. The combined financial burden of mental illness in the US—including medical expenses and lost productivity—is greater than the total economic burden of cancer. For those between the ages of 15 and 44 in the US and Canada, mental illnesses are the main cause of disability. However, only one in four adults and one in five kids and teenagers in need of mental health services receive the assistance they require.

Deinstitutionalization, according to some, has both beneficial and bad effects. Deinstitutionalization resulted in an 80% decrease in the number of public hospital beds' however, admissions to those beds increased by 90%. This research gave rise to the phrase "revolving door effect.". Individuals with severe and persistent mental illness are admitted to hospitals more frequently, despite having shorter hospital stays. The psychiatric units of general hospitals are quickly overloaded with the constant stream of patients being admitted and released. The number of people visiting emergency departments (EDs) for acutely disturbed individuals has increased by 400–500% in certain cities. Patients are frequently admitted to the emergency department (ED) and kept there until a bed becomes available for them to stay in or until the crisis resolves. Some people believe that there is a rise in suicide as a result of the boarding practice, which also irritates medical staff and leaves clients and their families feeling uncared for. In addition to better meeting client needs, having a sufficient number of psychiatric inpatient beds may even reduce violence, homelessness, and incarceration.

Recurring hospital admissions more frequently are made more difficult by shorter unplanned hospital stays. Even though they may not stabilize in a few days, people with severe and persistent mental illness may show signs of improvement. As a result, they are released into the community without the necessary skills to fit in. On the other hand, prearranged or scheduled brief hospital stays may help address this problem as they do not add to the revolving door phenomenon. Rehospitalization and decompensation are often the outcome. Furthermore, a lot of people struggle with both substance abuse and severe mental illness. Drug and alcohol abuse aggravates mental illness symptoms, which increases the likelihood of rehospitalization. In the current managed care setting, substance abuse problems cannot be addressed in the 3–5 days that are usually allocated for admissions.

In the United States today, 610,000 people—including 140,000 children—are homeless on any given night, making it a serious problem. Of those who are homeless, 257,300 people (or 33%) suffer from a severe mental illness or a long-term drug use problem. There are 110,000 people who are classified as chronically homeless' of them, 30% have a mental health disorder, and two-thirds have a primary substance abuse problem or another chronic health condition (Treatment Advocacy Center, 2019). Homeless and mentally ill people can be found in parks, bus and airport terminals, stairwells and alleys, prisons, and other public areas. Some seek refuge in halfway houses, shelters, or board and care facilities' others, who can afford it, book inexpensive hotel rooms. For many people with mental illness who end up on the streets, homelessness exacerbates their psychiatric issues, creating a vicious cycle.

A large number of issues facing mentally ill people who are homeless and those who come and go from psychiatric hospitals are caused by a dearth of sufficient community resources. States have not used the money they saved by closing state hospitals to fund community services and initiatives. The majority of funds allocated to mental health in the US are still used for inpatient psychiatric treatment' as a result, community mental health has never received the support system necessary to be successful. Effective community mental health services also need to be available, tailored to the needs of each individual, and culturally sensitive.

1.4.1. Objectives for the Future

More people than ever before are receiving treatment for mental illness. However, a sizable portion of the population remains untreated, notably, those who are homeless, incarcerated, or suffer from both mental illness and substance abuse. These kinds of statistics support the Healthy People 2020 mental health objectives put forth by the U.S. The Department of Human Resources. These goals were redesigned in January 2000 and January 2010 to improve the number of individuals who are identified, diagnosed, treated, and assisted in leading healthier lives. They were first created as Healthy People 2000. The goals also include lowering the suicide and homelessness rates, increasing employment rates for people with severe mental illnesses, and expanding the services available to adults and juveniles who are detained and suffering from mental health issues. For Healthy People 2030, a framework has been created and will be accessible in 2020.

Healthy People 2020 Mental Health Objectives:

- Reduce the suicide rate.
- Reduce suicide attempts by adolescents.
- Reduce the proportion of adolescents who engage in disordered eating behaviors in an attempt to control their weight.
- Reduce the proportion of persons who experience major depressive episode.
- Increase the proportion of primary care facilities that provide mental health treatment onsite or by paid referral.
- Increase the proportion of juvenile residential facilities that screen admissions for mental health problems.
- Increase the proportion of persons with serious mental illness who are employed.
- Increase the proportion of adults with mental health disorders who receive treatment.
- Increase the proportions of persons with co-occurring substance abuse and mental disorders who receive treatment for both disorders.
- Increase depression screening by primary care providers.
- Increase the number of homeless adults with mental health problems who receive mental health services.

1.4.2. Community-Based Care

The 2,000 community mental health centers that were planned to be constructed by 1980 had not been completed by the time of deinstitutionalization. Just 1,300 programs offered different kinds of psychosocial rehabilitation services by 1990. Community mental health centers either disregarded or provided inadequate care for individuals with severe and chronic mental illness. This implied that a large number of the general population's unmet needs were and still are those of people in need of services. Approximately half of all people with severe mental illness have not received any kind of treatment in the past 12 months, according to the Treatment Advocacy Center (2018). Individuals who have mild or minor mental illnesses are more likely to receive treatment, whereas those who have severe and long-lasting mental illnesses are less likely to do so. Consequences of nontreatment are cited by the Treatment Advocacy Center (2018) as:

- Homelessness;
- Psychiatric boarding;
- Arrest;
- Incarceration;
- Victimization;
- Suicidality;
- Familial violence;
- Danger to other.

Programs for community support services were created to address the needs of people with mental illness who were not housed in an institution. Along with symptom management and medication, these programs emphasize education, socialization, vocational needs, and rehabilitation. States, counties, and certain private organizations pay for these services. As a result, there are regional differences in the quantity and quality of services offered across the nation. For instance, there might be fewer people in need of mental health services and less funding available in rural areas. Despite having larger budgets, large metropolitan areas also have thousands of people in need of services' rarely is there enough money to cover all of the population's needs.

It was not well anticipated by the community-based system how much support individuals with severe and chronic mental illness would require. A 1:1 staff-to-client ratio is often necessary because teaching clients the skills they need to live independently in the community is time-consuming and labor-intensive. Many clients lack these skills. Additionally, learning these skills is made more challenging by the nature of some mental illnesses. For instance, a client experiencing hallucinations or "hearing voices" may find it difficult to follow directions or pay attention. Some clients have abrupt mood swings' they may find it impossible to get out of bed one day and then struggle to focus or pay attention the next few days. Community-based programs have advantages over inpatient treatment for many mental health patients, even with the system's shortcomings. In contrast to institutions, clients are able to stay in their communities, stay in touch with friends and family, and enjoy their personal freedom. Along with practical everyday living skills like cooking and shopping, people in institutions frequently lose hope and motivation. Treatment in the community will therefore continue to be a trend.

1.4.3. Cost Containment and Managed Care

In the US, the cost of Healthcare skyrocketed during the 1970s and 1980s. The goal of managed care is to intentionally regulate the relationship between the cost and quality of care received. People receive care in a managed care system according to need rather than wish. The people who evaluate the need for care are employed by the organization that is providing it. Health maintenance organizations, which were successful in certain areas with healthier populations of people, were the forerunners of managed care in the early 1970s.

To control the use of insurance funds, managed care organizations and utilization review firms created a new type of managed care in the 1990s that required providers to obtain approval before providing care. An attempt to deliver essential services while controlling costs was made possible by case management, also known as case-by-case care management. A case manager is assigned to each client, who is responsible for arranging for all forms of care the client may require. The idea behind this strategy is to reduce fragmented care from multiple sources, get rid of unnecessary service overlap, give care in the least restrictive setting possible, and save money for insurance companies. Actually, costs are frequently kept to a minimum by refusing services that are judged unnecessary or by replacing more costly medical care—like hospital stays—with less costly alternatives.

Because psychiatric disorders are long-term in nature, their treatment is expensive. The cost of a single, brief hospital stay can range from $20,000 to $30,000. There are also fewer reliable indicators of health or disease. For instance, a clinician dealing with a suicidal patient must trust the patient's report of suicidality' suicidal thoughts cannot be detected by lab testing or other diagnostic procedures. Insurance coverage for mental Healthcare differs from that for physical health care' specific annual maximums or allotted days of hospital stay are frequently in place. When the limits of private insurance are reached, treatment is paid for with state funds. State funding for mental health services becomes less available as states face financial challenges.

Behavioral Healthcare organizations under private ownership are responsible for managing mental health services, both in terms of providing services and controlling costs. Individuals who don't have access to private insurance must rely on their home counties to provide the money through taxes. The demand for these services and the funding necessary to provide them frequently far outpaces supply. Furthermore, a large number of people who suffer from mental illness refuse to receive treatment. Many times, these people are imprisoned or homeless. Getting everyone who needs treatment to receive it effectively and finding the money to pay for it are two of the biggest challenges facing society in the future.

Medicare and Medicaid are two insurance programs that are managed by the Healthcare Finance Administration. Medicare provides coverage to individuals 65 years of age or older, those with chronic kidney disease, and those with specific disabilities. Medicaid is a program for low-income individuals and families that is jointly funded by the federal and state governments. Medicaid is state-specific' each state sets its own eligibility requirements, service scope, and service payment rate. Medicaid covers recipients of SSI and SSDI until they turn 65, except a 24-month period during which recipients of SSDI are not eligible. On the other hand, SSI recipients are qualified right away. Regretfully, not all disabled individuals apply for disability benefits, and not all applicants are granted benefits. Thus, many individuals who suffer from severe and ongoing mental illness receive no benefits at all.

Mental health parity, or equality in insurance coverage for both physical and mental illnesses, is another funding concern. Insurance companies used to have spending limits on treatment for mental illness and drug addiction. Certain policies imposed an annual treatment dollar cap, while others restricted the number of days covered annually or throughout the insured person's life (as defined by the policy). The Mental Health Parity Act, passed by Congress in 1996, eliminated lifetime and annual dollar caps on mental Healthcare for employers with more than 50 employees. Substance abuse was exempt from this law, though, and businesses were still allowed to set annual caps on the number of hospital days and clinic visits. As a result, parity was not truly present. Furthermore, some insurers decide not to offer any mental health coverage, which removes the requirement for parity because parity is only necessary if mental health is covered. (American Nurses Association, 2014' Virani et al., 2017)

1.5. Psychiatric Nursing Practice

Linda Richards received her diploma from Boston's New England Hospital for Women and Children in 1873. She went on to develop educational initiatives in Illinois state-based mental hospitals and enhance nursing care in psychiatric hospitals. Because of her belief that "the mentally sick should be at least as well cared for as the physically sick," Richards is regarded as the first American psychiatric nurse.

Nurses were first trained to care for patients with mental illness at McLean Hospital in Belmont, Massachusetts, in 1882. The primary focus of custodial care was exercise, diet, and cleanliness. Nurses provided clients with psychiatric disorders with compassionate and tolerant care, adapting medical-surgical principles to their needs. With the development of somatic therapies for the treatment of mental disorders, the role of psychiatric nurses grew. Nurses had to use their medical-surgical skills more extensively for treatments like insulin shock therapy (1935), psychosurgery (1936), and electroconvulsive therapy (1937).

Nursing Mental Diseases, written by Harriet Bailey, was the first textbook for psychiatric nurses and was released in 1920. The first nursing school to offer a psychiatric nursing course was Johns Hopkins, which opened its doors in 1913. The National League for Nursing, which accredits nursing programs, did not mandate that schools include psychiatric nursing experience until 1950. Hildegard Peplau and June Mellow, two pioneering nursing theorists, influenced the field of psychiatric nursing practice. Interpersonal Relations in Nursing and Interpersonal Techniques: The Crux of Psychiatric Nursing were published by Peplau in 1952 and 1962, respectively. She wrote extensively about anxiety and detailed the phases and tasks of the therapeutic nurse-client relationship. The key component of her beliefs, the interpersonal dimension, serves as the basis for modern practice.

Mellow outlined her strategy of concentrating on clients' psychosocial needs and strengths in her 1968 book, Nursing Therapy. According to Mellow (1986), a nurse who practices therapy is especially qualified to work with patients who have serious mental illness in the context of their daily lives, emphasizing on the present moment to address each patient's psychosocial needs. The fields of psychiatric nursing benefited greatly from the contributions of Mellow and Peplau. Standards of care are created by the American Nurses Association (ANA) and are updated as necessary. Professional associations have established authoritative statements known as standards of care that outline the duties that nurses are responsible for fulfilling. They are not enforceable unless they are included in state board rules and regulations or the State Nurse Practice Act. These professional standards are used to identify safe and acceptable practices and evaluate the caliber of care in the event of legal issues or lawsuits. Specialty areas create standards for practice based on these standards.

The American Psychiatric Nurses Association (APNA) has standards of practice and standards of professional performance. These also outline the areas of practice and phenomena of concern for today's psychiatric–mental health nurse. The phenomena of concern describe the 13 areas of concern that mental health nurses focus on when caring for clients. The standards of care incorporate the phases of the nursing process, including specific types of interventions for nurses in psychiatric settings. They also outline standards for professional performance, quality of care, performance appraisal, education, collegiality, ethics, collaboration, research, and resource utilization.

Phenomena of concern for psychiatric–mental health nurses include:

- Promotion of optimal mental and physical health and well-being and prevention of mental illness;
- Impaired ability to function related to psychiatric, emotional, and physiologic distress;
- Alterations in thinking, perceiving, and communicating because of psychiatric disorders or mental health problems;
- Behaviors and mental states that indicate potential danger to self or others;
- Emotional stress related to illness, pain, disability, and loss;

- Symptom management, side effects, or toxicities associated with self-administered drugs, psychopharmacologic intervention, and other treatment modalities;
- The barriers to treatment efficacy and recovery posed by alcohol and substance abuse and dependence;
- Self-concept and body image changes, developmental issues, life process changes, and end-of-life issues;
- Physical symptoms that occur along with altered psychological status;
- Psychological symptoms that occur along with altered physiologic status;
- Interpersonal, organizational, sociocultural, spiritual, or environmental circumstances or events that have an effect on the mental and emotional well-being of the individual and family or community;
- Elements of recovery, including the ability to maintain housing, employment, and social support, that help individuals reengage in seeking meaningful lives;
- Societal factors such as violence, poverty, and substance abuse.

Areas of Practice

- Basic-Level Functions:
    - Counseling;
    - Interventions and communication techniques;
    - Problem-solving;
    - Crisis intervention;
    - Stress management;
    - Behavior modification.
- Milieu Therapy:
    - Maintain therapeutic environment;
    - Teach Skills;
    - Encourage communication between clients and others;
    - Promote growth through role modeling.
- Self-care Activities:
    - Encourage independence;
    - Increase self-esteem;
    - Improve function and health.
- Psychobiologic Interventions:
    - Administer medications;
    - Teach;
    - Observe.
- Health Teaching
- Case Management
- Health Promotion and Maintenance
- Advanced-Level Functions
    - Psychotherapy;
    - Prescriptive authority for drugs (in many states);
    - Consultation and liaison;
    - Evaluation;
    - Program development and management;
    - Clinical supervision.

1.6. Neurobiologic Theories and Psychopharmacology

Even though there is still much to learn about the causes of mental illness, science has made significant progress in the last 30 years in explaining how the brain functions and offering potential explanations for why some brains function differently than others.

These developments in neurobiologic research are having a significant impact on clinical practice and are constantly adding to the body of knowledge in the field of psychiatry. The psychiatric-mental health nurse needs to be somewhat knowledgeable about the current theories surrounding mental illness as well as the fundamentals of brain function. A summary of the main anatomical components of the nervous system and the neurotransmission process, which describes how they function. It outlines the main neurobiologic theories that are currently being proposed to explain mental illness, including those involving stress and the immune system, genetics and heredity, and infectious agents.

These neurobiologic theories are relevant to psychopharmacology, the use of drugs to treat mental illness. These drugs have a direct impact on the central nervous system (CNS), which in turn influences emotions, thought processes, behavior, and perceptions. The five types of medications used to treat mental illness are covered in this chapter, along with information on their mechanisms of action, adverse effects, and the roles that nurses play in client education and administration. While many psychiatric disorders can only be effectively treated with pharmaceutical interventions, adjunctive therapies like family therapy, psychotherapy, and cognitive and behavioral therapies can significantly improve treatment outcomes for patients. (American Nurses Association, 2014' Virani et al., 2017)

1.7. The Nervous System and How It Works

1.7.1. Central Nervous System

The brain, spinal cord, and related nerves that regulate voluntary movements make up the central nervous system (CNS). The brain stem, limbic system, cerebellum, and cerebrum make up the structural components of the brain. The locations of brain structures are displayed in Figures 1.1 and 1.2.

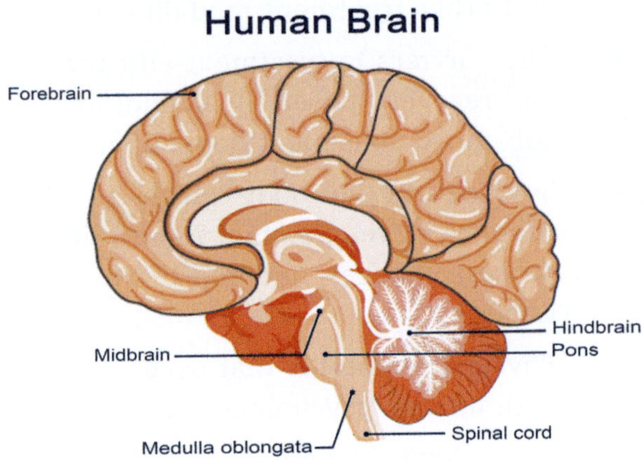

Figure 1.1. *Anatomy of the brain.*

Source: https://media.geeksforgeeks.org/wp-content/uploads/20231011151200/Human-Brain.png.

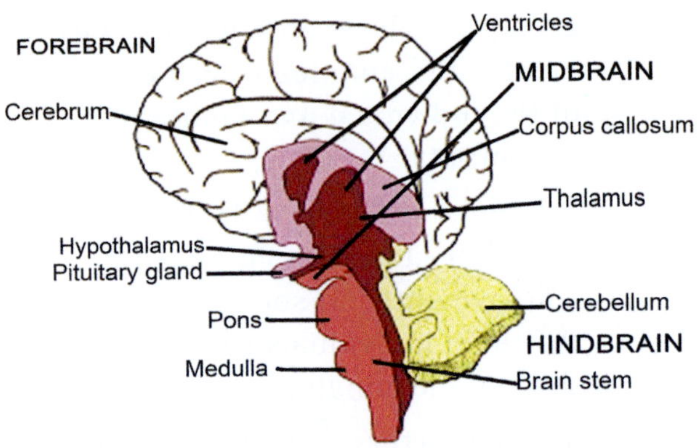

Figure 1.2. *The brain and its structures.*

Source: https://nbia.ca/wp-content/uploads/2014/03/brain-structure1-300x190.jpg.

1.7.1.1. Cerebrum

The pineal body, or gland, is situated between the two hemispheres of the cerebrum, while all other lobes and structures are present in both halves. An endocrine gland, the pineal body affects the function of the pituitary, islets of

Langerhans, parathyroid, adrenal, and gonad glands. The pathway that connects and coordinates the two hemispheres' functions is known as the corpus callosum. The left hemisphere is responsible for the regulation of the right side of the body and serves as the hub for analytical processes like reading, writing, and math. The left side of the body is under the control of the right hemisphere, which also houses the creative, intuitive, and artistic centers. The frontal, parietal, temporal, and occipital lobes comprise the four cerebral hemispheres. While some lobe functions are integrated, others are distinct. The organization of thought, movement, memories, emotions, and moral behavior is governed by the frontal lobes. The integration of all of this data facilitates problem-solving and decision-making while regulating arousal and focusing attention. There is a correlation between dementia, attention-deficit/hyperactivity disorder (ADHD), and schizophrenia with abnormalities in the frontal lobes. The parietal lobes aid in spatial orientation and interpret touch and taste sensations. The senses of smell, hearing, memory, and emotional expression are all centered in the temporal lobes. The coordination of language production and visual interpretation, including depth perception, is aided by the occipital lobes.

1.7.1.2. Cerebellum

The cerebellum, which sits beneath the cerebrum, is where postural corrections and movement coordination are centralized. It gathers and processes data from every part of the body, including the muscles, joints, organs, and other CNS components. Studies have indicated that disorders like Parkinson's disease and dementia are linked to impaired smooth coordinated movements due to neurotransmitter dopamine transmission inhibition in this region.

1.7.1.3. Brain Stem

The midbrain, pons, medulla oblongata, and the nuclei of cranial nerves III through XII are all part of the brain stem. The medulla, situated at the apex of the spinal cord, houses critical centers related to breathing and heart activity. The pons, which functions as a primary motor pathway, bridges the anatomical and functional gap located above the medulla and in front of the cerebrum. The cerebellum and pons are connected to the cerebrum by the midbrain. Its length is just 0 point 8 in (2 cm), and it contains the majority of the extrapyramidal and reticular activating systems. The reticular activating system affects awareness, consciousness, motor function, and sleep. The brain communicates with the spinal nerves regarding movement and coordination through the extrapyramidal system. The brain stem's locus coeruleus, a tiny cluster of norepinephrine-producing neurons, is linked to impulsive behavior, stress, and anxiety.

1.7.1.4. Limbic System

The limbic system comprises the thalamus, hypothalamus, hippocampus, and amygdala. It is situated above the brain stem, though some sources have different information about which structures are part of this system. The thalamus controls emotion, sensation, and activity. The hypothalamus is involved in the regulation of body temperature, appetite, hormones, sexual drive, and impulsive behavior that is linked to emotions of rage, excitement, or anger. Memory and emotional arousal are processes mediated by the amygdala and hippocampus. Several mental diseases, including dementia's memory loss and manic or psychotic behavior's poorly regulated emotions and impulses, have been linked to limbic system disturbances.

1.7.2. Neurotransmitters

Neurons, or nerve cells, are grouped together in networks by about 100 billion brain cells. Through a process known as neurotransmission, these neurons exchange information with one another by sending electrochemical signals from one neuron to another. The dendrites, which are projections from the cell body, transmit these electrical signals to the dendrites of the subsequent neuron via the soma, or cell body, the axon, which are long, extended structures, and the synapses, which are gaps between cells. In the nervous system, unique chemical messengers known as neurotransmitters facilitate the electrochemical messages that travel across the synapses between neural cells. The chemicals produced by the neuron that help with information transfer throughout the body are called neurotransmitters. They either inhibit or halt an activity in the cells (inhibitory) or excite or stimulate an activity in the cells (excitatory). Like a particular key shape fits into a lock, these neurotransmitters fit into specific receptor cells embedded in the dendritic membrane. Neurotransmitters are either carried back from the synapse to the axon to be stored for later use (reuptake) or metabolized and inactivated by enzymes, mainly monoamine oxidase (MAO), after they are released into the synapse and transmit the message to the receptor cells (Figure 1.3).

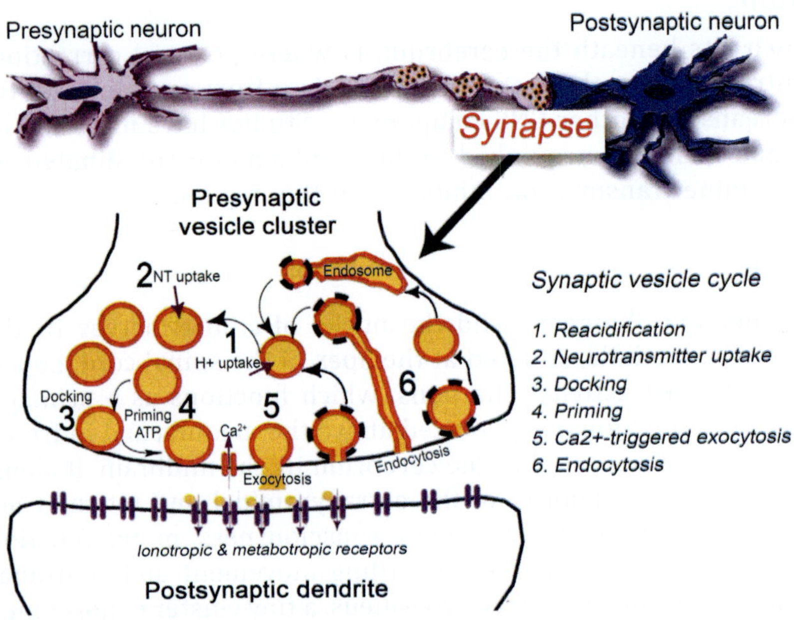

Figure 1.3. *Schematic illustration of (1) neurotransmitter (T) release' (2) binding of transmitter to postsynaptic receptor' termination of transmitter action by (3a) reuptake of transmitter into the presynaptic terminal, (3b) enzymatic degradation, or (3c) diffusion away from the synapse' and (4) binding of transmitter to presynaptic receptors for feedback regulation of transmitter release.*

Source: https://ars.els-cdn.com/content/image/3-s2.0-B9780123694379500104-f06-01-9780123694379.jpg.

The precise ratios of these neurotransmitters are required for message transmission across synapses. Research is starting to reveal variations in the concentration of specific neurotransmitters between the brains of individuals with specific mental illnesses and those without any symptoms of mental illness (Figure 1.4).

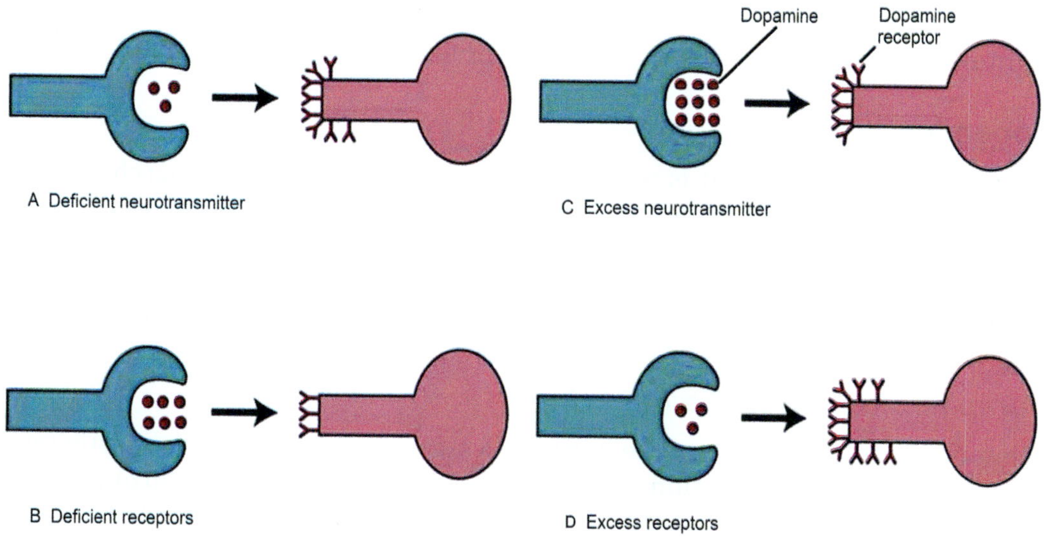

Figure 1.4. *Abnormal neurotransmission causing some mental disorders because of excess transmission or excess responsiveness of receptors.*

Source: Sheila L. Videbeck, Psychiatric-Mental Health Nursing, ISBN-10: 1-975116-37-2.

Table 1.1. *Major Neurotransmitters*

Type	Mechanism of Action	Physiologic Effects
Dopamine	Excitatory	Controls complex movements, motivation, cognition; regulates emotional response
Norepinephrine (noradrenaline)	Excitatory	Causes changes in attention, learning and memory, sleep and wakefulness, mood
Epinephrine (adrenaline)	Excitatory	Controls fight or flight response
Serotonin	Inhibitory	Controls food intake, sleep and wakefulness, temperature regulation, pain control, sexual behaviors, regulation of emotions
Histamine	Neuromodulator	Controls alertness, gastric secretions, cardiac stimulation, peripheral allergic responses
Acetylcholine	Excitatory or inhibitory	Controls sleep and wakefulness cycle; signals muscles to become alert
Neuropeptides	Neuromodulators	Enhance, prolong, inhibit, or limit the effects of principal neurotransmitters
Glutamate	Excitatory	Results in neurotoxicity if levels are too high
γ-Aminobutyric acid	Inhibitory	Modulates other neurotransmitters

Source: Sheila L. Videbeck, Psychiatric-Mental Health Nursing, ISBN-10: 1-975116-37-2.

It has been discovered that major neurotransmitters influence both the actions and adverse effects of psychotropic medications as well as mental disorders. The primary neurotransmitters, along with their effects and actions, are listed in Table 1.1. The most research has been done on dopamine and serotonin in relation to the diagnosis and treatment of mental illnesses. The main neurotransmitters linked to mental illnesses are covered in the sections that follow.

1.7.2.1. Dopamine

Dopamine is a neurotransmitter that is mostly found in the brain stem. Research has shown that dopamine regulates emotional responses, motivation, and complicated movements. It is made from the amino acid tyrosine, which is found in food, and is typically excitatory. Parkinson's disease and other psychoses, as well as movement disorders, are associated with dopamine. Antipsychotic drugs function by lowering dopamine activity and blocking dopamine receptors.

1.7.2.2. Norepinephrine and Epinephrine

The most common neurotransmitter in the nervous system, norepinephrine is mostly found in the brain stem and affects mood regulation, sleep and wakefulness patterns, learning and memory, attention, and wakefulness. Adrenaline and norepinephrine are other names for norepinephrine and its derivative, epinephrine, respectively. Several anxiety disorders have been linked to excess norepinephrine' deficiencies in this hormone may also be linked to depression, social disengagement, and memory loss. While some antidepressants prevent MAO from metabolizing norepinephrine, others block its reuptake. Although epinephrine is only found in small amounts in the brain, it regulates the peripheral nervous system's fight-or-flight response.

1.7.2.3. Serotonin

Tryptophan is a dietary amino acid that is converted into serotonin. Serotonin primarily has inhibitory effects and is involved in temperature regulation, sexual behavior, sleep and wakefulness, appetite control, and emotion regulation. Serotonin is involved in schizophrenia, anxiety, and mood disorders. It has been discovered to play a role in the withdrawn demeanor, hallucinations, and delusions associated with schizophrenia. Certain antidepressants prevent serotonin from being reabsorbed, which prolongs its half-life in the synapses and elevates mood.

1.7.2.4. Histamine

Research is being done on the function of histamine in mental illness. It plays a role in cardiac stimulation, regulation of stomach secretions, peripheral allergy reactions, and alertness. Certain psychotropic medications block histamine, which can cause drowsiness, hypotension, and weight gain.

1.7.2.5. Acetylcholine

The brain, spinal cord, and peripheral nervous system all contain the neurotransmitter acetylcholine, which is especially present at the neuromuscular junction of skeletal muscle. It could be inhibitory or excitatory. It is produced by the body from dietary choline, which is present in vegetables and red meat. It has been shown to have an impact on the sleep-wake cycle and to activate muscles. Research has indicated that individuals suffering from Alzheimer's disease have fewer neurons that secrete acetylcholine, while those with myasthenia gravis—a disorder affecting the muscles that results in muscle weakness due to impulses failing to cross the myoneural junction—have fewer acetylcholine receptors.

1.7.2.6. Glutamate

Glutamate is an excitatory amino acid that can have major neurotoxic effects at high levels. It has been implicated in the brain damage caused by stroke, hypoglycemia, sustained hypoxia or ischemia, and some degenerative diseases such as Huntington's or Alzheimer's.

1.7.2.7. Gamma-Aminobutyric Acid

The main inhibitory neurotransmitter in the brain is gamma-aminobutyric acid, also known as GABA. Rather than acting as a direct stimulus, it has been observed that GABA affects other neurotransmitter systems. Benzodiazepines and other drugs that boost GABA function are used to treat anxiety and promote sleep.

1.8. Brain Imaging Techniques

The only methods available to study the brain in the past were autopsies and surgery. But over the last 25 years, a number of brain imaging methods have been developed that make it possible to see the structure and functionality of the brain. These methods have assisted in linking particular brain regions to particular functions and are helpful in the diagnosis of certain brain disorders. Research to determine the causes of mental illnesses can also benefit from the use of brain imaging techniques. Table 1.2 lists and contrasts a number of these diagnostic methods.

Table 1.2. *Brain Imaging Technology*

Procedure	Imaging Method	Results	Duration
Computed tomography (CT)	Serial x-rays of brain	Structural image	20–40 minutes
Magnetic resonance imaging (MRI)	Radio waves from brain detected from magnet	Structural image	45 minutes
Positron emission tomography (PET)	Radioactive tracer injected into bloodstream and monitored as client performs activities	Functional	2–3 hours
Single-photon emission computed tomography (SPECT)	Same as PET	Functional	1–2 hours

Source: Sheila L. Videbeck, Psychiatric-Mental Health Nursing, ISBN-10: 1-975116-37-2.

1.8.1. Types of Brain Imaging Techniques

A precise x-ray beam is used in computed tomography (CT), also known as computed axial tomography, to create cross-sectional images (slices) layer by layer. In addition to storing the images on magnetic tape or film, a computer reconstructs the images on a monitor. Because CT can see the soft tissues of the brain, it is used to measure the size of the brain's ventricles and to diagnose primary tumors, metastases, and effusions. It has been observed that some individuals with schizophrenia have enlarged ventricles' this finding is linked to a worse prognosis and pronounced negative symptoms (Figure 1.5). During a CT scan, the patient must remain still on a table that resembles a stretcher for 20 to 40 minutes while the stretcher travels through a "ring" that resembles a tunnel to capture multiplex images.

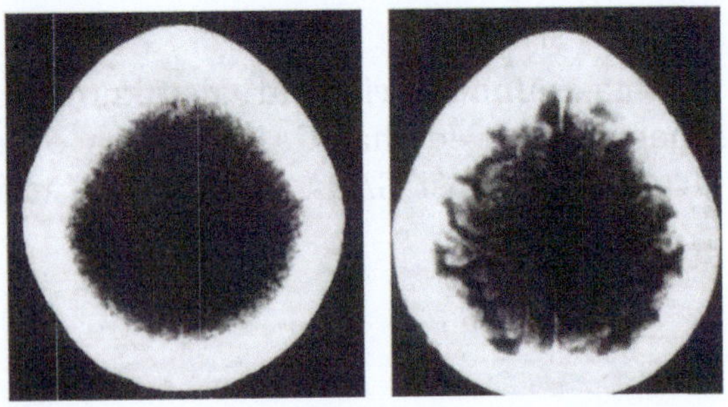

Figure 1.5. *Example of computed tomography of the brain of a patient with schizophrenia (right) compared with a normal control (left).*

Source: Sheila L. Videbeck, Psychiatric-Mental Health Nursing, ISBN-10: 1-975116-37-2.

A powerful magnet and radio waves are used to create an energy field for magnetic resonance imaging (MRI), a kind of body scan. An image or scan is created from the energy field. MRI can display blood flow patterns and tissue abnormalities like edema and provides greater tissue detail and contrast than CT scans. It can also be used to measure the thickness and size of brain structures' cortical thickness can be reduced by up to 7% in people with schizophrenia. An MRI takes about 45 minutes to complete, and the patient must lie in a small, closed chamber and remain motionless throughout. Patients who experience claustrophobia or elevated anxiety might need to be sedated before the procedure. MRIs are not permitted for patients who have pacemakers or metal implants, such as orthopedic devices or heart valves.

The function of the brain is examined using more sophisticated imaging methods like single-photon emission computed tomography (SPECT) and positron emission tomography (PET). After injecting radioactive materials into the bloodstream, the client's performance of cognitive tasks under the operator's guidance is tracked along with the substances' movement through the brain. While SPECT uses a single photon, PET uses two photons at once. While SPECT takes one to two hours, PET takes two to three hours and offers better resolution with sharper and clearer pictures. According to Gur and Gur (2017), the main purpose of PET and SPECT is research rather than the diagnosis and treatment of patients with mental illnesses. The ability to identify the amyloid plaques and tangles of Alzheimer's disease in living patients using the chemical markers FDDNP and PET is a recent breakthrough' previously, these conditions could only be diagnosed through autopsy. According to these scans, patients with Alzheimer's disease have less cerebral blood flow and less brain metabolism of glucose. Some people with schizophrenia also show reduced blood flow to the brain (Figure 1.6).

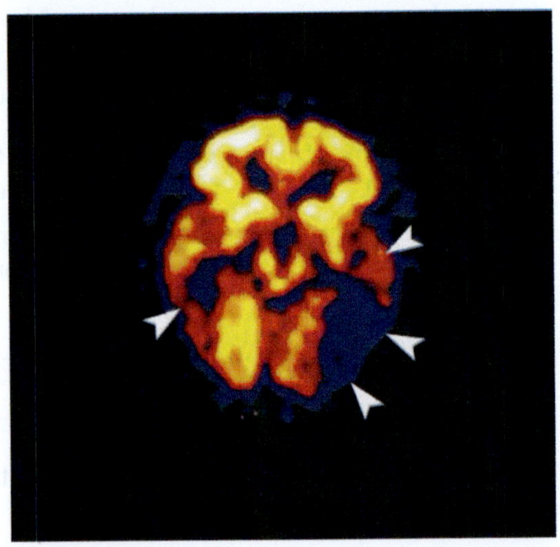

Figure 1.6. *Example of axial (horizontal) positron emission tomography of a male patient with Alzheimer's disease, showing defects (arrowheads) in metabolism in the regions of the cerebral cortex of the brain.*

Source: Sheila L. Videbeck, Psychiatric-Mental Health Nursing, ISBN-10: 1-975116-37-2.

1.8.2. Limitations of Brain Imaging Techniques

Although imaging techniques such as PET and SPECT have helped bring about tremendous advances in the study of brain diseases, they have some limitations:

- The use of radioactive substances in PET and SPECT limits the number of times a person can undergo these tests. There is the risk that the client will have an allergic reaction to the substances. Some clients may find receiving intravenous doses of radioactive material frightening or unacceptable.
- Imaging equipment is expensive to purchase and maintain, so availability can be limited. A PET camera costs about $2.5 million' a PET scanning facility may take up to $6 million to establish.
- Some persons cannot tolerate these procedures because of fear or claustrophobia.
- Researchers are finding that many of the changes in disorders such as schizophrenia are at the molecular and chemical levels and cannot be detected with current imaging techniques.

1.9. Neurobiologic Causes of Mental Illness

1.9.1. Genetics and Heredity

In contrast to numerous physical ailments that have been determined to be inherited, like Duchenne muscular dystrophy, Huntington's disease, and cystic fibrosis, the causes of mental illnesses appear to be complex. Present theories and research suggest that many mental illnesses could be associated with a particular gene or set of genes, but that nongenetic factors also play a significant role and that genetics is not the only cause. One of the most exciting findings to date is the 2007 discovery of variations in the gene SORL1, which may have a role in late-onset Alzheimer's disease. The search for genetic connections to other illnesses, such as mood disorders and schizophrenia, is still ongoing. This is the focus of the ongoing research of the National Human Genome Research Institute, funded by the National Institutes of Health and the U.S. Department of Energy. Commencing in 1988, this global research endeavor is the most extensive of its kind. All of the human DNA has been identified, and research is still being done to find the traits and illnesses that are associated with each gene (encoding). The project also discusses the social, legal, and ethical ramifications of research on human genetics. Ethical, Legal, and Social Implications, or ELSI, is a program that focuses on issues related to genetics research, clinical integration of new genetic technologies, privacy and justice in the use and interpretation of genetic information, and professional and public education.

Three types of studies are commonly conducted to investigate the genetic basis of mental illness:

- **Twin Studies:** They are used to compare the rates of certain mental illnesses or traits in monozygotic (identical) twins, who have an identical genetic makeup, and dizygotic (fraternal) twins, who have a different genetic makeup. Fraternal twins have the same genetic similarities and differences as nontwin siblings.
- **Adoption Studies:** They are used to determine a trait among biologic versus adoptive family members.

- **Family Studies:** They are used to compare whether a trait is more common among first-degree relatives (parents, siblings, and children) than among more distant relatives or the general population.

Although some genetic links have been found in certain mental disorders, studies have not shown that these illnesses are solely genetically linked. Investigation continues about the influence of inherited traits versus the influence of the environment—the "nature versus nurture" debate.

1.9.2. Stress and the Immune System (Psychoimmunology)

Many paths are being explored by researchers to identify potential causes of mental illness. A relatively new field of research called psychoimmunology looks at how the body's immune system is impacted by psychosocial stressors. Many diseases may arise as a result of a weakened immune system, especially in populations where genetic susceptibility already exists. There hasn't been any success in connecting a particular stressor to a particular disease thus far. Nonetheless, neurotransmitters can be influenced by the brain and immune system. Mood dysregulation and depression are common when the inflammatory response plays a critical role in diseases like multiple sclerosis or lupus erythematosus.

1.9.3. Infection as a Possible Cause

An infection's role in mental illness is a topic of study for certain researchers. The majority of studies on viral theories have concentrated on schizophrenia, but none have offered precise or convincing proof as of yet. The possibility that a virus may actually change human genes, the existence of a virus with an affinity for CNS tissues, and the exposure of a mother to a virus during a critical stage of the fetus's nervous system development are among the theories being developed and investigated. It has been suggested that inflammation may causally contribute to the pathology of schizophrenia because prenatal infections may affect the fetus's developing brain. (American Nurses Association, 2014' Virani et al., 2017)

1.10. The Nurse's Role in Research and Education

The implications for clients and their families remain vague and nonspecific despite the abundance of research reports in the fields of neurobiology, genetics, and heredity. A lot of the time, clients and their families find it difficult to understand or contradicting when reading media reports about new research and studies. In addition to making sure that clients and families are aware of developments in these areas, the nurse must assist them in differentiating between facts and conjecture. If and how new research might impact a client's course of treatment or prognosis, the nurse can explain it. When you need information or have questions answered, the nurse is a great resource. (American Nurses Association, 2014' Virani et al., 2017).

1.11. Psychopharmacology

For many clients suffering from mental disorders, medication management is a critical matter that has a substantial impact on treatment outcomes. The sections that follow cover various drug classes (psychotropic drugs) used to treat mental illnesses, including stimulants, mood stabilizers, antipsychotics, antidepressants, and anxiolytics. It is important for nurses to be aware of the interactions, side effects, and contraindications of these medications as well as the nursing interventions needed to support patients in adhering to their prescribed regimens. Nurses must understand a few terms that are used when talking about drugs and drug therapy. A drug's maximal therapeutic effect is referred to as its efficacy. The term "potency" refers to the quantity of a medication required to produce the desired maximum effect' high-potency medications are effective at lower dosages, while low-potency medications require larger dosages. The half-life of a drug is the amount of time it takes for half of it to leave the bloodstream. It might be necessary to administer medications three or four times a day for those with shorter half-lives, but once a day for those with longer half-lives. Five times the half-life of a drug is the amount of time it takes for it to fully exit the body after being stopped.

The U.S. Food and Drug Administration (FDA) is responsible for supervising the testing and marketing of medications for public safety. Clinical drug trials for novel drugs and medication effectiveness and side effect monitoring are examples of these activities. Every drug is approved by the FDA for use in a specific population and for a specific disease. Sometimes a medication works well for a different illness than the one for which it was originally tested and approved by the FDA. We refer to this as off-label use. One instance is the prescription of certain anticonvulsant medications (approved to stop seizures) for the off-label purpose of helping patients with bipolar disorder by stabilizing their mood. The frequency and seriousness of medication side effects are also observed by the FDA. The FDA may issue a black box warning if a drug is found to have serious or potentially fatal side effects, even though these side effects are uncommon. This means that a box that is highlighted and placed apart from the text on package inserts must warn of any serious or potentially fatal side effects.

1.11.1. Principles that Guide Pharmacologic Treatment

The following are several principles that guide the use of medications to treat psychiatric disorders:

- A medication is selected based on its effect on the client's target symptoms such as delusional thinking, panic attacks, or hallucinations. The medication's effectiveness is evaluated largely by its ability to diminish or eliminate the target symptoms.
- Many psychotropic drugs must be given in adequate dosages for some time before their full effects are realized. For example, tricyclic antidepressants can require 4 to 6 weeks before the client experiences optimal therapeutic benefit.
- The dosage of medication is often adjusted to the lowest effective dosage for the client. Sometimes a client may need higher dosages to stabilize his or her target symptoms, while lower dosages can be used to sustain those effects over time.
- As a rule, older adults require lower dosages of medications than younger clients to experience therapeutic effects. It may also take longer for a drug to achieve its full therapeutic effect in older adults.
- Psychotropic medications are often decreased gradually (tapering) rather than abruptly. This is because of potential problems with rebound (temporary return of symptoms), recurrence (of the original symptoms), or withdrawal (new symptoms resulting from

discontinuation of the drug).

- Follow-up care is essential to ensure compliance with the medication regimen, to make needed adjustments in dosage, and to manage side effects.
- Compliance with the medication regimen is often enhanced when the regimen is as simple as possible in terms of both the number of medications prescribed and the number of daily doses.

1.11.2. Antipsychotic Drugs

The delusions and hallucinations associated with schizophrenia, schizoaffective disorder, and the manic phase of bipolar disorder are examples of psychotic symptoms that are treated with antipsychotic medications, formerly known as neuroleptics. Antipsychotics are used off-label to treat aggression, anxiety, sleeplessness, and delusions, hallucinations, and other disruptive behaviors that can occasionally accompany Alzheimer's disease. Antipsychotic medications function by preventing dopamine receptors from being occupied. Clinical applications for them date back to the 1950s. In addition to being the main medical treatment for schizophrenia, they are also used to treat acute manic episodes, psychotic depression, and drug-induced psychosis. Sometimes, modest doses of traditional antipsychotics help clients with dementia who exhibit psychotic symptoms. Elderly patients with psychosis related to dementia may have higher mortality rates when taking second-generation antipsychotics. For brief psychotic symptoms, like those experienced by certain clients with borderline personality disorder, short-term antipsychotic therapy may be helpful. For both conventional and atypical antipsychotic medications, Table 1.3 provides the available dosage forms, typical daily oral dosages, and extreme dosage ranges. When working with elderly adults or kids who have psychoses, extreme behavior management issues, or aggression, the low end of the extreme range is usually utilized.

Table 1.3. *Antipsychotic Drugs*

Generic (Trade) Name	Forms	Daily Dosage*	Extreme Dosage Ranges*
Conventional or first-generation antipsychotics			
Phenothiazines			
Chlorpromazine (Thorazine)	T, L, INJ	200–1,600	25–2,000
Perphenazine (Trilafon)	T, L, INJ	16–32	4–64
Fluphenazine (Prolixin)	T, L, INJ	2.5–20	1–60
Thioridazine (Mellaril)	T, L	200–600	40–800
Mesoridazine (Serentil)	T, L, INJ	75–300	30–400
Trifluoperazine (Stelazine)	T, L, INJ	6–50	2–80
Thioxanthene			
Thiothixene (Navane)	C, L, INJ	6–30	6–60
Butyrophenones			
Haloperidol (Haldol)	T, L, INJ	2–20	1–100
Droperidol (Inapsine)	INJ	2.5	
Dibenzazepine			
Loxapine (Loxitane)	C, L, INJ	60–100	30–250
Dihydroindolone			
Molindone (Moban)	T, L	50–100	15–250
Atypical or second-generation antipsychotics			
Clozapine (Clozaril)	T	150–500	75–700
Fazaclo (clozapine)	DT	150–500	75–700
Risperidone (Risperdal)	T, L, DT	2–8	1–16
Olanzapine (Zyprexa)	T	5–15	5–20
Quetiapine (Seroquel)	T	300–600	200–750
Ziprasidone (Geodon)	C, INJ	40–160	20–200
Paliperidone (Invega)	T	6	3–12
Iloperidone (Fanapt)	T	12–24	2–24
Asenapine (Saphris)	T (SL)	10–20	10–20
Lurasidone (Latuda)	T	40–80	20–160
Third-generation antipsychotics			
Aripiprazole (Abilify)	T	15–30	10–40
Cariprazine (Vraylar)	C	3–6	1.5–6
Brexpiprazole (Rexulti)	T	1–3	5–4

*Values are in milligrams per day for oral doses only. C, capsule' DT, orally disintegrating tablet' INJ, injection for IM (usually prn) use' L, liquid for oral use' SL, sublingual' T, tablet.

Source: Sheila L. Videbeck, Psychiatric-Mental Health Nursing, ISBN-10: 1-975116-37-2.

1.11.2.1. Mechanism of Action

All antipsychotics primarily function by inhibiting dopamine receptors in the nervous system' however, the exact therapeutic mechanism of action is still unknown. There are five subcategories of dopamine receptors: D1, D2, D3, D4, and D5. D2, D3, and D4 have been linked to mental health issues. The first-generation, or conventional, antipsychotic medications are strong D2, D3, and D4 antagonists. Because the D2 receptors are blocked, this not only makes them effective in treating the target symptoms but also causes many extrapyramidal side effects (discussion to follow). The lower frequency of extrapyramidal side effects may be explained by the relatively weak D2 blockers found in more recent, atypical or second-generation antipsychotic medications like clozapine (Clozaril). Furthermore, certain antidepressants and second-generation antipsychotics both prevent serotonin from being reabsorbed, which makes them more effective in treating the depressive symptoms of schizophrenia. The most recent second-generation agents are lurasidone (Latuda), asenapine (Saphris), iloperidone (Fanapt), and paliperidone (Invega). Although paliperidone (Invega) is an extended-release medication, it shares chemical similarities with risperidone (Risperdal). This indicates that the client can typically take one dose per day, which could contribute to higher compliance. Since asenapine (Saphris) is a sublingual tablet, patients need to wait 10 to 15 minutes after taking the medication before consuming any food or liquids.

Dopamine system stabilizers, the third generation of antipsychotics, are currently under development. These medications are believed to stabilize dopamine output, meaning that when dopaminergic transmission is too high, they decrease it, or they preserve or enhance it. As a result, symptoms are controlled without some of the negative effects associated with other antipsychotic drugs. The first medication of this kind, aripiprazole (Abilify), received FDA approval for use in 2002. The more recent third-generation antipsychotics are brexpiprazole (Rexulti) and cariprazine (Vraylar). These medications are used to treat depression, bipolar disorder, schizophrenia, and manic episodes. Sedation, weight gain, akathisia, headache, anxiety, and nausea are the most frequent side effects.

Depot injection is a time-release intramuscular medication that comes in six different antipsychotics for maintenance therapy. Due to the slow absorption of two first-generation antipsychotics due to the use of sesame oil as the injection vehicle, fewer administrations of the medication are required to maintain the intended therapeutic effects. Decanoate haloperidol (Haldol) has a duration of 4 weeks, and decanoate fluphenazine (Prolixin) has a duration of 7 to 28 days. Depot injections must be administered every two to four weeks to maintain the therapeutic effect of these medications once the patient's condition has stabilized with oral doses. These second-generation antipsychotics, olanzapine pamoate (Zyprexa Relprevv), paliperidone (Invega Sustenna), and risperidone (Risperdal Consta), encapsulate the active drug within polymer-based microspheres that break down gradually in the body, releasing the drug gradually at a controlled rate. Every two weeks, 25 milligrams of risperidone (Consta). The dosage of Invega Sustenna is 117 mg every four weeks. 210 mg or 405 mg of Zyprexa Relprevv can be administered every two weeks or every four weeks. After an injection, Zyprexa Relprevv may result in postinjection delirium/sedation syndrome, which can cause sedation, agitation, confusion, disorientation, and cognitive impairment. This condition can then progress to ataxia, convulsions, weakness, and hypertension, all of which may result in cardiac arrest. Due to the insolubility of aripiprazole particles, Abilify

Maintena, a third-generation antipsychotic, is slowly absorbed into the bloodstream. As a result, the patient must be monitored closely by a medical professional for three hours following the injection and remain symptom-free and alert before being released. Abilify Maintena 400 mg is administered once a month following the start of oral medication.

1.11.2.2. Side Effects

Extrapyramidal Side Effects

The primary adverse effects of antipsychotic medications are extrapyramidal symptoms (EPSs), which are severe neurologic symptoms. These consist of akathisia, pseudoparkinsonism, and acute dystonia. Even though these reactions are frequently referred to as EPSs, they all have unique characteristics. Differentiating between the reactions can be challenging because a client may experience all of them during therapy. EPSs are brought on by the blockade of D2 receptors in the brain stem's midbrain region. Acute dystonia, pseudoparkinsonism, and akathisia all have similar treatments that involve reducing the dosage of the antipsychotic, switching to a different antipsychotic, or giving anticholinergic medication. First-generation antipsychotic drugs cause more EPSs than second-generation antipsychotic drugs, with ziprasidone (Geodon) rarely causing EPSs. Atypical antipsychotic medications are frequently prescribed because of their lower incidence of EPSs, even though anticholinergic drugs also have side effects.

Acute dystonia is characterized by sudden, severe muscular rigidity and cramping, a stiff or thick tongue that makes swallowing difficult, and, in extreme situations, laryngospasm and breathing problems. Dystonia is more common in males, clients under 40, those on high-potency medications like thiothixene and haloperidol, and in the first week of treatment. Muscle group spasms or stiffness can result in oculogyric crisis (eyes rolled back in a locked position), opisthotonus (tightness throughout the body with the head back and an arched neck), and torticollis (twisted head and neck). For the client, acute dystonic reactions can be excruciating and terrifying. Treatment with anticholinergic medications, such as intramuscular diphenhydramine (Benadryl) or intramuscular benztropine mesylate (Cogentin), usually produces fast relief.

Table 1.4 lists the drugs and their routes and dosages used to treat EPSs. The addition of a regularly scheduled oral anticholinergic, such as benztropine, may allow the client to continue taking the antipsychotic drug with no further dystonia. Recurrent dystonic reactions would necessitate a lower dosage or a change in the antipsychotic drug.

Table 1.4. *Drugs Used to Treat Extrapyramidal Side Effects*

Generic (Trade) Name	Oral Dosages (mg)	IM/IV Doses (mg)	Drug Class
Amantadine (Symmetrel)	100 bid or tid	–	Dopaminergic agonist
Benztropine (Cogentin)	1–3 bid	1–2	Anticholinergic
Biperiden (Akineton)	2 tid–qid	2	Anticholinergic
Diazepam (Valium)	5 tid	5–10	Benzodiazepine
Diphenhydramine (Benadryl)	25–50 tid or qid	25–50	Antihistamine
Lorazepam (Ativan)	1–2 tid	–	Benzodiazepine
Procyclidine (Kemadrin)	2.5–5 tid	–	Anticholinergic
Propranolol (Inderal)	10–20 tid; up to 40 qid	–	Beta-Blocker
Trihexyphenidyl (Artane)	2–5 tid	–	Anticholinergic

bid, two times a day' IM, intramuscularly' IV, intravenous' qid, four times a day' tid, three times a day.

Source: Sheila L. Videbeck, Psychiatric-Mental Health Nursing, ISBN-10: 1-975116-37-2.

A common term for drug-induced parkinsonism, also known as pseudoparkinsonism, is EPS. A stiff, hunched posture, mask-like facial features, reduced arm swing, a shuffling, festinating gait (with small steps), cogwheel rigidity (ratchet-like joint movements), drooling, tremor, bradycardia, and coarse pill-rolling movements of the thumb and fingers when at rest are among the symptoms that are similar to those of Parkinson disease. Amantadine, a dopamine agonist that increases the transmission of dopamine blocked by the antipsychotic drug, or switching to an antipsychotic with a lower incidence of EPS are two treatment options for Parkinsonism. The client describes akathisia as an overwhelming need to move around. The client exhibits signs of restlessness, anxiety, and agitation' they frequently walk or stand rigidly and don't make natural gestures. Often, clients stop taking their antipsychotic medication due to this inward restlessness and inability to relax or sit still. Treatment options for akathisia include adding an oral drug such as a benzodiazepine, beta-blocker, or anticholinergic, or modifying antipsychotic medication.

Neuroleptic Malignant Syndrome

A potentially lethal idiosyncratic response to an antipsychotic (or neuroleptic) medication is known as neuroleptic malignant syndrome (NMS). The main signs and symptoms of NMS include pallor, diaphoresis, elevated enzyme levels, especially creatine phosphokinase, stiffness, high fever, and autonomic instability, which includes unstable blood pressure, pallor, and diaphoresis. NMS patients are frequently silent, confused, and prone to fits of agitation or stupor. All antipsychotics appear to have the potential to result in NMS' however, the risk is heightened by high dosages of drugs with high potencies. NMS may happen at any time, but it usually manifests itself during the first two weeks of treatment or following a dosage increase.

The risk factors for NMS are concurrent medical illnesses, malnutrition, and dehydration. The client will receive supportive medical care to treat dehydration and hyperthermia until their physical condition stabilizes, along with the immediate discontinuation of all antipsychotic medications. Following NMS, the client and the doctor must have a thorough discussion about the relative risks and potential benefits of therapy before deciding whether to treat the patient with additional antipsychotic medications.

Tardive Dyskinesia

The most common cause of tardive dyskinesia (TD), a syndrome characterized by involuntary movements that never go away, is prolonged use of traditional antipsychotic medications. Approximately 20% to 30% of patients undergoing long-term treatment experience TD symptoms, with the exact etiology still unknown. Involuntary movements of the tongue, truncal musculature, upper and lower extremities, and facial and neck muscles are among the symptoms of TD. Typical facial expressions include lip-smacking, blinking, grimacing, tongue thrusting and protruding, and other excessive and needless movements. Once TD develops, it cannot be reversed, though antipsychotic medication dosage reduction or cessation can halt the disease's progression. Regretfully, antipsychotic drugs have the potential to conceal the initial symptoms of TD' that is, higher antipsychotic drug dosages will momentarily mask the initial symptoms. But as the TD symptoms get worse, they "break through" the antipsychotic drug's effects.

The first medications to treat TD were approved by the FDA in 2017: deutetrabenazine (Austedo, Teva) and valbenazine (Ingrezza). These medications are inhibitors of the vesicular monoamine transporter 2 (VMAT2). These medications are thought to lessen the activity of monoamines like dopamine, serotonin, and norepinephrine, which in turn lessens the atypical movements linked to TD and Huntington chorea. The recommended daily dosage ranges for valbenazine and deutetrabenazine are 40–80 mg and 12–48 mg, respectively. These medications induce akathisia, restlessness, QT prolongation, and somnolence. Furthermore, valbenazine may result in headaches, nausea, vomiting, and balance issues. In patients with Huntington chorea, utetrabenazine can also result in NMS, as well as elevated depression and suicidal thoughts. When using antipsychotics, the main objective is to prevent TD. This can be achieved by adjusting medication, minimizing maintenance dosages, and routinely checking the client for the onset of TD using a standardized assessment tool like the Abnormal Involuntary Movement Scale. Clients who require antipsychotic medication despite having symptoms of TD are frequently prescribed one of the atypical antipsychotic medications, which have not been shown to cause or exacerbate TD.

Anticholinergic Side Effects

Antipsychotics frequently cause orthostatic hypotension, dry mouth, constipation, urinary hesitancy or retention, blurred near vision, dry eyes, photophobia, nasal congestion, and impaired memory as anticholinergic side effects. These side effects typically go away in three to four weeks, but they never totally go away. The client may experience more issues with anticholinergic side effects if they are taking anticholinergic medications for EPSs. Hard candies or calorie-free drinks can help relieve dry mouth, and incorporating grains and fruit into the diet, drinking enough water, and using stool softeners can help avoid constipation.

Other Side Effects

Antipsychotic medications also raise prolactin levels in the blood. In addition to menstrual irregularities, decreased libido, erectile and orgasmic dysfunction, and breast enlargement and tenderness in both sexes, elevated prolactin may also raise the risk of breast cancer. It might also be a factor in weight gain. The majority of antipsychotic drugs can cause weight gain, but ziprasidone (Geodon) is an exception. Most second-generation antipsychotic medications cause weight gain. The most notable weight increases occur when using clozapine (Clozaril) and olanzapine (Zyprexa). Since 2004, the FDA has required pharmaceutical companies to include a warning on the label about the increased risk of hyperglycemia and diabetes when using atypical antipsychotics. Although the precise cause of this weight gain is unknown, some clients report increased appetite, binge eating, cravings for carbohydrates, changes in food preferences, and decreased satiety as a result of it. Histamine antagonism stimulates appetite, prolactin elevation may activate feeding centers, and there may be an as-yet-unidentified interplay of various neurotransmitter and receptor interactions that alter appetite, energy intake, and feeding behavior. Genetics can also predispose clients to weight gain and metabolic syndrome, according to Penninx and Lange's (2018) research. A group of illnesses known as metabolic syndrome raises the risk of heart disease, diabetes, and stroke.

The syndrome is diagnosed when three or more of the following are present:

- **Obesity**—excess weight, increased body mass index (BMI), and increased abdominal girth because of fat deposits;
- Increased Blood Pressure;
- High Blood Sugar Level;
- **High Cholesterol**—with at least 150 mg/dL of triglyceride' less than 40 mg/dL of high-density lipoprotein for women and 50 mg/dL for men.

Individuals with schizophrenia are frequently obese, which raises their risk of cardiovascular disease and type 2 diabetes. Furthermore, there is a lower chance that clients with severe, ongoing mental illness will exercise or consume low-fat, nutritionally balanced diets' this pattern reduces the possibility that they will be able to prevent weight gain or shed excess weight. Shorter life expectancy is caused by an increased risk of heart disease, so it is advised that clients taking antipsychotics participate in an educational program to control their weight and lower their BMI. But it can be a challenging task. Gill, Zechner, Zambo, Swarbrick, and Murphy (2016) discovered that when staff members offered information and helpful support when needed, clients performed better. Where cognitive difficulties existed, information about physical activity requirements and a healthy diet were adjusted to accommodate the client. Social support rooted in the community was offered to assist clients in gradually implementing the necessary adjustments in their homes.

The majority of antipsychotic medications have comparatively mild negative effects on the heart, including tachycardia, palpitations, and postural hypotension. Prolonged QT interval prolongation is another side effect of some antipsychotic medications, including thioridazine (Mellaril), droperidol (Inapsine), and mesoridazine (Serentil). Over 500 ms is regarded as a dangerous QT interval, linked to sudden death and potentially fatal dysrhythmias. An ECG may show torsade de pointes, or a rapid heartbeat of 150 to 250 beats per minute, due to the prolonged QT interval, a rare but possible condition that gives the ECG a "twisted" appearance. While droperidol is most frequently used as an adjuvant to anesthesia or to induce sedation, thioridazine and mesoridazine are used to treat psychosis. Although sertindole, also known as Select, was used to treat psychosis in Europe, its use was later discontinued due to the high number of cardiac dysrhythmias and fatalities it caused.

Clozapine has a potentially fatal side effect called agranulocytosis, but it has fewer traditional side effects than most antipsychotic medications. Leukopenia, fever, malaise, ulcerative sore throat, and other symptoms appear suddenly. This side effect might appear up to 24 weeks after therapy starts and might not show up right away. Initially, in order to receive the following week's supply of clozapine, patients had to have a weekly white blood cell (WBC) count greater than 3,500/mm^3. For the first six months, all clients are required to have weekly WBCs drawn. If the client's WBC and absolute neutrophil count (ANC) are 3,500/mm^3 and 2,000/mm^3, respectively, these lab tests may be checked every two weeks for the first six months, and then every four weeks after that. This reduced monitoring necessitates ongoing clozapine therapy. Any therapy stoppage necessitates a return to more frequent monitoring for a predetermined amount of time. For four weeks following the cessation of clozapine, weekly monitoring of the WBC and ANC is necessary.

1.11.2.3. Client Teaching

When a client is taking antipsychotic medication, the nurse advises them about potential side effects and suggests that they report any concerns to their doctor rather than stopping the medication. The nurse gives the patient advice on how to keep up with their medication schedule and manage any unpleasant side effects. Eating sugar-free hard candies and drinking sugar-free beverages relieve dry mouth. Sugary drinks and candies high in calories should be avoided by the client as they increase the risk of dental cavities, cause weight gain, and provide little relief from dry mouth. Constipation can be avoided or relieved by exercising, drinking more water, and eating more bulk-forming foods. While laxatives should be avoided by the client, stool softeners are acceptable. The client may be photosensitive, making sunburn more likely, so sunscreen use is advised.

Clients ought to keep an eye on how sleepy or drowsy they are feeling. They should refrain from operating a vehicle and engaging in other potentially hazardous activities until their reflexes and response times appear normal. If the client misses a dose of their antipsychotic medication and it's only been three or four hours, they can catch up on it. The client may skip the missed dose if it is more than four hours past due or if the next dose is about to expire. The nurse advises patients who struggle to remember to take their medication to use a pillbox that can be prefilled with precise dosages for the day or week, or to use a chart to record doses when taken.

1.11.3. Antidepressant Drugs

Antidepressant medications are mainly used to treat psychotic depression, anxiety disorders, major depressive illness, and the depressed phase of bipolar disorder. Antidepressant medications are used off-label to treat a variety of conditions, such as chronic pain, migraines, peripheral and diabetic neuropathies, sleep apnea, dermatological conditions, panic attacks, and eating disorders. The two neurotransmitters that control mood, arousal, attention, sensory processing, and appetite—serotonin and norepinephrine—interact with antidepressants in some way, though the exact mode of action is unclear.

Antidepressants are divided into four groups:

- Tricyclic and the related cyclic antidepressants;
- Selective serotonin reuptake inhibitors (SSRIs);
- MAO inhibitors (MAOIs);
- Other antidepressants such as desvenlafaxine (Pristiq), venlafaxine (Effexor), bupropion (Wellbutrin), duloxetine (Cymbalta), trazodone (Desyrel), and nefazodone (Serzone).

Table 1.5 lists the dosage forms, usual daily dosages, and extreme dosage ranges.

Table 1.5. *Antidepressant Drugs*

Generic (Trade) Name	Forms	Usual Daily Dosages*	Extreme Dosage Ranges*
Selective serotonin reuptake inhibitors			
Fluoxetine (Prozac)	C, L	20–60	10–80
Fluvoxamine (Luvox)	T	150–200	50–300
Paroxetine (Paxil)	T	20–40	10–50
Sertraline (Zoloft)	T	100–150	50–200
Citalopram (Celexa)	T, L	20–40	20–60
Escitalopram (Lexapro)	T	10–20	5–30
Cyclic compounds			
Imipramine (Tofranil)	T, C, INJ	150–200	50–300
Desipramine (Norpramin)	T, C	150–200	50–300
Amitriptyline (Elavil)	T, INJ	150–200	50–300
Nortriptyline (Pamelor)	C, L	75–100	25–150
Doxepin (Sinequan)	C, L	150–200	25–300
Trimipramine (Surmontil)	C	150–200	50–300
Protriptyline (Vivactil)	T	15–40	10–60
Maprotiline (Ludiomil)	T	100–150	50–200
Mirtazapine (Remeron)	T	15–45	15–60
Amoxapine (Asendin)	T	150–200	50–250
Clomipramine (Anafranil)	C, INJ	150–200	50–250
Other compounds			
Bupropion (Wellbutrin)	T	200–300	100–450
Venlafaxine (Effexor)	T, C	75–225	75–375
Desvenlafaxine (Pristiq)	T	50–100	50 every other day–400
Trazodone (Desyrel)	T	200–300	100–600
Nefazodone (Serzone)	T	300–600	100–600
Duloxetine (Cymbalta)	C	60	30–90
Vilazodone (Viibryd)	T	20–4	10–40
Monoamine oxidase inhibitors			
Phenelzine (Nardil)	T	45–60	15–90
Tranylcypromine (Parnate)	T	30–50	10–90
Isocarboxazid (Marplan)	T	20–40	10–60

*Values are in milligrams per day for oral doses only. C, capsule' INJ, injection for IM use' L, liquid' T, tablet.

Source: Sheila L. Videbeck, Psychiatric-Mental Health Nursing, ISBN-10: 1-975116-37-2.

Even though they have anticholinergic side effects, orthostatic hypotension (a drop in blood pressure on rising), and varying degrees of sedation, cyclic compounds were the first choice of medications to treat depression for many years after they became available in the 1950s. Furthermore, cyclic antidepressants have the potential to be fatal if overdosed. During that same period, the MAOIs were discovered to have a positive effect on people with depression. Although the MAOIs have a low incidence of sedation and anticholinergic effects, they must be used with extreme caution for several reasons:

- A life-threatening side effect, hypertensive crisis, may occur if the client ingests foods containing tyramine (an amino acid) while taking MAOIs.
- Because of the risk of potentially fatal drug interactions, MAOIs cannot be given in combination with other MAOIs, tricyclic antidepressants, meperidine (Demerol), CNS depressants, many antihypertensives, or general anesthetics.
- MAOIs are potentially lethal in overdose and pose a potential risk in clients with depression who may be considering suicide.

Since fluoxetine (Prozac) was first made available in 1987, selective serotonin reuptake inhibitors (SSRIs) have supplanted cyclic medications as the first line of treatment for depression due to their equal effectiveness and lack of unpleasant side effects. For the treatment of obsessive compulsive disorder (OCD), clomipramine and SSRIs work well. Once fluoxetine has stabilized a client's depression, the first and only medication that can be administered once a week as maintenance therapy is Prozac Weekly. It has an enteric coating that delays the release of the medication's 90 milligrams of fluoxetine into the bloodstream.

1.11.3.1. Preferred Drugs for Clients at High Risk for Suicide

When treating depressed clients, suicide is always the first thing that needs to be considered. SSRIs, venlafaxine, nefazodone, and bupropion, as opposed to cyclic compounds and MAOIs, do not carry the risk of a fatal overdose, making them generally better options for individuals who are highly impulsive or suicidal. However, only mild and moderate depression can benefit from SSRIs. Even after antidepressant treatment is started, the risk of suicide needs to be assessed. The possibility of a suicide attempt rises if the client experiences increased energy but persists in having suicidal thoughts. Furthermore, because it frequently takes weeks for the drugs to fully take effect, patients may lose hope and grow weary of waiting to feel better, which can lead to suicidal thoughts and actions. SSRIs are linked to an increased risk of suicide in children and adolescents, according to an FDA warning.

1.11.3.2. Mechanism of Action

Although the exact mechanism by which antidepressants work as a medication is unknown, their effects on the central nervous system are well understood. The brain's monoamine neurotransmitter systems—in particular, norepinephrine and serotonin—are the main site of interaction. These two neurotransmitters aid in controlling arousal, alertness, attention, mood, sensory processing, and appetite. They are released throughout the brain. Following release, norepinephrine, serotonin, and dopamine are reabsorbed into presynaptic neurons, eliminating them from the synapses. These three neurotransmitters are reloaded for later release or are broken down by the MAO enzyme after reuptake. The SSRIs inhibit serotonin reuptake, the MAOIs interfere with enzyme metabolism, and the cyclic antidepressants and venlafaxine primarily inhibit norepinephrine reuptake and partially inhibit serotonin. This is not a full explanation, though, as antidepressants are rarely helpful until taken for several weeks, whereas the inhibition of MAO and the blockade of serotonin and norepinephrine reuptake happen in a matter of hours. It could take four to six weeks for cyclic compounds to start working, two to four weeks for MAOIs, and two to three weeks for SSRIs. The way these medications work is thought to be an "initiating event" that leads to eventual therapeutic effectiveness when neurons respond more slowly and serotonin becomes available at the synapses.

1.11.3.3. Side Effects of Selective Serotonin Reuptake Inhibitors

When it comes to side effects, SSRIs are less common than cyclic compounds. Many common side effects, including anxiety, agitation, akathisia (motor restlessness), nausea, insomnia, and sexual dysfunction—specifically, decreased sexual drive or trouble getting an erection or orgasm—can result from enhanced serotonin transmission. Additionally, even though SSRIs cause less weight gain than other antidepressants, weight gain is a problem that arises and persists during antidepressant therapy. Usually, taking medicine with food helps reduce nausea. Benzodiazepines or beta-blockers like propranolol (Inderal) are commonly used to treat akathisia. Even if the patient takes the medication in the morning, insomnia might still be an issue' in such cases, a low-dose trazodone or sedative-hypnotic may be necessary. Headaches, sweating, diarrhea, hand tremor, and sedation—especially with paroxetine [Paxil]—are less frequent adverse effects. Treatment for headaches and diarrhea is typically symptomatic. Continued sedation and sweating are probably signs that you should switch to a different antidepressant.

1.11.3.4. Side Effects of Cyclic Antidepressants

The newer miscellaneous compounds and SSRIs are less likely to cause side effects than cyclic compounds. The degree of adverse effects varies amongst the medications in this category, but overall, they belong to the same groups. The anticholinergic effects of cyclic antidepressants, which block cholinergic receptors, include dry mouth, constipation, urinary hesitancy or retention, dry nasal passages, and blurred near vision. More severe anticholinergic side effects, especially in older adults, can include ileus, delirium, and agitation. Orthostatic hypotension, tachycardia, sedation, and weight gain are other frequent side effects. Although patients may grow tolerant to anticholinergic effects, these side effects are frequently the cause of patient withdrawal from medication. Sexual dysfunction is often reported by patients on cyclic compounds that are comparable to issues with SSRIs. It is frequently stated that sexual dysfunction and weight gain are the causes of noncompliance.

1.11.3.5. Side Effects of Monoamine Oxidase Inhibitors

Daytime drowsiness, sleeplessness, weight gain, dry mouth, orthostatic hypotension, and sexual dysfunction are among the most typical side effects of MAOIs. Treatment for sedation and insomnia is challenging and may involve switching to a different medication. The possibility of a potentially fatal hypertensive crisis with MAOIs is especially concerning if the patient consumes tyramine-containing food or uses sympathomimetic medications. Since the tyramine in some foods must be broken down by the enzyme MAO, inhibiting it raises serum tyramine levels, which can lead to severe hypertension, hyperpyrexia, tachycardia, diaphoresis, tremulousness, and cardiac dysrhythmias. Meperidine is one of the opiate derivatives that may interact fatally with MAOIs, along with SSRIs, some cyclic compounds, buspirone (BuSpar), and dextromethorphan. The client outlines the foods to avoid and must be able to adhere to a tyramine-free diet. Research is presently being conducted to find out if a transdermal patch containing selegiline could effectively treat depression without the side effects of dietary tyramine and oral MAOIs.

1.11.3.6. Side Effects of Other Antidepressants

The antidepressants mirtazapine, trazodone, and nefazodone frequently cause drowsiness among the other or novel medication classes. Headaches are frequently brought on by both trazodone and nefazodone. Nausea and dry mouth are additional side effects of nevazodone. There is a chance that bupropion, venlafaxine, and desvenlafaxine will make you feel queasy, agitated, and sleepless. Dizziness, perspiration, or sedation are additional side effects of venlafaxine. With one significant exception—that is, razodone can result in priapism, a prolonged and excruciating erection that requires immediate medical attention and drug withdrawal—sexual dysfunction is far less common with the newer antidepressants. Impotence is another side effect of pruritus.

1.11.3.7. Drug Interactions

When an SSRI and an MAOI are taken concurrently, a rare but potentially dangerous medication interaction known as serotonin syndrome (or serotonergic syndrome) may occur. The client may also experience it if they take one of these medications too soon after finishing therapy with the other. Put differently, before starting therapy with another drug, the person's system must be cleared of the first one. In severe cases, agitation, sweating, fever, tachycardia, hypotension, rigidity, hyperreflexia, and even coma and death are among the symptoms. These signs resemble those of an overdose on SSRIs.

1.11.3.8. Client Teaching

Unless sedation is an issue, patients should take SSRIs first thing in the morning' paroxetine is known to cause sedation most of the time. A client may take an SSRI up to eight hours after missing a dose if they forget to take it. Clients should ideally take cyclic compounds at night in a single daily dose to reduce side effects. If a client forgets to take a dose of a cyclic compound, the dose should be skipped for that day or taken within three hours of the missed dose. Until the sedative effects are determined, clients should drive carefully or engage in activities requiring quick, alert reflexes. Patients on MAOIs should be informed that if they disregard specific dietary guidelines, they may experience a potentially fatal hyperadrenergic crisis. A written list of foods to stay away from while taking MAOIs should be given to them. The nurse should advise patients not to take any additional medication, including over-the-counter preparations, without first consulting their doctor or pharmacist. Patients using MAOIs run the risk of experiencing major or even fatal drug interactions.

1.11.4. Mood-Stabilizing Drugs

Mood-stabilizing medications are used to treat acute manic episodes, prevent or lessen the highs and lows associated with bipolar illness, and stabilize the patient's mood. The most well-known mood stabilizer is lithium. Several anticonvulsants, especially valproic acid (Depakote, Depakene) and carbamazepine (Tegretol) are also useful mood stabilizers. For mood stabilization, other anticonvulsants like lamotrigine (Lamictal), topiramate (Topamax), oxcarbazepine (Trileptal), and gabapentin (Neurontin) are also used. Clonazepam, also known as Klonopin, is occasionally used to treat acute manic episodes. The topic of antianxiety medications includes clonazepam.

1.11.4.1. Mechanism of Action

Lithium has a wide range of neurobiologic effects, but little is known about how it works in bipolar disorder. The reuptake of some neurotransmitters, including dopamine, acetylcholine, norepinephrine, and serotonin, is normalized by lithium. It acts intracellularly rather than within neuronal synapses, reducing norepinephrine release by competing with calcium. It also directly affects G-proteins and specific enzyme subsystems, including phosphatidylinositol and cyclic adenosine monophosphates. One of the first-line treatments for bipolar disorder is lithium. Anticonvulsants' off-label use as mood stabilizers raises questions about their exact mode of action. It is well known that topiramate and valproic acid raise GABA levels, which are inhibitory neurotransmitters. It is believed that valproic acid and carbamazepine work by blocking the kindling process, which stabilizes mood. This is known as the snowball effect, which is observed when mild seizure activity appears to accumulate into more frequent and severe seizures. Anticonvulsants increase the threshold to stop these small seizures in seizure management. It is believed that, when triggered by more frequent minor episodes, the same kindling process may also take place in the development of full-blown mania. This could also account for the anticonvulsant's efficacy in treating and preventing mania.

1.11.4.2. Dosage

There are no parenteral forms of lithium' it is only available in tablets, capsules, liquid, and sustained-release forms. Lithium dosage effectiveness is established by measuring serum lithium levels and evaluating the patient's clinical response to the medication. 900 to 3,600 mg should be taken daily' more crucially, the serum lithium level should be around 1 mEq/L. Less than 0.5 mEq/L of serum lithium is rarely therapeutic, and more than 1.5 mEq/L is typically regarded as toxic. While the therapeutic dosage is being determined, the lithium level should be checked every two to three days. After that, it should be checked once a week. The level may only need to be checked once a month or less frequently if the client's condition is stable. There are three different forms of carbamazepine: liquid, tablet, and chewable tablet. The typical dosage range is 800–1,200 mg/day' the highest dosage range is 200–2,000 mg/day. Valproic acid comes in liquid, tablet, and capsule forms. It can also be purchased as a sprinkle. The recommended daily dosage for valproic acid is 1,000–1,500 mg' an extreme range is 750–3,000 mg. Therapeutic levels of both of these anticonvulsants are tracked in serum drug levels, which are measured 12 hours after the last dose of the medication.

1.11.4.3. Side Effects

Mild nausea or diarrhea, anorexia, fine hand tremor, polydipsia, polyuria, a metallic taste in the mouth, and fatigue or lethargy are typical side effects of lithium therapy. Acne and weight gain are later side effects of lithium therapy that cause clients distress. When taking propranolol, the fine tremor is frequently relieved, and taking the medication with food may help with nausea. Gaining weight and being lethargic are hard to control or minimize, and they often result in noncompliance. Lithium has toxic side effects that include extreme diarrhea, vomiting, fatigue, weak muscles, and loss of coordination. If left untreated, these symptoms deteriorate and may result in death, a coma, or renal failure. If toxic signs appear, stop taking the medication right away. Dialysis might be necessary if lithium levels are higher than 3 mEq/L. Side effects of valproic acid and carbamazepine include dry mouth, drowsiness, and blurred vision. Furthermore, valproic acid may result in weight gain, alopecia, and hand tremor, while carbamazepine may cause rashes and orthostatic hypotension. Dizziness, sedation, weight loss (instead of gain), and a higher risk of renal calculi are all brought on by topiramate. It's crucial to routinely check blood levels for patients taking lithium and anticonvulsants. To check plasma levels 12 hours after the last dose, the time of the last dose needs to be precise. Taking these drugs with food reduces nausea. Until fatigue, blurred vision, dizziness, or lethargy have passed, the client should not try to drive.

1.11.5. Antianxiety Drugs (Anxiolytics)

Antianxiety medications, also known as anxiolytic medications, are used to treat alcohol withdrawal, depression, obsessive compulsive disorder (OCD), insomnia, anxiety, and anxiety disorders. Among the most commonly prescribed medications in today's world are antianxiety drugs. Numerous medications belonging to various categories have been employed to address anxiety and sleeplessness. The most commonly prescribed medications are benzodiazepines because they have been shown to be the most effective in treating anxiety. In addition, doctors may prescribe benzodiazepines for their anticonvulsant and muscle relaxant properties. Since buspirone is a nonbenzodiazepine and is frequently used to treat anxiety, it is included in this section. Some medications that may be used to treat anxiety include propranolol, hydroxyzine (Vistaril), and clonidine (Catapres), but they are not covered in this discussion because they are much less effective.

1.11.5.1. Mechanism of Action

GABA is the primary inhibitory neurotransmitter in the brain, and benzodiazepines mediate its effects. Activation of GABA receptors hyperpolarizes neurons and is therefore inhibitory because GABA receptor channels admit the anion chloride into neurons only. By attaching to a particular location on the GABA receptor, benzodiazepines exert their effects. By functioning as a partial agonist at serotonin receptors and reducing serotonin turnover, buspirone is thought to produce its anxiolytic effects. Different benzodiazepines have different half-lives, are metabolized in different ways, and work differently to treat anxiety and insomnia. After a single dose, the dosages, half-lives, and onset time are listed in Table 1.6. Longer half-lived drugs can accumulate in the body and cause "next-day sedation" effects, but they also require less frequent dosing and have fewer rebound effects between doses. Drugs with shorter half-lives, on the other hand, have rebound effects and need more frequent dosages but do not build up in the body or cause sedation the following day.

Table 1.6. *Antianxiety (Anxiolytic) Drugs*

Generic (Trade) Name	Daily Dosage Range	Half-Life (h)	Speed of Onset
Benzodiazepines			
Alprazolam (Xanax)	0.75–1.5	12–15	Intermediate
Chlordiazepoxide (Librium)	15–100	50–100	Intermediate
Clonazepam (Klonopin)	1.5–20	18–50	Intermediate
Clorazepate (Tranxene)	15–60	30–200	Fast
Diazepam (Valium)	4–40	30–100	Very fast
Flurazepam (Dalmane)	15–30	47–100	Fast
Lorazepam (Ativan)	2–8	10–20	Moderately slow
Oxazepam (Serax)	30–120	3–21	Moderately slow
Temazepam (Restoril)	15–30	9.5–20	Moderately fast
Triazolam (Halcion)	0.25–0.5	2–4	Fast
Nonbenzodiazepine			
Buspirone (BuSpar)	15–30	3–11	Very slow

Source: Sheila L. Videbeck, Psychiatric-Mental Health Nursing, ISBN-10: 1-975116-37-2.

Temazepam (Restoril), triazolam (Halcion), and flurazepam (Dalmane) are most often prescribed for sleep rather than for relief of anxiety. Diazepam (Valium), chlordiazepoxide (Librium), and clonazepam are often used to manage alcohol withdrawal as well as to relieve anxiety.

1.11.5.2. Side Effects

The primary issue with benzodiazepines is that they can lead to physical dependence, even though this isn't a true side effect. When a drug is stopped, significant discontinuation symptoms appear' these symptoms frequently mirror the initial symptoms that the patient sought treatment for. Clients with long-term benzodiazepine use, such as those with panic disorder or generalized anxiety disorder, should be particularly concerned about this. Psychological dependence on benzodiazepines is not uncommon' patients either think they can't manage their anxiety without the drugs or fear that their symptoms will return. This may result in the abuse or overuse of these medications. Buspirone doesn't result in this kind of bodily reliance.

The side effects most commonly reported with benzodiazepines are those associated with CNS depression, such as drowsiness, sedation, poor coordination, and impaired memory or clouded sensorium. When used for sleep, clients may complain of next-day sedation or a hangover effect. Clients often develop a tolerance to these symptoms, and they generally decrease in intensity. Common side effects from buspirone include dizziness, sedation, nausea, and headache. Elderly clients may have more difficulty managing the effects of CNS depression. They may be more prone to falls from the effects on coordination and sedation. They may also have more pronounced memory deficits and may have problems with urinary incontinence, particularly at night.

Patients need to understand that antianxiety medications only treat the symptoms of anxiety, such as sleeplessness or anxiety, rather than the underlying issues that lead to the condition. When taking benzodiazepines, the effects of alcohol are greatly increased' one drink can have the same effects as three drinks. Therefore, when taking benzodiazepines, clients should abstain from alcohol. When attempting activities like driving or going to work, clients should be aware of decreased response time, slower reflexes, and possible sedative effects of these drugs. Withdrawal from benzodiazepines can be lethal. The patient should never stop taking benzodiazepines suddenly or without a doctor's supervision once they have begun a course of therapy.

1.11.6. Stimulants

Due to their strong effects on CNS stimulation, stimulant medications—more especially, amphetamines—were first used to treat psychiatric disorders in the 1930s. Although those uses are rare in modern practice, they were once used to treat obesity and depression. Many people abuse dextroamphetamine, also known as dexedrine, to get high or stay up late. These days, the main conditions for which stimulants are used are narcolepsy (unwanted but insatiable episodes of daytime sleepiness that interfere with daily life), ADHD in children and adolescents, and residual attention deficit disorder in adults. Amphetamine (Adderall), dextroamphetamine (Dexedrine), and methylphenidate (Ritalin) are the three main stimulant medications used to treat ADHD. Because pemoline (Cylert) may cause liver problems, it is not often used for ADHD. Methylphenidate makes up 90% of the stimulant medication prescribed to children with ADHD among these medications. Antidepressants have been used to treat between 10% and 30% of ADHD patients who do not respond well to stimulant medications. As the first non-stimulant drug created especially for ADHD, atomoxetine (Strattera), a selective norepinephrine reuptake inhibitor, was approved in 2003 for the treatment of ADHD.

1.11.6.1. Mechanism of Action

Since methylphenidate and amphetamines release neurotransmitters (dopamine, serotonin, and adrenaline) from presynaptic nerve terminals rather than directly acting as agonists on postsynaptic receptors, they are frequently referred to as indirectly acting amines. They also prevent these neurotransmitters from being reabsorbed. While pemoline primarily affects dopamine and therefore has less effect on the sympathetic nervous system, methylphenidate produces milder CNS stimulation than amphetamines. Initially, it was believed that treating ADHD in children with methylphenidate and pemoline caused the opposite effect of most stimulants, which is a calming or slowing of brain activity. This is untrue, as the child's ability to block out distractions and control their own behavior is enhanced due to the stimulation of the brain's inhibitory centers. By preventing norepinephrine from being reabsorbed into neurons, atomoxetine helps increase the amount of this neurotransmitter in synapses, which aids in the transmission of electrical impulses throughout the brain.

1.11.6.2. Dosage

Adult patients with narcolepsy are treated with divided doses of 20–200 mg/day of methylphenidate and dextroamphetamine. Adults with narcolepsy may develop a tolerance to the stimulants, necessitating higher dosages in order to maintain improvement. Sustained-release versions of stimulant drugs are also offered, enabling once-daily dosing. People with ADHD do not exhibit tolerance. The dosages used to treat ADHD in children differ greatly depending on the doctor, the child's age, weight, and behavior, as well as the family's tolerance of the child's actions. The typical dosage ranges for these stimulants are listed in Table 1.7. The child's stimulants must be given to them in school by the school nurse or another authorized adult. Preparations for sustained release remove the requirement for extra dosage at school.

Table 1.7. *Drugs Used to Treat Attention-Deficit/Hyperactivity Disorder*

Generic (Trade) Name	Dosage
Stimulants	
Methylphenidate (Ritalin)	Adults: 20–200 mg/day, orally, in divided doses Children: 10–60 mg/day, orally, in 2–4 divided doses
Sustained release (Ritalin-SR, Concerta, Metadate-CD)	20–60 mg/day, orally, single dose
Transdermal patch (Daytrana)	Adults and children: 15 mg patch worn for 9 hours/day
Dextroamphetamine (Dexedrine)	Adults: 20–200 mg/day, orally, in divided doses Children: 5–40 mg/day, orally, in 2 or 3 divided doses
Sustained release (Dexedrine-SR)	10–30 mg/day, orally, single dose
Amphetamine (Adderall)	5–40 mg/day, orally, in divided doses
Sustained release (Adderall-SR)	10–30 mg/day, orally, single dose
Pemoline (Cylert)	Children: 37.5–112.5 mg/day, orally, single dose in the morning
Selective norepinephrine reuptake inhibitor	
Atomoxetine (Strattera)	0.5–1.5 mg/kg/day, orally, single dose

Source: Sheila L. Videbeck, Psychiatric-Mental Health Nursing, ISBN-10: 1-975116-37-2.

1.11.6.3. Side Effects

The most typical stimulant side effects include nausea, irritability, anorexia, and weight loss. Chocolate, sugar, and caffeine should be avoided by the client as they may exacerbate these symptoms.

Palpitations, dry mouth, dizziness, and blurred vision are less frequent adverse effects. The most frequent long-term issue with stimulants is the suppression of certain children's growth and weight. By taking "drug holidays" on weekends, holidays, or during summer vacation, which helps restore normal eating and growth patterns, this can usually be avoided. Atomoxetine may result in nausea, vomiting, lethargy, and upset stomach in addition to decreased appetite. Stimulants have the potential to be abused, though this is rarely an issue for young people. Stimulant dosages taken after meals may lessen nausea and anorexia. Drinks devoid of caffeine are advised, and customers should stay away from chocolate and high sugar content. Because even a 10-day supply of the medication can be fatal, it is crucial to keep it out of the child's reach.

1.11.7. Disulfiram (Antabuse)

When disulfiram and alcohol are combined, the body reacts negatively because disulfiram is a sensitizing agent. The only purpose of this agent is to discourage alcohol consumption in those undergoing alcoholism treatment. For those who are not impulsive and are driven to refrain from drinking, it can be helpful. A person taking disulfiram may experience the following symptoms five to ten minutes after consuming alcohol: a throbbing headache, sweating, dry mouth, nausea, vomiting, dizziness, and weakness, as well as facial and body flushing from vasodilation. Chest pain, dyspnea, severe hypotension, confusion, and even death are possible in extreme cases. The symptoms appear quickly and go away in 30 to 2 hours. Disulfiram is most effective in people whose liver enzyme levels are within or near normal range because the liver metabolizes it.

Aldehyde dehydrogenase is an enzyme involved in the metabolism of ethanol, and disulfiram inhibits it. After that, acetaldehyde levels are raised five to ten times higher than usual, which causes the disulfiram–alcohol reaction. The sympathetic nervous system's decreased norepinephrine and adrenaline levels, which are brought on by dopamine β-hydroxylase inhibition, intensify this reaction. If a patient is taking disulfiram, education is crucial. When used by a client taking disulfiram, many common products like shaving cream, aftershave lotion, cologne, deodorant, and over-the-counter medications like cough preparations contain alcohol and can cause the same reaction as drinking alcohol. The customer needs to make sure they carefully read product labels and choose alcohol-free products. Individuals using disulfiram have also reported experiencing tremor, impotence, halitosis, fatigue, and drowsiness as side effects. Disulfiram may also cause problems with the client's other medications, including barbiturates, long-acting benzodiazepines like diazepam and chlordiazepoxide, phenytoin (Dilantin), isoniazid, and warfarin (Coumadin). Sometimes doctors will prescribe acamprosate (Campral) to patients who are recovering from alcohol addiction or abuse. It helps lessen the emotional and physical discomfort, such as anxiety, sweating, and disturbed sleep, that comes with the first few weeks or months of sobriety. The recommended dosage is two 333 mg tablets three times a day. Renal impairments prevent the use of this medication. The mild side effects include flatulence, diarrhea, nausea, and pruritus. (American Nurses Association, 2014' Virani et al., 2017)

A Closer Look

Psychiatric Nurse

Psychiatric nurses specialize in caring for patients with mental health disorders, providing them with holistic and compassionate care throughout their treatment journey. These nurses possess a diverse skill set that enables them to assess, diagnose, and treat individuals experiencing a wide range of mental health conditions, including anxiety disorders, mood disorders, psychotic disorders, substance use disorders, and personality disorders. One of the primary responsibilities of psychiatric nurses is to conduct comprehensive psychiatric assessments, which involve gathering information about patients' mental health history, symptoms, and current functioning. Based on these assessments, they collaborate with other members of the healthcare team to develop individualized care plans tailored to each patient's unique needs and goals. Psychiatric nurses also play a crucial role in administering psychiatric medications and monitoring their effectiveness and side effects. They educate patients and their families about their medications, helping them understand the importance of adherence and providing support to address any concerns or questions. In addition to medication management, psychiatric nurses are skilled in delivering various therapeutic interventions, including individual counseling, group therapy, and cognitive-behavioral therapy (CBT). They create safe and supportive environments where patients can explore their thoughts and feelings, learn coping skills, and work towards recovery and improved mental well-being. Furthermore, psychiatric nurses advocate for their patients' rights and access to quality mental healthcare. They collaborate with interdisciplinary teams to ensure that patients receive comprehensive and coordinated care that addresses not only their psychiatric needs but also any co-occurring medical or social issues. Overall, psychiatric nurses play a vital role in supporting individuals with mental health disorders, helping them navigate challenges, manage symptoms, and work towards recovery and improved quality of life. Through their expertise, empathy, and commitment to excellence in care, psychiatric nurses make a meaningful difference in the lives of their patients and their families.

Summary

- Psychiatric-Mental Health Nursing (PMHN) is a specialized field within nursing that focuses on promoting mental health, preventing mental illness, and providing care and support for individuals experiencing psychiatric disorders or mental health challenges.
- Mental illness includes disorders that affect mood, behavior, and thinking, such as depression, schizophrenia, anxiety disorders, and addictive disorders.
- The cerebrum is divided into two hemispheres' all lobes and structures are found in both halves except for the pineal body, or gland, which is located between the hemispheres. The pineal body is an endocrine gland that influences the activities of the pituitary gland, islets of Langerhans, parathyroids, adrenals, and gonads.
- The brain stem includes the midbrain, pons, and medulla oblongata and the nuclei for cranial nerves III through XII. The medulla, located at the top of the spinal cord, contains vital centers for respiration and cardiovascular functions.
- The limbic system is an area of the brain located above the brain stem that includes the thalamus, hypothalamus, hippocampus, and amygdala (although some sources differ regarding the structures this system includes).
- Neurotransmitters are the chemical substances manufactured in the neuron that aid in the transmission of information throughout the body. They either excite or stimulate an action in the cells (excitatory) or inhibit or stop an action (inhibitory).
- Norepinephrine, the most prevalent neurotransmitter in the nervous system, is located primarily in the brain stem and plays a role in changes in attention, learning and memory, sleep and wakefulness, and mood regulation.
- Serotonin is derived from tryptophan, a dietary amino acid. The function of serotonin is mostly inhibitory, and it is involved in the control of food intake, sleep and wakefulness, temperature regulation, pain control, sexual behavior, and regulation of emotions.
- Computed tomography (CT), also called computed axial tomography, is a procedure in which a precise x-ray beam takes cross-sectional images (slices) layer by layer. A computer reconstructs the images on a monitor and also stores the images on magnetic tape or film.
- In magnetic resonance imaging (MRI), a type of body scan, an energy field is created with a huge magnet and radio waves. The energy field is converted to a visual image or scan. MRI produces more tissue detail and contrast than CT and can show blood flow patterns and tissue changes such as edema.
- Antipsychotic drugs, formerly known as neuroleptics, are used to treat the symptoms of psychosis, such as the delusions and hallucinations seen in schizophrenia, schizoaffective disorder, and the manic phase of bipolar disorder.
- Extrapyramidal symptoms (EPSs),serious neurologic symptoms, are the major side effects of antipsychotic drugs. They include acute dystonia, pseudoparkinsonism, and akathisia.
- Antipsychotic drugs also increase blood prolactin levels. Elevated prolactin may cause breast enlargement and tenderness in men and women' diminished libido, erectile and orgasmic dysfunction, and menstrual irregularities' and increased risk for breast cancer.

- The nurse informs clients taking antipsychotic medication about the types of side effects that may occur and encourages clients to report such problems to the physician instead of discontinuing the medication.
- Antidepressant drugs are primarily used in the treatment of major depressive illness, anxiety disorders, the depressed phase of bipolar disorder, and psychotic depression.

References

1. Allison, S., Bastiampillai, T., Licinio, J., Fuller, D. A., Bidargaddi, N., & Sharfstein, S. S. (2018). When should governments increase the supply of psychiatric beds? *Molecular Psychiatry, 23*(4), 796–800.
2. American Nurses Association, & American Psychiatric Nurses Association. (2014). *Psychiatric–Mental Health Nursing: Scope and Standards of Practice* (2nd ed.). Nursebooks.org.
3. Arms, T., Bostic, T., & Cunningham, P. (2014). Educational intervention to increase detection of metabolic syndrome in patients at community mental health centers. *Journal of Psychosocial Nursing and Mental Health Services, 52*(9), 32–36.
4. Baly, M. (1982). A leading light. *Nursing Mirror, 155*(19), 49–51.
5. Coakley, C., Bolton, P., Flaherty, L., et al. (2012). The incidence of metabolic risk factors in an inpatient psychiatric setting. *Journal of Psychosocial Nursing and Mental Health Services, 50*(3), 24–30.
6. Debost, J. P., Larsen, J. T., Munk-Olsen, T., Mortensen, P. B., Meyer, U., & Petersen, L. (2017). Joint effects of exposure to prenatal infection and peripubertal psychological trauma in schizophrenia. *Schizophrenia Bulletin, 43*(1), 171–179.
7. Doona, M. (1984). At least as well cared for ... Linda Richards and the mentally ill. *Image: The Journal of Nursing Scholarship, 16*(2), 51–56.
8. Gill, K. J., Zechner, M., Zambo, A. E., Swarbrick, M., & Murphy, A. (2016). Wellness for life: A pilot of an interprofessional intervention to address metabolic syndrome in adults with serious mental illnesses. *Psychiatric Rehabilitation Journal, 39*(2), 147–153.
9. Gollaher, D. (1995). *Voice for the Mad: The Life of Dorothea Dix*. Free Press.
10. Gur, R. E., & Gur, R. C. (2017). Functional brain imaging in schizophrenia. In B. J. Sadock, V. A. Sadock, & P. Ruiz (Eds.), *Comprehensive Textbook of Psychiatry* (Vol. 1, 10th ed., pp. 1475–1488). Lippincott, Williams, & Wilkins/Wolters Kluwer.
11. Kim, A. P., Baker, D. E., & Levien, T. L. (2018). VMAT2 inhibitors: New drugs for treatment of tardive dyskinesia. *Consultant Pharmacist, 33*(4), 201–209.
12. Kroll, D. S., Karno, J., Mullen, B., Shah, S. B., Pallin, D. J., & Gitlin, D. F. (2018). Clinical severity alone does not determine disposition decisions for patients in the emergency department with suicide risk. *Psychosomatics, 59*(4), 388–393.
13. McMillan, I. (1997). Insight into Bedlam: One hospital's history. *Journal of Psychosocial Nursing and Mental Health Services, 3*(6), 28–34.
14. Medford-Davis, L. N., & Beall, R. C. (2017). The changing healthcare policy environment and behavioral health services delivery. *Psychiatric Clinics of North America, 40*(3), 533–540.

15. Mellow, J. (1986). A personal perspective of nursing therapy. *Hospital and Community Psychiatry, 37*(2), 182–183.

16. Meyers, K. J., Upadhyaya, H. P., Landry, J. L., Chhabra-Khanna, R., Falk, D. M., Seetharama Rao, B., & Jones, M. E. (2017). Postinjection delirium/sedation syndrome in patients with schizophrenia receiving olanzapine long-acting injection: Results from a large observational study. *British Journal of Psychiatry Open, 3*(4), 186–192.

17. National Alliance for the Mentally Ill. (2018). *Mental Health Parity Laws*. Retrieved from: https://www.nami.org/parity-report-grades-states-on-parity-laws/ (accessed on 7 September 2024).

18. National Institutes of Health. (2018). *Mental Illness Statistics*. Retrieved from: https://www.nimh.nih.gov/statistics/mental-illness.shtml (accessed on 7 September 2024).

19. Penninx, B. W. J. H., & Lange, S. M. M. (2018). Metabolic syndrome in psychiatric patients: Overview, mechanisms, and implications. *Dialogues in Neuroscience, 20*(1), 63–73.

20. Raison, C. L., & Miller, A. H. (2017). Pathogen-host defense in the evolution of depression: Genetics, bioregional differences, and female preponderance. *Neuropsychopharmacology, 42*(1), 5–27.

21. Rosenblatt, A. (1984). Concepts of the asylum in the care of the mentally ill. *Hospital and Community Psychiatry, 35*, 244–250.

22. Stahl, S. M. (2017). *Essential Psychopharmacology: The Prescriber's Guide* (6th ed.). Cambridge University Press.

23. Treatment Advocacy Center. (2018). *Consequences of Non-Treatment*. Retrieved from: https://www.treatmentadvocacycenter.org/key-issues/consequences-of-non-treatment (accessed on 7 September 2024).

24. Treatment Advocacy Center. (2019). *How Many People with Serious Mental Illness Are Homeless?* Retrieved from: https://www.treatmentadvocacycenter.org/fixing-the-system/features-and-news/2596-how-many-people-with-serious-mental-illness-are-homeless (accessed on 7 September 2024).

25. U.S. Census Bureau. (2010). *2010 Census Survey Results*. Retrieved from: http://www.census.gov (accessed on 7 September 2024).

26. U.S. Department of Health and Human Services. (2010). *Healthy People 2020*. DHHS.

27. Virani, A. S., Bezchlibnyk-Butler, K. Z., & Jeffries, J. J. (2017). *Clinical Handbook of Psychotropic Drugs* (22nd ed.). Hogrefe Publishing.

Chapter

PSYCHOSOCIAL THEORIES AND THERAPY

2

Contents

Introduction

Psychosocial theories and therapy in mental health provide a comprehensive framework for understanding and addressing the complex interplay between psychological, social, and environmental factors that influence mental health and well-being. Rooted in various theoretical perspectives, psychosocial approaches aim to promote resilience, facilitate personal growth, and enhance the quality of life for individuals experiencing mental health challenges. One of the foundational theories in psychosocial therapy is psychodynamic theory, which emphasizes the role of unconscious processes, early childhood experiences, and interpersonal relationships in shaping an individual's thoughts, feelings, and behaviors. Psychodynamic therapy seeks to explore and resolve underlying conflicts and patterns of behavior through insight, reflection, and interpretation, fostering self-awareness and emotional healing. Another prominent theory is cognitive-behavioral theory, which focuses on the reciprocal relationship between thoughts, emotions, and behaviors. Cognitive-behavioral therapy (CBT) aims to identify and challenge maladaptive beliefs and behaviors, replace negative cognitive patterns with more adaptive ones, and develop practical coping skills to manage stress, anxiety, depression, and other mental health concerns effectively.

Additionally, social learning theory highlights the importance of observational learning, modeling, and reinforcement in shaping behavior. Therapeutic interventions based on social learning principles focus on enhancing social skills, problem-solving abilities, and coping strategies through role-playing, behavior rehearsal, and feedback.

Furthermore, humanistic-existential theories emphasize the significance of self-awareness, personal agency, and existential meaning in promoting psychological well-being. Humanistic-existential therapies, such as person-centered therapy and existential therapy, prioritize the client's subjective experience, autonomy, and inherent capacity for growth and self-actualization, fostering a supportive therapeutic relationship conducive to self-exploration and personal development.

Overall, psychosocial theories and therapy in mental health offer a diverse array of conceptual frameworks and therapeutic approaches tailored to the unique needs and preferences of individuals seeking support for their mental health concerns. By addressing psychological, social, and environmental factors holistically, psychosocial interventions strive to empower individuals, enhance their resilience, and promote their overall mental health and well-being.

Orientation and Directional Terms

Term	Definition	Illustration
Cognitive-behavioral therapy (CBT)	Cognitive behavioral therapy (CBT) is a form of psychological treatment that has been demonstrated to be effective for a range of problems including depression, anxiety disorders, alcohol and drug use problems, marital problems, eating disorders, and severe mental illness.	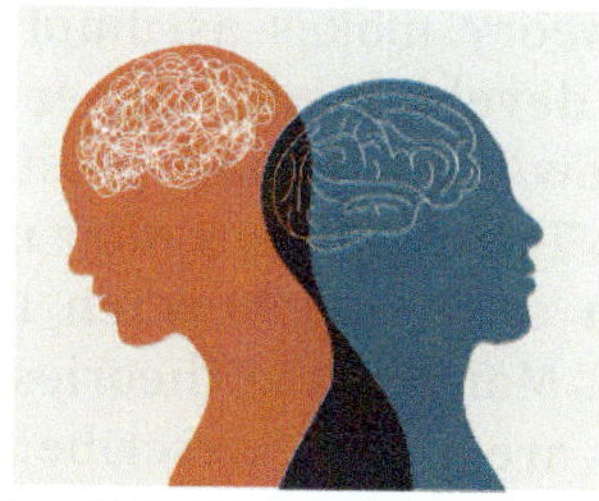
Social learning theory	Social learning theory suggests that social behavior is learned by observing and imitating the behavior of others. Psychologist Albert Bandura developed social learning theory open_in_new as an alternative to the earlier work of fellow psychologist B.F. Skinner, known for his influence on behaviorism.	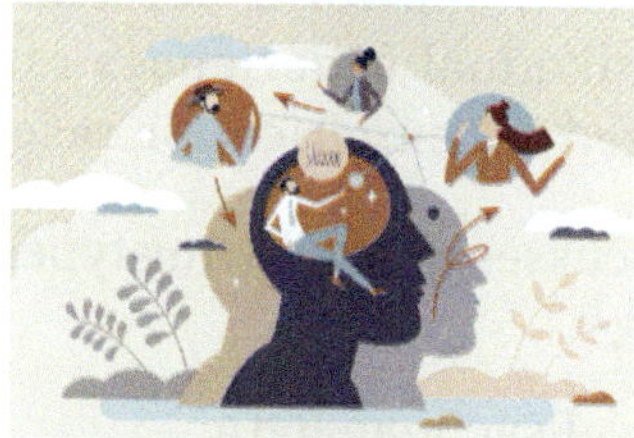
Psychoanalytic	Psychoanalytic was developed in order to clarify the causes of the disorders and to restore mental health. This is possible by enabling the ego to become aware of the id's needs that have been repressed into the unconscious and to find a realistic solution to resolve the conflicts.	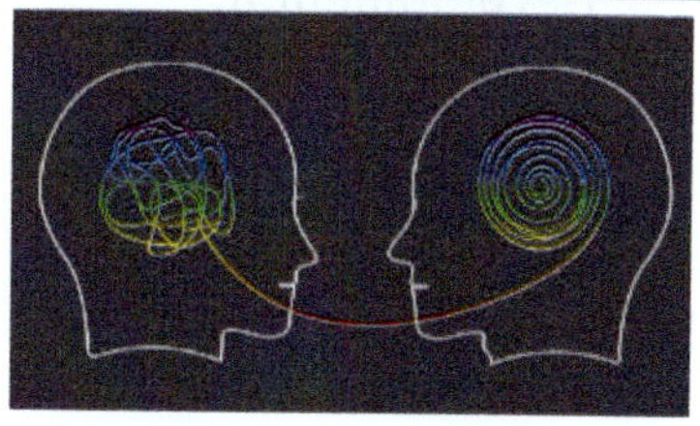
Primary care physician (PCP)	Primary care physician (PCP) is a doctor who helps you manage all aspects of your health. They help you stay healthy and get better when you are sick. PCPs have a wide range of responsibilities, from regular checkups to diagnosing and treating illnesses, injuries and other health conditions.	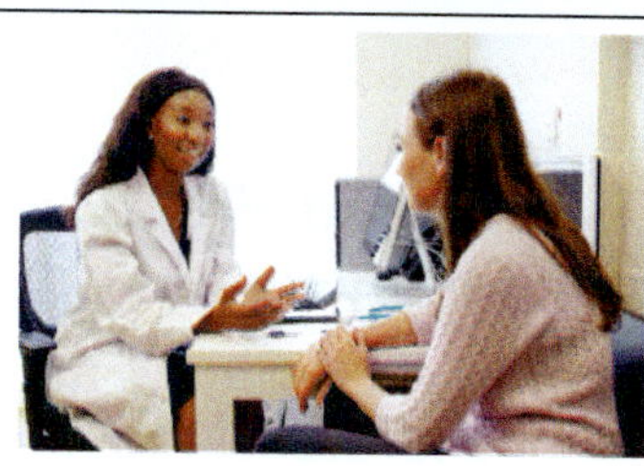
Family therapy	Family therapy is a form of talk therapy that focuses on the improvement of relationships among family members. It can also help treat specific mental health or behavioral conditions, such as substance use disorder or oppositional defiant disorder.	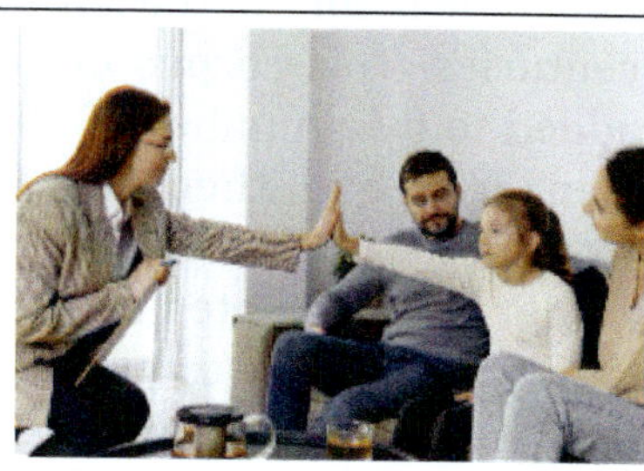

2.1. Psychosocial Theories

Numerous theories make an effort to explain mental illness, health, and behavior in people. Every theory makes assumptions about how normal development happens based on the worldview, beliefs, and presumptions of the theorist. These theories offer methods that the clinician can employ when interacting with patients. Many of the theories covered in this chapter are better described as conceptual models or frameworks because they developed from individual experiences rather than being supported by empirical or research evidence.

Discusses the following types of psychosocial theories:

- Psychoanalytic;
- Developmental;
- Interpersonal;
- Humanistic;
- Behavioral;
- Existential.

2.1.1. Psychoanalytic Theories

2.1.1.1. Sigmund Freud: The Father of Psychoanalysis

The majority of his life was spent in Vienna, where Sigmund Freud (1856–1939) created psychoanalytic theory in the late 19th and early 20th centuries. This corpus of knowledge has been added to by a number of other renowned psychoanalysts and theorists, but Freud is without a doubt its founder. Many theorists and practitioners later created their own theories and treatment philosophies because they disagreed with much of Freud's psychoanalytic theory (Figure 2.1).

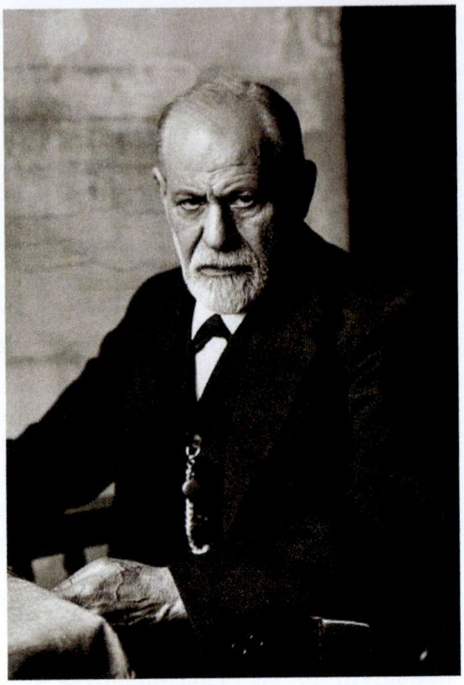

Figure 2.1. *Sigmund Freud—the father of psychoanalysis.*

Source: https://en.m.wikipedia.org/wiki/File:Sigmund_Freud_1926.jpg.

The idea that all human behavior is caused and explicable is supported by psychoanalytic theory (deterministic theory). According to Freud, a lot of human behavior is motivated by suppressed (from conscious awareness) sexual impulses and desires. His work with a few clients—all women—who exhibited strange behaviors like speech and vision problems, eating disorders, and limb paralysis—provided him with the first ideas and explanations of human behavior. Freud saw these symptoms as "hysterical" or neurotic behaviors in women since there was no recognized physiological basis for them. After working with these women for several years, Freud concluded that a large number of their issues were brought on by early trauma or an inability to fulfill the necessary stages of psychosexual development. These women suppressed their traumatic experiences, unfulfilled needs, and sexual desires. These unresolved conflicts led to the "hysterical" or neurotic behaviors that were observed are:

- **Personality Components:** The ego, superego, and id. Three elements comprised Freud's conceptualization of personality structure: the id, ego, and superego (Freud, 1923, 1962). The aspect of a person's nature known as the id is what represents fundamental or innate desires like aggressiveness, pleasure-seeking behavior, and sexual impulses. Instant gratification is a goal of the id, which also leads to impulsive, thoughtless behavior and disregard for social norms. The superego is the aspect of a person's nature that contrasts sharply with the id because it represents moral and ethical ideas, values, and social and familial expectations. The mediating or balancing force between the id and the superego is the third element, the ego. The ego stands for responsible and flexible behavior that enables an individual to lead a fulfilling life. According to Freud's theory, anxiety arises from the ego's endeavors to harmonize the impetuous impulses of the id with the strict regulations of the superego.
- **Behavior Motivated by Subconscious Thoughts and Feelings:** According to Freud (1923, 1962), there are three levels of awareness at which the human personality functions: conscious, preconscious, and unconscious. The perceptions, ideas, and feelings that are present in an individual's awareness—such as being aware of joy or remembering a loved one—are referred to as conscious. Although a person's subconscious thoughts and feelings are not conscious to them at the moment, they are retrievable with some effort' an adult may remember actions, feelings, or thoughts from their childhood. The domain of ideas and emotions that drive an individual despite their complete ignorance of them is known as the unconscious. This category includes some innate drives or motivations as well as the majority of defense mechanisms (see discussion to follow). Following Freud's theories, the unconscious is where traumatic memories that are too painful to recall are suppressed. Freud believed that much of what we do and say is motivated by our subconscious thoughts or feelings (those in the preconscious or unconscious level of awareness). A Freudian slip is a term we commonly use to describe slips of the tongue—for example, saying "You look portly today" to an overweight friend instead of "You look pretty today." Freud believed that these slips are not accidents or coincidences, but rather are indications of subconscious feelings or thoughts that accidentally emerge in casual day-to-day conversation.
- **Freud's Dream Analysis:** According to Freud, a person's dreams are a reflection of their subconscious and often carry a deep symbolic or hidden meaning. One of the main psychoanalytic techniques is dream analysis, which entails talking about

a client's dreams to ascertain their actual significance and meaning. For instance, a client may describe experiencing terrifying dreams about snakes chasing her regularly. According to Freud, who would see the snake as a phallic symbol that represents the penis, the woman may be afraid of intimate relationships with men. Free association is another technique used to access subconscious thoughts and feelings. In this technique, the therapist asks the client to quickly respond with the first thought that comes to mind after uttering a word in an attempt to elicit the true thoughts and feelings of the client. Such rapid reactions, according to Freud, would probably reveal suppressed or subconscious feelings or thoughts.

Table 2.1. *Ego Defense Mechanisms*

Compensation	Overachievement in one area to offset real or perceived deficiencies in another area • Napoleon complex: diminutive man becoming emperor • Nurse with low self-esteem working double shifts so that her supervisor will like her
Conversion	Expression of an emotional conflict through the development of a physical symptom, usually sensorimotor in nature • Teenager forbidden to see X-rated movies is tempted to do so by friends and develops blindness, and the teenager is unconcerned about the loss of sight
Denial	Failure to acknowledge an unbearable condition; failure to admit the reality of a situation or how one enables the problem to continue • Diabetic person eating chocolate candy • Spending money freely when broke • Waiting 3 days to seek help for severe abdominal pain
Displacement	Ventilation of intense feelings toward persons less threatening than the one who aroused those feelings • Person who is mad at the boss yells at his or her spouse • Child who is harassed by a bully at school mistreats a younger sibling
Dissociation	Dealing with emotional conflict by a temporary alteration in consciousness or identity • Amnesia that prevents recall of yesterday's auto accident • Adult remembers nothing of childhood sexual abuse
Fixation	Immobilization of a portion of the personality resulting from unsuccessful completion of tasks in a developmental stage • Never learning to delay gratification • Lack of a clear sense of identity as an adult
Identification	Modeling actions and opinions of influential others while searching for identity, or aspiring to reach a personal, social, or occupational goal • Nursing student becoming a critical care nurse because this is the specialty of an instructor she admires
Intellectualization	Separation of the emotions of a painful event or situation from the facts involved; acknowledging the facts but not the emotions • Person shows no emotional expression when discussing serious car accident

Introjection	Accepting another person's attitudes, beliefs, and values as one's own • Person who dislikes guns becomes an avid hunter, just like a best friend
Projection	Unconscious blaming of unacceptable inclinations or thoughts on an external object • Man who has thought about same-gender sexual relationship but never had one beats a man who is gay • Person with many prejudices loudly identifies others as bigots
Rationalization	Excusing own behavior to avoid guilt, responsibility, conflict, anxiety, or loss of self-respect • Student blames failure on teacher being mean • Man says he beats his wife because she does not listen to him
Reaction formation	Acting the opposite of what one thinks or feels • Woman who never wanted to have children becomes a supermom • Person who despises the boss tells everyone what a great boss she is
Regression	Moving back to a previous developmental stage to feel safe or have needs met • A 5-year-old asks for a bottle when new baby brother is being fed • Man pouts like a 4-year-old if he is not the center of his girlfriend's attention
Repression	Excluding emotionally painful or anxiety-provoking thoughts and feelings from conscious awareness • Woman has no memory of the mugging she suffered yesterday • Woman has no memory before age 7, when she was removed from abusive parents
Resistance	Overt or covert antagonism toward remembering or processing anxiety-producing information • Nurse is too busy with tasks to spend time talking to a dying patient. • Person attends court-ordered treatment for alcoholism but refuses to participate
Sublimation	Substituting a socially acceptable activity for an impulse that is unacceptable • Person who has quit smoking sucks on hard candy when the urge to smoke arises • Person goes for a 15-minute walk when tempted to eat junk food
Substitution	Replacing the desired gratification with one that is more readily available • Woman who would like to have her own children opens a day care center
Suppression	Conscious exclusion of unacceptable thoughts and feelings from conscious awareness • Student decides not to think about a parent's illness to study for a test • Woman tells a friend she cannot think about her son's death right now
Undoing	Exhibiting acceptable behavior to make up for or negate unacceptable behavior • Person who cheats on a spouse brings the spouse a bouquet of roses • Man who is ruthless in business donates large amounts of money to charity

Source: Sheila L. Videbeck, Psychiatric-Mental Health Nursing, ISBN-10: 1-975116-37-2.

- **Ego Defense Mechanisms:** According to Freud, the self, or ego, employs ego defense mechanisms in an effort to defend itself and deal with primal urges or emotionally upsetting ideas, sensations, or experiences. Table 2.1 provides an explanation of defense mechanisms. For instance, a person who has been given a six-month cancer diagnosis and told not to discuss his condition with others is utilizing denial as a defense mechanism, which is the inability to acknowledge the truth of the circumstance. A cancer patient may be utilizing the reaction formation defense mechanism to shield his emotions if he is consistently happy. People frequently require assistance to see reality because most defense mechanisms function at the unconscious level of awareness, meaning they are often unaware of what they are doing.
- **Five Stages of Psychosexual Development:** Freud's theory of childhood development

was predicated on the idea that libido, or sexual energy, was what motivated people to act in certain ways. According to his theory, children go through five phases of psychosexual development: genital (11–13 years), phallic/oedipal (3-5 years), latency (5–11 years or 13 years), oral (birth to 18 months), and anal (18–36 months). These phases are outlined in Table 2.2, along with the related developmental assignments. When a person finds it difficult to move from one stage to the next, stops at a specific point, or regresses to an earlier stage, psychopathology results. For his time, Freud's candid examination of sexual impulses, especially in children, was regarded as shocking (Freud, 1923, 1962).

Table 2.2. *Freud's Developmental Stages*

Phase	Age	Focus
Oral	Birth to 18 months	Major site of tension and gratification is the mouth, lips, and tongue; includes biting and sucking activities. Id is present at birth. Ego develops gradually from rudimentary structure present at birth.
Anal	18–36 months	Anus and surrounding area are major source of interest. Voluntary sphincter control (toilet training) is acquired.
Phallic/oedipal	3–5 years	Genital is the focus of interest, stimulation, and excitement. Penis is organ of interest for both sexes. Masturbation is common. Penis envy (wish to possess penis) is seen in girls; oedipal complex (wish to marry opposite-sex parent and be rid of same-sex parent) is seen in boys and girls.
Latency	5–11 or 13 years	Resolution of oedipal complex. Sexual drive channeled into socially appropriate activities such as school work and sports. Formation of the superego.
Genital	11–13 years	Final stage of psychosexual development. Begins with puberty and the biologic capacity for orgasm; involves the capacity for true intimacy.

Source: Adapted from Freud, S. (1962). The ego and the id (J. Strachey, Trans). In The standard edition of the complete psychological works of Sigmund Freud. New York, NY: W. W. Norton & Company. (Original work published 1923.).

- **Transference and Countertransference:** The ideas of transference and countertransference were created by Freud. When a client projects attitudes and feelings from previous relationships onto the therapist, this is known as transference (Freud, 1923, 1962). In a therapeutic relationship, transference patterns are unconsciously and automatically occurring. An adolescent female client, for instance, might respond to the nurse in the same way that she does to her parents if the nurse is roughly the same age as the teen's parents. She may react sarcastically or with strong feelings of rebellion' these are really reactions to her experiences with her parents, not the nurse. When a therapist projects past attitudes or emotions onto a client, it's known as countertransference. For instance, a female nurse who is extremely frustrated with an adolescent client and has teenage children may respond by sounding stern or reprimanding. By counter transferring her own attitudes and feelings toward her children onto the client, the nurse is doing just that. By analyzing their own emotions and reactions, applying self-awareness, and consulting with colleagues, nurses can manage countertransference.

2.1.1.2. Current Psychoanalytic Practice

The main goals of psychoanalysis are to identify the unconscious and repressed thoughts, feelings, and conflicts that the client believes to be the source of their anxiety, as well as to assist the client in understanding and resolving these conflicts and anxieties. The methods of free association, dream interpretation, and behavior analysis are employed by the analytic therapist. Today, psychoanalysis is still used, albeit sparingly. For several years, the analysis is conducted in weekly or more frequent sessions. Because it is expensive and not covered by traditional health insurance plans, it is sometimes referred to as "therapy for the rich."

2.1.2. Developmental Theories

2.1.2.1. Erik Erikson and Psychosocial Stages of Development

German-born psychoanalyst Erik Erikson (1902–1994) expanded on the work of Sigmund Freud on personality development throughout life, emphasizing the stages of social and psychological development. Erikson defined eight psychosocial stages of development in his 1950 book Childhood and Society. The person has to finish a life task that is critical to their wellbeing and mental health at each level. The virtues of life—hope, purpose, fidelity, love, caring, and wisdom—can be attained through these endeavors (Erikson, 1963). Table 2.3 describes the stages, life tasks, and virtues.

Table 2.3. *Erikson's Stages of Psychosocial Development*

Stage	Virtue	Task
Trust vs. mistrust (infant)	Hope	Viewing the world as safe and reliable; relationships as nurturing, stable, and dependable
Autonomy vs. shame and doubt (toddler)	Will	Achieving a sense of control and free will
Initiative vs. guilt (preschool)	Purpose	Beginning development of a conscience; learning to manage conflict and anxiety
Industry vs. inferiority (school age)	Competence	Emerging confidence in own abilities; taking pleasure in accomplishments
Identity vs. role confusion (adolescence)	Fidelity	Formulating a sense of self and belonging
Intimacy vs. isolation (young adult)	Love	Forming adult, loving relationships, and meaningful attachments to others
Generativity vs. stagnation (middle adult)	Care	Being creative and productive; establishing the next generation
Ego integrity vs. despair (maturity)	Wisdom	Accepting responsibility for oneself and life

Source: Sheila L. Videbeck, Psychiatric-Mental Health Nursing, ISBN-10: 1-975116-37-2.

Numerous fields continue to employ Erikson's eight psychosocial phases of development. According to him, psychological development happens in phases that build upon one another, with each stage requiring the accomplishment of a prior stage and a life task. For instance, the infant must learn to develop fundamental trust (the positive outcome), such as that he or she will be fed and taken care of, during the infant stage (birth to 18 months). Establishing trust is crucial, as mistrust, which is the unfavorable consequence of this phase, will hinder an individual's growth all through their life.

2.1.2.2. Jean Piaget and Cognitive Stages of Development

Jean Piaget (1896–1980) studied how children's cognitive abilities and intelligence grow. According to his theory, a child's level of functioning increases with each passing stage, and human intelligence develops in a sequential manner based on age. Piaget was adamant in his schema that maturation and biological changes were the causes of cognitive development.

Piaget's four stages of cognitive development are as follows:

- **Sensorimotor**—birth to 2 years: The child develops a sense of self as separate from the environment and the concept of object permanence, that is, tangible objects do not cease to exist just because they are out of sight. He or she begins to form mental images.
- **Preoperational**—2 to 6 years: The child develops the ability to express self with language, understands the meaning of symbolic gestures, and begins to classify objects.
- **Concrete Operations**—6 to 12 years: The child begins to apply logic to thinking, understands spatiality and reversibility, and is increasingly social and able to apply rules' however, thinking is still concrete.
- **Formal Operations**—12 to 15 years and beyond The child learns to think and reason in abstract terms, further develops logical thinking and reasoning and achieves cognitive maturity.

According to Piaget's theory, people reach cognitive maturity between the middle and late stages of adolescence. According to some of Piaget's detractors, cognitive development is more individualized and less rigid than his theory implies. The theory of Piaget is helpful when working with kids. If the nurse is aware of the child's cognitive development stage, she or he may be able to communicate with them more effectively. Additionally, the way that children are taught is frequently designed with their cognitive development in mind.

2.1.3. Interpersonal Theories

2.1.3.1. Harry Stack Sullivan: Interpersonal Relationships and Milieu Therapy

American psychiatrist Harry Stack Sullivan (1892–1949) added the importance of interpersonal relationships to the theory of personality development. According to Sullivan, a person's personality encompasses more than just their individual traits, especially in terms of their social interactions. He believed that unsatisfactory or inadequate relationships lead to anxiety, which he believed to be the root cause of all emotional issues (Sullivan, 1953). Sullivan's most significant contribution to the field of mental health is most likely his explanation of the value and significance of interpersonal relationships in one's life.

- **Five Life Stages:** Sullivan identified five developmental phases, each concentrating on a different type of interpersonal relationship: infancy, childhood, juvenile, preadolescence, and adolescence. In addition, he listed three cognitive modes of experience that develop over time and proposed a connection between mental illnesses and the survival of an early mode. The prototaxic mode, which is typical of childhood and infancy, consists of isolated, fleeting experiences that are unrelated to one another. Schizophrenia adults display enduring prototaxic experiences. Early childhood is when the parataxic mode starts as the child starts to link experiences chronologically. The child might interpret the events as coincidences or random occurrences and be unable to rationally explain them. Though he or she might not be aware of it, the child tries to calm themselves by reliving happy memories. Sullivan described someone who is in the parataxic mode as having paranoid thoughts and verbal blunders. The syntaxic mode, which first manifests in school-age children and becomes more prevalent in preadolescence, is characterized by the ability to analyze experiences in a range of contexts and by the person's ability to view himself and the world in the context of the environment. The dominance of the syntactic mode is one way to characterize maturity (Sullivan, 1953) (Table 2.4).

Table 2.4. *Sullivan's Life Stages*

Stage	Ages	Focus
Infancy	Birth to onset of language	Primary need exists for bodily contact and tenderness. Prototaxic mode dominates (no relation between experiences). Primary zones are oral and anal. If needs are met, infant has sense of well-being; unmet needs lead to dread and anxiety.
Childhood	Language to 5 years	Parents are viewed as source of praise and acceptance. Shift to parataxic mode; experiences are connected in sequence to each other. Primary zone is anal. Gratification leads to positive self-esteem. Moderate anxiety leads to uncertainty and insecurity; severe anxiety results in self-defeating patterns of behavior.
Juvenile	5–8 years	Shift to the syntaxic mode begins (thinking about self and others based on analysis of experiences in a variety of situations). Opportunities for approval and acceptance of others. Learn to negotiate own needs. Severe anxiety may result in a need to control or in restrictive, prejudicial attitudes.
Preadolescence	8–12 years	Move to genuine intimacy with friend of the same sex. Move away from family as source of satisfaction in relationships. Major shift to syntaxic mode occurs. Capacity for attachment, love, and collaboration emerges or fails to develop.
Adolescence	Puberty to adulthood	Lust is added to interpersonal equation. Need for special sharing relationship shifts to the opposite sex. New opportunities for social experimentation lead to the consolidation of self-esteem or self-ridicule. If the self-system is intact, areas of concern expand to include values, ideals, career decisions, and social concerns.

Source: Adapted from Sullivan, H. S. (1953). The interpersonal theory of psychiatry. New York, NY: W. W. Norton & Company.

2.1.3.2. Therapeutic Community or Milieu.

Sullivan thought that the development of fulfilling interpersonal relationships should be the aim of treatment. For the client, the therapist offers a corrective interpersonal relationship. The phrase "participant observer" was first used by Sullivan to describe the therapist's job, which entails both participation in and observation of the development of the relationship. Although the term "therapeutic community" was not widely used until Maxwell Jones published The Therapeutic Community in 1953, Sullivan is also credited with creating the first milieu or therapeutic community for young men with schizophrenia in 1929. The idea of a therapeutic milieu or community views client interaction as advantageous, and treatment places a strong emphasis on this client-to-client interaction. Up until this point, it was thought that the only crucial aspect of the patient's treatment was their interaction with the psychiatrist. Sullivan and later Jones noted that in a secure, therapeutic environment, client interactions yielded significant advantages for the clients. Sullivan originated the idea of milieu therapy, which entailed clients interacting with one another to work on daily problems as a group, practice interpersonal relationship skills, and provide feedback to one another about their behavior.

One of the main treatment modalities in the acute hospital setting was milieu therapy. However, inpatient hospital stays are frequently too brief in today's healthcare setting for patients to form deep connections with one another. As a result, there is minimal discussion of milieu therapy. One of the nurse's main responsibilities, in addition to ensuring every client's safety and protection and encouraging social interaction, is still managing the milieu.

2.1.3.3. Hildegard Peplau: Therapeutic Nurse–Patient Relationships

Building on Sullivan's interpersonal theories, Hildegard Peplau (1909–1999' Figure 2.2) was a nursing theorist and clinician who also saw the nurse's role as a participant observer. The four phases of the therapeutic nurse-patient relationship are orientation, identification, exploitation, and resolution. Peplau developed this concept (Table 2.5).

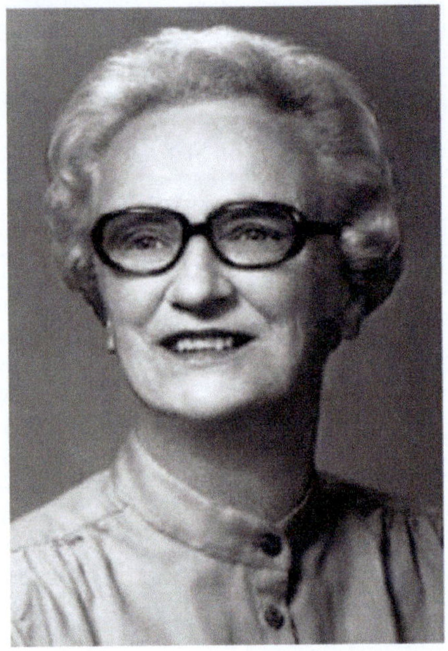

Figure 2.2. *Hildegard Peplau, who developed the phases of the nurse–client therapeutic relationship that has made great contributions to the foundation of nursing practice today.*

Source: Sheila L. Videbeck, Psychiatric-Mental Health Nursing, ISBN-10: 1-975116-37-2.

During these phases, the client accomplishes certain tasks and makes relationship changes that help the healing process (Peplau, 1952):

- The orientation phase is directed by the nurse and involves engaging the client in treatment, providing explanations and information, and answering questions.

- The identification phase begins when the client works interdependently with the nurse, expresses feelings, and begins to feel stronger.
- In the exploitation phase, the client makes full use of the services offered.
- In the resolution phase, the client no longer needs professional services and gives up dependent behavior. The relationship ends.

Table 2.5. *Peplau's Stages and Tasks of Relationships*

Stage	Tasks
Orientation	Patient's problems and needs are clarified. Patient asks questions. Hospital routines and expectations are explained. Patient harnesses energy toward meeting problems. Patient's full participation is elicited.
Identification	Patient responds to persons he or she perceives as helpful. Patient feels stronger. Patient expresses feelings. Interdependent work with the nurse occurs. Roles of both patient and nurse are clarified.
Exploitation	Patient makes full use of available services. Goals such as going home and returning to work emerge. Patient's behaviors fluctuate between dependence and independence.
Resolution	Patient gives up dependent behavior. Services are no longer needed by patient. Patient assumes power to meet own needs, set new goals, and so forth.

Source: Adapted from Peplau, H. (1952). Interpersonal relations in nursing. New York, NY: G. P. Putnam's Sons.

Peplau's concept of the nurse-client relationship, with tasks and behaviors characteristic of each stage, has been modified but remains in use today.

- **Roles of the Nurses in the Therapeutic Relationship:** Peplau also wrote about the roles of the nurses in the therapeutic relationship and how these roles help meet the client's needs. The primary roles she identified are as follows:
    - **Stranger**—offering the client the same acceptance and courtesy that the nurse would to any stranger;
    - **Resource Person**—providing specific answers to questions within a larger context;
    - **Teacher**—helping the client learn either formally or informally;
    - **Leader**—offering direction to the client or group;
    - **Surrogate**—serving as a substitute for another, such as a parent or sibling;
    - **Counselor**—promoting experiences leading to health for the client, such as expression of feelings.

Peplau also believed that the nurse could take on many other roles, including consultant, tutor, safety agent, mediator, administrator, observer, and researcher. These were not defined in detail but were "left to the intelligence and imagination of the readers" (Peplau, 1952).

- **Four Levels of Anxiety:** According to Peplau, anxiety is the body's first reaction to a psychic threat. She distinguished between mild, moderate, severe, and panic anxiety (Table 2.6). These form the basis for working in a range of contexts with clients who experience anxiety.

Table 2.6. *Anxiety Levels*

Mild	Moderate	Severe	Panic
Sharpened senses	Selectively attentive	Perceptual field reduced to one detail or scattered details	Perceptual field reduced to focus on self
Increased motivation	Perceptual field limited to the immediate task	Cannot complete tasks	Cannot process environmental stimuli
Alert	Can be redirected	Cannot solve problems or learn effectively	Distorted perceptions
Enlarged perceptual field	Cannot connect thoughts or events independently	Behavior geared toward anxiety relief and is usually ineffective	Loss of rational thought
Can solve problems	Muscle tension	Feels awe, dread, or horror	Personality disorganization
Learning is effective	Diaphoresis	Doesn't respond to redirection	Doesn't recognize danger
Restless	Pounding pulse	Severe headache	Possibly suicidal
Gastrointestinal "butterflies"	Headache	Nausea, vomiting, diarrhea	Delusions or hallucination possible
Sleepless	Dry mouth	Trembling	Can't communicate verbally
Irritable	Higher voice pitch	Rigid stance	Either cannot sit (may bolt and run) or is totally mute and immobile
Hypersensitive to noise	Increased rate of speech	Vertigo	
	Gastrointestinal upset	Pale	
	Frequent urination	Tachycardia	
	Increased automatisms (nervous mannerisms)	Chest pain	
		Crying	
		Ritualistic (purposeless, repetitive) behavior	

Source: Adapted from Peplau, H. (1952). Interpersonal relations in nursing. New York, NY: G. P. Putnam's Sons.

- A person with mild anxiety can learn new behaviors and solve problems because they are more aware of their surroundings and have sharper senses. The individual's perceptual field, or range of available stimuli, is unbounded.
- Reduced perceptual field (focusing only on the current task) and the inability to learn new behaviors or solve problems without help are characteristics of moderate anxiety. The person can be guided to the task by someone else.
- Feelings of terror or dread are part of severe anxiety. The individual exhibits tachycardia, diaphoresis, and chest pain in addition to being unable to be directed toward a task and focusing only on sporadic details. Someone who suffers from extreme anxiety might visit the emergency room, thinking they are having a heart attack.

- Loss of rational thought, delusions, hallucinations, and total physical immobility and muteness are all possible symptoms of panic anxiety. The individual may dash off and run in all directions, frequently putting themselves in danger.

2.1.4. Humanistic Theories

Humanism signifies a profound departure from the psychoanalytic perspective that sees each person as an impulse-driven, neurotic with repressed psychic issues, as well as from the emphasis on and analysis of the client's prior experiences. Humanism emphasizes the good aspects of individuals, their potential for change, and the development of self-worth. Humanists give greater weight to the present and future while still taking into account an individual's past experiences.

2.1.4.1. Abraham Maslow: Hierarchy of Needs

American psychologist Abraham Maslow (1921–1970) specialized in examining an individual's needs and motivations. He was different from earlier theorists in that he stressed health rather than just illness and problems, and he concentrated on the individual as a whole rather than just one aspect of them. When Maslow (1954) developed the hierarchy of needs, he arranged and depicted the fundamental drives or needs that drive human behavior using a pyramid. The physiological needs of food, water, shelter, sexual expression, and pain relief are the most fundamental needs that must be satisfied first. The needs for safety and security, such as freedom from harm or threatened deprivation, protection, and security, are covered in the second level. The needs for love and belonging, which include acceptance, friendship, and long-term intimacy, make up the third level. Esteem needs, such as the need for respect from others and respect from oneself, are a part of the fourth level. Self-actualization, or the need for justice, beauty, and truth, is the highest level.

According to Maslow's theory, an individual's behavior would be dominated by their basic needs at the base of the pyramid until those needs were satisfied, at which point the needs at a higher level would take precedence. For instance, unfulfilled needs for food and shelter can take precedence over all other concerns in life, to the point where a hungry person will risk harm and social rejection to obtain food. A person who has fulfilled every need in the hierarchy and reached their full potential in life is referred to as self-actualization by Maslow. Very few people ever reach complete self-actualization. Individual differences in motivation—which isn't always constant throughout life—are explained by Maslow's theory. A person may decline to a less motivated state as a result of traumatic life events or poor health. For instance, a 35-year-old woman functioning at the "love and belonging" level may regress to the "safety" level to receive cancer treatment and protect her own health. This theory aids nurses in comprehending how clients' intentions and actions shift during times of crisis.

2.1.4.2. Carl Rogers: Client-Centered Therapy

A humanistic American psychologist, Carl Rogers (1902–1987) created a novel approach to client-centered therapy by emphasizing the therapeutic alliance. One of the first to refer to patients as clients instead of patients was Rogers. Client-centered therapy places more emphasis on the client's role as the key to healing than that of the therapist. According to Rogers, every individual has a unique perspective on the world and is the best judge of their own experiences (Rogers, 1961). According to Rogers, patients perform "the work of healing," and they are capable of recovering on their own in the presence of a caring and supportive therapist-client relationship. The best people to understand and interpret their own experiences, rebuild self-worth, and move closer to self-actualization are the clients.

The therapist takes a person-centered approach, a supportive role, rather than a directive or expert role, because Rogers viewed the client as the expert on his or her life. The therapist must promote the client's self-esteem as much as possible through three central concepts:

- **Unconditional Positive Regard**—a nonjudgmental caring for the client that is not dependent on the client's behavior;
- **Genuineness**—realness or congruence between what the therapist feels and what he or she says to the client;
- **Empathetic Understanding**—in which the therapist senses the feelings and personal meaning of the client and communicates this understanding to the client.

The client's self-esteem is boosted and their need for defensive behavior is reduced when they receive unconditional positive regard. The natural process of self-actualization can proceed as long as the client continues to accept who they are. According to Rogers, human nature also has an innate drive toward self-actualization, or the pursuit of positive change and self-improvement. Every one of us has a high regard for ourselves and a strong desire to reach self-actualization from birth. A person maintains feelings of self-worth and moves closer to self-actualization when they have supportive and nurturing relationships with other people, which is healthy. It is unhealthy for the person to experience frequent confrontations with others or be in relationships that do not support them' this causes them to lose their self-worth, become defensive, and lose their tendency toward self-actualization.

2.1.5. Behavioral Theories

Reaction against introspection models that concentrated on the structure and functions of the mind gave rise to behaviorism. A branch of psychology known as behaviorism is concerned with observable behaviors and how to modify them externally. It does not attempt to elucidate the workings of the mind. Behaviorists think that a system of incentives and penalties can modify behavior. For adults, a steady paycheck serves as a continual source of reinforcement, encouraging them to keep showing up for work each day and strive for excellence. It encourages constructive behavior at work. Someone is most likely to quit working if they stop getting paid. A driver is likely to keep speeding if they consistently speed (negative behavior) and are not stopped. The driver is probably going to slow down if they get a speeding ticket (a negative reinforcer). However, the driver is likely to start speeding again if they are not caught for it during the following four weeks (the negative reinforcer is removed).

2.1.5.1. Ivan Pavlov: Classical Conditioning

Ivan Pavlov developed his theory of classical conditioning through laboratory experiments involving dogs. This theory states that behavior can be modified by conditioning with external or environmental stimuli. Dogs salivated (response) when they saw or smelled food (stimulus), according to Pavlov's observations from his dog experiments. The goal of Pavlov's (1849–1936) training was to modify this salivating reaction or behavior. The dogs would salivate when he produced the food after ringing a bell (a new stimulus) to elicit the desired response. Pavlov repeatedly performed the bell ringing and the food presentation. He could eventually ring the bell, at which point the dogs would start to salivate even in the absence of food. The dogs' new response to hearing the bell was to salivate, which they had "conditioned" into doing. It was a conditioned response, or classical conditioning, that had changed their behavior.

2.1.5.2. B.F. Skinner: Operant Conditioning

One of the most influential behaviorists was B.F. Skinner (1904–1990), an American psychologist. He created the theory of operant conditioning, which holds that prior experiences—especially those that were repeatedly reinforced—are the primary source from which people learn new behaviors. While some criticize his theories for failing to take into account the role that needs, wants, or thoughts play in driving behavior, his contributions have produced many significant ideas that are still applied today. Although Skinner accepted that needs and feelings play a role in motivation, he only saw behavior as something that could be observed, examined, and either learned or unlearned. According to him, thoughts and feelings that go along with a behavior can also be altered. What mattered was altering the conduct.

The following principles of operant conditioning described by Skinner (1974) form the basis for behavior techniques in use today:

- All behavior is learned.
- Consequences result from behavior—broadly speaking, reward and punishment.
- Behavior that is rewarded with reinforcers tends to recur.
- Positive reinforcers that follow a behavior increase the likelihood that the behavior will recur.
- Negative reinforcers that are removed after a behavior increase the likelihood that the behavior will recur.
- Continuous reinforcement (a reward every time the behavior occurs) is the fastest way to increase that behavior, but the behavior will not last long after the reward ceases.
- Random intermittent reinforcement (an occasional reward for the desired behavior) is slower to produce an increase in behavior, but the behavior continues after the reward ceases.

In behavior modification therapy, which aims to strengthen a desired behavior or response by reinforcement, either positive or negative, these behavioral principles of rewarding or reinforcing behaviors are used to assist people in changing their behavior. For instance, if assertiveness is the desired behavior, the group leader gives the client attention and positive feedback whenever the client uses assertiveness techniques in a communication group. This is an example of positive reinforcement.

When a behavior occurs, a stimulus is immediately removed as part of negative reinforcement, increasing the likelihood that the behavior will occur again. To alleviate anxiety, a client may offer to speak first in a group if they experience anxiety while waiting to speak. Operant principles may be applied in a group home context to implement a token economy, which engages residents in carrying out daily tasks. Every resident has a chart that lists desired behaviors, like taking a shower, getting dressed, and rising on time. The chart is marked daily when the desired behavior is exhibited. Every time one of the desired behaviors is exhibited, the resident receives a token or reward at the end of the day or week. The tokens can be redeemed by the resident for things like TV time, snacks, or a lenient curfew.

Behavioral approaches can be used to treat conditioned reactions, such as phobias or anxieties. Clients with phobias can benefit from systematic desensitization to get over their unreasonable anxieties and panic attacks. The client is asked to enumerate, in order of least to most anxiety-provoking, all circumstances involving the phobic object. To reduce and manage anxiety, the client learns and puts relaxation techniques into practice. After being in the least anxiety-inducing scenario, he or she applies the relaxation techniques to control the ensuing anxiety. The patient is progressively exposed to an increasing number of anxiety-inducing circumstances until they can handle the most stressful scenario.

A wide range of issues can be solved with behavioral techniques. Gaining weight is the aim of anorexia nervosa treatment. When therapy starts, a behavioral contract is formed between the patient and the doctor or therapist. At first, the client is confined to the hospital unit and has limited unsupervised time. The contract might state that the client will receive more unsupervised time or time off the unit if they gain a specific amount of weight, like 0 point 2 kg per day, as long as the weight gain continues. Goals for working with kids who have attention-deficit/hyperactivity disorder include getting them to finish their schoolwork, taking turns talking, and other things. When a task is finished, the child receives a sticker or "star". The child gets rewarded after earning a certain amount of stars.

2.1.6. Existential Theories

According to existential theorists, behavioral abnormalities arise from an individual's lack of self-awareness or awareness of their surroundings. A self-alienated person experiences loneliness, sadness, and helplessness. Harsh self-criticism combined with a lack of self-awareness keeps the person from engaging in fulfilling relationships. Self-imposed constraints prevent the person from having the freedom to select from all available options. Existential theorists contend that the individual is caving into external pressures and desires while evading personal accountability. All existential therapies aim to assist the client in finding their true self. They stress taking personal accountability for one's thoughts, emotions, actions, and decisions. These treatments encourage the patient to look forward to the future while living completely in the present. Carl Rogers and existential therapists are occasionally grouped together. Existential therapies are summarized in Table 2.7.

2.1.6.1. Cognitive Therapy

Cognitive therapy, which focuses on immediate thought processing—how an individual perceives or interpret their experiences and determine how they feel and behave—is a common tool used by existential therapists. For instance, when someone perceives a circumstance as hazardous, they become anxious and attempt to flee. According to Beck (1976), basic emotions such as sadness, elation, anxiety, and anger are responses to perceptions of gain, danger, and wrongdoing by others. Aaron Beck is recognized for having invented cognitive therapy for depression sufferers.

Table 2.7. *Existential Therapies*

Therapy	Therapist	Therapeutic Process
Rational emotive therapy	Albert Ellis	A cognitive therapy using confrontation of "irrational beliefs" that prevent the individual from accepting responsibility for self and behavior
Logotherapy	Viktor E. Frankl	A therapy designed to help individuals assume personal responsibility (the search for meaning [*logos*] in life is a central theme)
Gestalt therapy	Frederick S. Perls	A therapy focusing on the identification of feelings in the here and now, which leads to self-acceptance
Reality therapy	William Glasser	Therapeutic focus is need for identity through responsible behavior; individuals are challenged to examine ways in which their behavior thwarts their attempts to achieve life goals

Source: Sheila L. Videbeck, Psychiatric-Mental Health Nursing, ISBN-10: 1-975116-37-2.

2.1.6.2. Rational Emotive Therapy

Eleven "irrational beliefs" that people use to justify their unhappiness were recognized by Albert Ellis, the creator of rational emotive therapy. An instance of an illogical belief is the notion that "if I love someone, they must love me back just as much". Ellis asserted that the person who holds onto this blatantly false belief will be extremely unhappy and will place the blame on the person who rejects them. Ellis also thinks that humans have "automatic thoughts" that make them unhappy in particular circumstances. To help people recognize these automatic thoughts, he developed the ABC technique: A stands for the activating stimulus or event, C for the excessive or inappropriate response, and B for the mental space that needs to be filled in by the automatic thought.

2.1.6.3. Viktor Frankl and Logotherapy

The people he saw in Nazi concentration camps during World War II served as the basis for Viktor Frankl's beliefs. His curiosity about the reasons behind some people's survival and others' demise led him to the conclusion that survivors were able to find purpose in their lives despite living in abject poverty. Thus, logotherapy's main theme is the pursuit of meaning, or logos. The ideas developed by Viktor Frankl are frequently employed by therapists and counselors who assist clients with spirituality and bereavement.

2.1.6.4. Gestalt Therapy

Identifying a person's feelings and thoughts in the present moment is a key component of Gestalt therapy, which was established by Frederick "Fritz" Perls. According to Perls, having self-awareness results in accepting oneself and taking ownership of one's own ideas and emotions. Gestalt therapists frequently utilize writing and reading exercises, journaling, and other techniques to help their clients let go of the past and concentrate on the present to help their clients become more self-aware.

2.1.6.5. Reality Therapy

William Glasser created reality therapy, an approach that concentrates on an individual's behavior and how it hinders them from reaching their life aspirations. He formulated this approach after working with individuals exhibiting delinquent behavior, struggling in school, and experiencing emotional issues. Glasser asserted that individuals who were not successful often blamed external factors for their problems rather than taking personal responsibility. He believed that they needed to establish their own identities by exhibiting responsible behavior. Reality therapy encourages clients to analyze how their behavior impedes their efforts to achieve their life objectives.

2.1.7. Crisis Intervention

A crisis is a life-changing event that causes an intense emotional reaction in the person experiencing it. People go through a crisis when they face a situation in life or a stressor that they are unable to effectively handle by using their usual coping mechanisms. The stages of a crisis are as follows, according to Caplan (1964): (1) the person is exposed to a stressor, feels anxious, and tries to cope by using customary coping mechanisms' (2) anxiety increases when these mechanisms are ineffective' (3) the person makes every effort to deal with the stressor, including trying new coping mechanisms' and (4) when coping mechanisms fail, the person experiences disequilibrium and severe distress.

Crises occur in response to a variety of life situations and events and fall into three categories:

- Maturational crises, sometimes called developmental crises, are predictable events in the normal course of life, such as leaving home for the first time, getting married, having a baby, and beginning a career.
- Situational crises are unanticipated or sudden events that threaten the individual's integrity, such as the death of a loved one, the loss of a job, and physical or emotional illness in the individual or family member.
- Adventitious crises, sometimes called social crises, include natural disasters like floods, earthquakes, or hurricanes' war' terrorist attacks' riots' and violent crimes such as rape or murder.

Keep in mind that not every crisis-causing event is of a "negative" nature. Although they are frequently desired by the individual, life events like marriage, retirement, and childbirth can nevertheless provide incredibly difficult obstacles. Aguilera (1998) distinguished three variables that impact an individual's likelihood of experiencing a crisis: the person's interpretation of the incident, the presence of emotional support, and the availability of sufficient coping strategies. When an individual in distress requests aid, these three elements serve as a framework for a successful intervention. It is possible to help the person see the situation or problem in a different light, such as a chance for development or transformation as opposed to a danger. One way to lessen feelings of isolation or overwhelm is to help the person find new sources of support or use the support they already have. Ultimately, helping the person acquire new coping mechanisms will help end the current crisis and provide new coping abilities for the future.

Crisis is defined as self-limiting, meaning that it typically lasts for 4 to 6 weeks rather than forever. One of three options is used to resolve the crisis at the end of that period. In the first two, the person either regains the level of functioning they had before the crisis or starts to function at a higher level' both are beneficial outcomes for the person. The third resolution, which is detrimental to the person, is that the person's functioning stabilizes at a level below precrisis functioning. When the problem (crisis response and precipitating event or issue) is well-defined, there is a greater chance of favorable results. Similarly, better results are linked to early intervention.

People who are going through a crisis are typically in distress and are inclined to ask for assistance. To ease their discomfort, they are willing to try new coping mechanisms and are prepared to learn them. This is the best opportunity for a successful intervention. Based on the individual's assessment, crisis intervention employs a range of techniques. Directive interventions include giving the person new information, knowledge, or meaning' increasing their level of self-awareness by giving them feedback on their behavior' and guiding their behavior by making recommendations or offering courses of action. These interventions are intended to evaluate the person's health status and encourage problem-solving. Supportive interventions include encouraging the person to recognize and talk about their feelings, acting as a sounding board for them, and reaffirming their value to address their needs for sympathetic understanding. The most successful methods and approaches incorporate a mix of these various forms of intervention.

2.2. Treatment Modalities

2.2.1. Benefits of Community Mental Health Treatment

Because they affect all areas of medicine, nursing, and related health disciplines, recent changes in Healthcare and reimbursement have an impact on mental health treatment. When it comes to treating mental illness, inpatient treatment is frequently the last rather than the first option. The current approach is based on the idea that clients would benefit more from staying in the community and receiving outpatient treatment whenever possible, not to mention that it would be more economical. Often, a client can engage in therapy while still working and maintaining relationships with friends, family, and other support networks. Additionally, outpatient therapy recognizes that a person's behavior patterns and personality, including coping mechanisms, communication modalities, and self-esteem, evolve gradually throughout a lifetime and are not amenable to change during a brief inpatient treatment stay. When someone is extremely psychotic, extremely depressed and suicidal, going through alcohol or drug withdrawal, or acting in ways that call for close supervision in a secure setting, they should be admitted to the hospital.

2.2.2. Individual Psychotherapy

One way to help someone change is through individual psychotherapy, which examines the person's thoughts, feelings, attitudes, and behavior. It entails the client and therapist having a one-on-one relationship. This type of therapy is typically sought after by those who want to better understand who they are and how they behave, change on a personal level, enhance their relationships with others, or find solace from emotional suffering. Similar to a nurse-client relationship, the client-therapist relationship goes through three stages: introduction, working, and termination. To ensure that the client receives the most benefit from therapy, it may be necessary to move quickly into the working phase due to cost-containment measures mandated by health maintenance organizations and other insurers.

The success of this kind of therapy is largely dependent on the therapist-client relationship. For therapy to be successful, the client and the therapist must get along. The formal training, life experience, and practice model of therapists differ. The choice of therapist holds great significance for the client's successful outcome. The client is responsible for choosing a therapist whose theoretical stance and therapeutic approach align with their needs and goals. To find a good fit, the client might also need to try a few different therapists. Theoretical views held by therapist have a significant impact on their therapeutic approach (covered previously in this chapter). An existential therapist, for instance, places more emphasis on the client's sense of self-responsibility than an interpersonal theory-trained therapist does on relationships. Recommending a therapist or group of therapists may be within the purview of the nurse or other healthcare professional who knows the patient well. Additionally, he or she might assist the client in comprehending the services provided by other therapists.

When choosing a therapist, the client should be thorough and inquire about the therapist's specialization and method of treatment. Because state laws govern the practice and licensing of therapists, there can be variations in the requirements for practicing psychotherapy, obtaining a license, and even whether a license is necessary. Some therapists practice exclusively within the state's legal boundaries despite having little to no formal training, credentials, or experience. A client can check the legal credentials of a therapist with the state licensing board' local phone books contain listings for state government agencies. Customers can find out from the Better Business Bureau whether they have a complaint about a specific therapist that needs to be looked into. A client can also inquire about a therapist's credentials and ethical standards by giving the local mental health services agency a call or by getting in touch with their primary care physician.

2.2.3. Groups

A group is any number of people who come together in person to complete tasks that call for cooperation, teamwork, or collaboration. Every individual within a group can influence and be influenced by other members of the group. The term "group content" describes what is said within the group, such as discussions of the project that needs to be finished, feelings and emotions, or instructional materials. The term "group process" describes how the group and its individual members behave, such as how they sit, how they speak, who speaks to whom, how quiet they are, and other things. Both the process and the content are ongoing throughout the group's existence.

2.2.3.1. Stages of Group Development

A group can be formed with the specific intention of fulfilling a goal within a given time frame. For example, a work group might be formed to finish a project assigned to it, or a therapy group might meet to discuss depression management techniques. These groups progress through discernible phases. Pregroup phases involve member selection, identification of the group's mission or purpose, and discussion of group structure. Group rules, such as who can join the group after it starts, how to handle absences and expectations for members, are all included in the structure of the group. It also specifies the location and frequency of meetings, names a group leader, and sets expectations for members. As soon as the group meets for the first time, the first stage of group development begins. Participants introduce themselves, the group goal is discussed, rules and expectations for participation are reviewed, and a leader may be chosen (if not already done). As the group members assess their comfort levels in the group environment, they start to "check out" the leader and each other. When members start to concentrate on the goal or task the group is attempting to complete, the working stage of group development starts. In a work group working on a specific project, this could happen quite quickly, but in a therapy group, it might take two or three sessions to build enough trust before members can open up about difficult situations or personal feelings. In this stage, many group traits could be observed. The degree to which members collaborate to achieve the goal is known as group cohesiveness. Cohesion is a desirable quality in a group and is linked to successful group dynamics. It is demonstrated by members who respect one another's contributions to the group, see themselves as we, and share accountability for the group's tasks. Members of a cohesive group are less likely to be afraid of reprisals or rejection when they feel free to voice any opinions, no matter how strong or weak. A group's outcome could suffer if its members are "overly cohesive," meaning that agreement and uniformity become the group's unspoken goals. If a therapy group is too close-knit, its members may not provide each other with the necessary feedback. Critical thinking and original problem-solving are unlikely to occur in a work group, which could lessen the significance of the group's output.

Members of some groups compete with one another, displaying rivalry. This could have a favorable impact on the group's result if the competition encourages compromise, better group performance, and personal development for each member. Nevertheless, competition frequently backfires on the group when disagreements go unresolved, members grow resentful, or the focus of the group is shifted from achieving its goals to squabbling and power struggles. Before the group disbands, the last phase, or termination, of the group takes place. Depending on the group's goal, the review of the group's work focuses on either the growth of the individual members or the group's accomplishments.

It can be challenging to track the phases of group growth in active groups because members come and go at different times. Instead, new members' involvement in the group changes as they become more involved, feel welcomed by the group, and participate in its activities. A self-help organization with explicit goals, Alcoholics Anonymous, is an example of this kind of group. Alcoholics Anonymous members are free to attend meetings as frequently or as infrequently as they like' ongoing groups may still exhibit competitiveness or group cohesiveness.

2.2.3.2. Group Leadership

A formal leader, or identified leader, is a person appointed to lead a group. A formal leader in therapy and education groups is typically chosen based on background, training, and experience. While some work groups choose a leader during the first meeting, others have formal leaders appointed beforehand. In most support and self-help groups, there are no formal leaders' instead, everyone is treated equally. A group with a recognized formal leader or one that is "leaderless" may produce an informal leader. Informal leaders are typically individuals who are acknowledged by others as possessing the skills, background, or qualities that other members find admirable or valuable. Successful group facilitators give equal attention to the group's process and its content. The group leader's responsibilities include providing comments and recommendations, urging everyone to participate (even the more reserved members to do so and setting boundaries for those who could take up too much time), elucidating ideas, feelings, and thoughts, summarizing the group's progress and achievements, and assisting the group in moving through the stages of development.

2.2.3.3. Group Roles

The roles that individuals play within a group are called roles. Not every member is conscious of their "role behavior," so the group may need to talk about how to handle members who behave differently. While certain roles help the group work more efficiently, others may have a negative impact on the group's performance. Information seekers, opinion seekers, information providers, energizers, coordinators, harmonizers, encouragers, and elaborators are among the roles that foster growth. The roles of monopolizer, aggressor, dominator, critic, recognition seeker, and passive follower are among those that hinder growth.

2.2.3.4. Group Therapy

Clients engage in group therapy sessions with other participants. Members of the group are expected to contribute to the group's success to help others, and they are also expected to benefit from others' contributions. There are established group guidelines that everyone must follow. These guidelines change based on the kind of group. Joining a group enables the client to pick up critical interpersonal skills as well as fresh perspectives on issues and strategies for coping with or resolving them. For instance, through engaging with other participants, clients frequently get input on how other people view and respond to them and their actions. For many clients with mental illnesses, who frequently struggle with interpersonal skills, this is vital information.

The therapeutic results of group therapy (Yalom & Leszcz, 2005) include the following:

- Gaining new information, or learning;
- Gaining inspiration or hope;
- Interacting with others;
- Feeling acceptance and belonging;
- Becoming aware that one is not alone and that others share the same problems;
- Gaining insight into one's problems and behaviors and how they affect others;
- Giving of oneself for the benefit of others (altruism).

Therapy groups vary with different purposes, degrees of formality, and structures. Our discussion includes psychotherapy groups, family therapy, family education, education groups, support groups, and self-help groups.

- **Psychotherapy Groups:** A psychotherapy group's objective is for its participants to become more aware of their behavior and to alter it for the better through group interaction and communication. Groups can be based on a particular medical diagnosis, like depression, or a specific problem, like enhancing social skills or controlling anxiety. To help group members understand how their behavior with others relates to fundamental personality traits, the group uses processes and techniques. Members discover they can assist other members in achieving their objectives and that they have obligations to other members. Groups for psychotherapy frequently have a formal structure and are led by one or two therapists. Creating the group's rules is one responsibility of the group leader or the group as a whole. These guidelines address privacy, being on time, showing up, and socializing with other members outside of scheduled group activities.

Open groups and closed groups are the two different categories of groups. Open groups are continuous, never-ending, and let participants come and go as needed. Closed groups are designed to retain the same participants for a predetermined number of meetings. If the group is closed, its members determine how to handle departing members as well as potential new member additions (Yalom and Leszcz, 2005).

- **Family Therapy:** A type of group therapy called family therapy involves the client's family members as well. The objectives include realizing how the client's psychopathology is influenced by family dynamics, utilizing the family's innate strengths and functional resources, reorganizing unhelpful family behavioral patterns, and enhancing family problem-solving techniques (Spitz and Spitz, 2017). Family therapy is a useful tool for treating and diagnosing a range of mental health conditions. Even though one family member is typically initially seen as the one in need of assistance and experiencing problems, it is frequently revealed during the therapeutic process that other family members are also experiencing emotional challenges.
- **Family Education:** A novel 12-week Family-to-Family Education Course led by qualified family members was created by the National Alliance for the Mentally Ill (NAMI). The curriculum emphasizes clinical depression, obsessive compulsive disorder, panic disorder, bipolar disorder, and schizophrenia. In addition to teaching family members the knowledge and skills they need to cope better, the course covers the clinical treatment of these illnesses. The focus on power and action in the social sphere and emotional understanding and healing in the personal sphere are among the unique aspects of this educational program. Additionally, NAMI offers Provider Education Programs that are instructed by two consumers, two family members, and a mental health professional who is also a consumer or family member. This training is intended to assist providers in understanding the struggles that families and clients face and in appreciating the bravery and tenacity required to cope with and recover from mental illness (National Alliance for the Mentally Ill, 2018).
- **Education Groups:** An education group's objective is to enlighten its participants on a particular topic, such as assertiveness training, medication management, or stress management. The group facilitator is an expert in the subject and could be a therapist, nurse, or other medical professional. Education groups typically have a set schedule of meetings and a fixed number of participants who stay with the group the entire time. After the group leader has given the material, participants can practice new skills or ask questions. Within a medication management group, the facilitator may talk about prescription regimens and potential side effects, check clients for side effects, and, in certain cases, even give the medication (e.g., depot injections of fluphenazine [Prolixin] decanoate or haloperidol [Haldol] decanoate).
- **Support Groups:** Support groups are set up to assist people who

are dealing with a similar issue in managing it. To encourage members to feel comfortable expressing themselves, the group facilitator fosters an environment of acceptance by probing members' thoughts and feelings. Support groups frequently give their members a safe space to talk about common issues and possible solutions as well as to express their feelings of annoyance, boredom, or unhappiness. The guidelines for support groups are different from those for psychotherapy in that communication and socializing between members is not only permitted but also encouraged outside of meetings. Certain groups may have a rule about confidentiality that is decided by the members. Support groups are often free-flowing, allowing participants to join and leave as needed. Common support groups include those for cancer or stroke victims, persons with AIDS, and family members of someone who has committed suicide. One national support group, Mothers Against Drunk Driving, is for family members of someone killed in a car accident caused by a drunk driver.

- **Self-Help Groups:** A self-help group is not a formal or structured therapy group' rather, its members share a common experience. While some self-help groups are arranged by professionals, the majority are run by participants without a designated leader. There are numerous self-help groups accessible. Some are regionally based and publish meeting announcements in regional newspapers. Some have national headquarters and websites, such as Alcoholics Anonymous, Parents Without Partners, Gamblers Anonymous, and Al-Anon (a support group for alcoholics' spouses and partners). The majority of self-help groups have a confidentiality policy that prohibits discussing or revealing to third parties what is seen or said during meetings. People only use their first names in many 12-step programs, like Alcoholics Anonymous and Gamblers Anonymous, to protect their identities (though in some situations, group members do know one another's names).

2.2.4. Complementary and Alternative Therapies

A federal government organization dedicated to conducting scientific research on complementary and alternative medicine (CAM) is the National Center for Complementary and Integrative Health (NCCIH). Formerly known as the National Center for Complementary and Alternative Medicine, this organization is a division of the Department of Health and Human Services and is a part of the National Institutes of Health. Treatments used in conjunction with conventional medicine practices (the medical model) are included in complementary medicine. Therapies employed instead of traditional medical care are included in alternative medicine. To ascertain the efficacy and safety of these practices, NCCIH carries out clinical research on how St. Investigating complementary and alternative medicine would include looking into using John's wort as a depression remedy rather than antidepressant medication. Complementary medicine research includes studies on the use of antidepressant drugs and chiropractic massage in the treatment of depression. Integrative medicine integrates complementary and alternative medicine (CAM) therapies that have been shown to be safe and effective by science. (National Center for Complementary and Integrative Health, 2017)

NCCIH studies a wide variety of complementary and alternative therapies:

- Alternative medical systems include homeopathic medicine and naturopathic medicine in Western cultures, and traditional Chinese medicine, which includes herbal and nutritional therapy, restorative physical exercises (yoga and tai chi), meditation, acupuncture, and remedial massage.
- Mind–body interventions include meditation, prayer, mental healing, and creative therapies that use art, music, or dance.
- Biologically based therapies use substances found in nature, such as herbs, food, and vitamins. Dietary supplements, herbal products, medicinal teas, aromatherapy, and a variety of diets are included.
- Manipulative and body-based therapies are based on the manipulation or movement of one or more parts of the body, such as therapeutic massage and chiropractic or osteopathic manipulation.
- Energy therapies include two types of therapy: biofield therapies, intended to affect energy fields that are believed to surround and penetrate the body, such as therapeutic touch, qi gong, and Reiki, and bioelectric-based therapies involving the unconventional use of electromagnetic fields, such as pulsed fields, magnetic fields, and alternating current or direct current fields. Qi gong is part of Chinese medicine that combines movement, meditation, and regulated breathing to enhance the flow of vital energy and promote healing. Reiki (which in Japanese means "universal life energy") is based on the belief that when spiritual energy is channeled through a Reiki practitioner, the patient's spirit and body are healed.

Reluctance to disclose CAM use to a psychiatrist or primary care physician may exist among clients. As a result, it's critical that nurses inquire directly and impartially about clients in terms use of vitamins, herbs, and other health practices.

2.2.5. Psychiatric Rehabilitation

To enable individuals with severe and persistent mental illness to live in the community, psychiatric rehabilitation services are provided. These initiatives are frequently referred to as community support services or community support initiatives. Psychiatric rehabilitation emphasizes the client's assets rather than just their disease. The customer takes an active role in designing the program. The goal of the programs is to assist the client in effectively managing their illness and its symptoms, obtaining the necessary resources, and reintegrating into the community.

These programs help clients with everyday living tasks like grocery shopping, transportation, cooking, budgeting, and personal hygiene. It is acknowledged that strong interpersonal ties and social support are essential for effective community living. Programs for psychiatric rehabilitation offer chances for socialization, like drop-in centers and locations where patients can go to be with people in a secure, encouraging setting. For clients who wish to look for and keep a job, there are resources such as job coaching, training, vocational referrals, and support. Community support programs also assist the client in getting medical care when necessary and educate the client about their illness and course of treatment. It is crucial to actively involve the client in determining the objectives of their rehabilitation. What medical professionals consider to be a patient's needs and what the patient believes to be valuable frequently diverge. Providing services that address each client's top priorities can greatly enhance their quality of life and aid in their rehabilitation and general well-being. Community mental health service programs are increasingly offering peer mentoring, advocacy, and counseling, with encouraging outcomes (Scanlon, Hancock, and Honey, 2017). Although they are less widespread, consumer-run mental health programs are becoming more and more prevalent.

2.3. The Nurse and Psychosocial Interventions

An essential part of the nursing process is intervention. Nurses can improve a client's social and psychological functioning as well as their communication, interpersonal skills, and social skills by implementing psychosocial interventions. Psychosocial interventions are frequently used by nurses in all practice settings, not just mental health, to help meet the needs of clients and achieve outcomes. A medical-surgical nurse, for instance, might have to employ interventions that combine behavioral principles, like providing positive reinforcement or establishing boundaries with manipulative behavior.

For example, a client with diabetes tells the nurse,

- "I promise to have just one bite of cake. Please! It's my grandson's birthday cake." (manipulative behavior)
- The nurse might use behavioral limit setting by saying,
- "I can't give you permission to eat the cake. Your blood glucose level will go up if you do, and your insulin can't be adjusted properly."
- When a client first attempts to change a colostomy bag but needs some assistance, the nurse might give positive feedback and say,
- "You gave it a good effort. You were able to complete the task with a little assistance."

Understanding the theories and treatment modalities presented can help the nurse select appropriate and effective intervention strategies.

A Closer Look

Psychotherapy

Psychotherapy is a collaborative and evidence-based treatment approach that aims to address a wide range of emotional, psychological, and behavioral issues. Grounded in the therapeutic relationship between a trained therapist and their client, psychotherapy offers a supportive and confidential space for individuals to explore their thoughts, feelings, and experiences. Through various therapeutic techniques and interventions, psychotherapy helps individuals gain insight into their emotions, behaviors, and patterns of thinking, leading to positive changes and personal growth.

One of the most widely used approaches to psychotherapy is cognitive-behavioral therapy (CBT), which focuses on identifying and challenging negative thought patterns and behaviors. By teaching clients practical skills and strategies to cope with stress, manage emotions, and modify maladaptive behaviors, CBT helps individuals develop more adaptive ways of thinking and behaving, leading to improved mental health outcomes. Another approach, psychodynamic therapy, delves into unconscious processes and unresolved conflicts stemming from early life experiences. Through exploration of past relationships and childhood experiences, psychodynamic therapy aims to uncover underlying emotional issues and facilitate insight and healing.

Interpersonal therapy (IPT) is another effective form of psychotherapy that focuses on improving interpersonal relationships and communication skills. By addressing specific interpersonal issues and conflicts, IPT helps individuals navigate challenging social interactions and improve the quality of their relationships, leading to enhanced emotional well-being. Additionally, humanistic and existential therapies emphasize personal growth, self-awareness, and authenticity, encouraging individuals to explore their values, meaning, and purpose in life. The duration and frequency of psychotherapy sessions vary depending on individual needs, treatment goals, and the specific approach used. Some individuals may benefit from short-term, focused therapy to address specific issues or crises, while others may engage in longer-term therapy to explore deeper-seated emotional issues and achieve lasting change. Regardless of the duration, the therapeutic process is characterized by collaboration, empathy, and mutual respect between the therapist and client.

Psychotherapy can be conducted in various settings, including individual therapy, group therapy, couples therapy, and family therapy, allowing for flexibility and customization based on individual preferences and needs. Moreover, advances in technology have expanded access to psychotherapy through online therapy platforms and teletherapy services, making mental health support more accessible and convenient. Psychotherapy offers a powerful and transformative path to healing and personal growth. By providing a safe and supportive environment for self-exploration and reflection, psychotherapy empowers individuals to overcome challenges, build resilience, and live more fulfilling lives. (Yalom & Leszcz, 2005)

Summary

- Psychoanalytic theory supports the notion that all human behavior is caused and can be explained (deterministic theory). Freud believed that repressed (driven from conscious awareness) sexual impulses and desires motivate much human behavior.
- Psychoanalysis focuses on discovering the causes of the client's unconscious and repressed thoughts, feelings, and conflicts believed to cause anxiety and on helping the client gain insight into and resolve these conflicts and anxieties.
- Behaviorism grew out of a reaction to introspection models that focused on the contents and operations of the mind. Behaviorism is a school of psychology that focuses on observable behaviors and what one can do externally to bring about behavior changes.
- Individual psychotherapy is a method of bringing about change in a person by exploring his or her feelings, attitudes, thinking, and behavior. It involves a one-to-one relationship between the therapist and the client.
- A group may be established to serve a particular purpose in a specified period such as a work group to complete an assigned project or a therapy group that meets with the same members to explore ways to deal with depression.
- The goal of a psychotherapy group is for members to learn about their behavior and to make positive changes in their behavior by interacting and communicating with others as members of a group. Groups may be organized around a specific medical diagnosis, such as depression, or a particular issue, such as improving interpersonal skills or managing anxiety.
- The National Alliance for the Mentally Ill (NAMI) developed a unique 12-week Family-to-Family Education Course taught by trained family members. The curriculum focuses on schizophrenia, bipolar disorder, clinical depression, panic disorder, and obsessive-compulsive disorder.
- In a self-help group, members share a common experience, but the group is not a formal or structured therapy group. Although professionals organize some self-help groups, many are run by members and do not have a formally identified leader.
- Psychiatric rehabilitation involves providing services to people with severe and persistent mental illness to help them live in the community. These programs are often called community support services or community support programs.
- Intervention is a crucial component of the nursing process. Psychosocial interventions are nursing activities that enhance the client's social and psychological functioning and improve social skills, interpersonal relationships, and communication.

References

1. Aguilera, D. C. (1998). *Crisis Intervention: Theory and Methodology* (7th ed.). Mosby.
2. Beck, A. T. (1976). *Cognitive Therapy and The Emotional Disorders.* International Universities Press.

3. Berne, E. (1964). *Games People Play*. Grove Press.
4. Caplan, G. (1964). *Principles of Preventive Psychiatry*. Basic Books.
5. Crain, W. C. (1980). *Theories of Development: Concepts and Application*. Prentice Hall.
6. Erikson, E. H. (1963). *Childhood and Society* (2nd ed.). Norton.
7. Frankl, V. E. (1959). *Man's Search for Meaning: An Introduction to Logotherapy*. Beacon Press.
8. Freud, S. (1962). The ego and the id (J. Strachey, Trans.). In *The standard Edition of the Complete Psychological Works of Sigmund Freud*. W. W. Norton & Company. (Original work published 1923.)
9. Glasser, W. (1965). *Reality Therapy: A New Approach to Psychiatry*. Harper & Row.
10. Maslow, A. H. (1954). *Motivation and Personality*. Harper & Row.
11. Miller, P. H. (1983). *Theories of Developmental Psychology*. W. H. Freeman.
12. Millon, T. (1967). *Theories of Psychopathology*. W. B. Saunders.
13. Nathan, H. J., Poulin, P., Wozny, D., Taljaard, M., Smyth, C., Gilron, I., & Shergill, Y. (2017). Randomized trial of the effect of mindfulness-based stress reduction on pain-related disability, pain intensity, health-related quality of life, and A1C in patients with painful diabetic neuropathy. *Clinical Diabetes, 35*(5), 294–304.
14. National Alliance for the Mentally Ill. (2018). *NAMI Family-to-Family*. Retrieved from: https://www.nami.org/Find-Support/NAMI-Programs/NAMI-Family-to-Family (accessed on 7 September 2024).
15. National Center for Complementary and Integrative Health. (2017). *Complementary, Alternative, or Integrative Health: What's in a Name?* Retrieved from: https://nccih.nih.gov/health/integrative-health (accessed on 7 September 2024).
16. Peplau, H. (1952). *Interpersonal Relations in Nursing*. G. P. Putnam's Sons.
17. Perls, F. S., Hefferline, R. F., & Goodman, P. (1951). *Gestalt Therapy: Excitement and Growth in the Human Personality*. Dell Publishing.
18. Rogers, C. R. (1961). *On Becoming a Person: A Therapist's View of Psychotherapy*. Houghton Mifflin.
19. Scanlon, J. N., Hancock, N., & Honey, A. (2017). Evaluation of a peer-delivered, transitional, and post-discharge support program following psychiatric hospitalization. *BMC Psychiatry, 17*(1), 307.
20. Skinner, B. F. (1974). *About Behaviorism*. Alfred A. Knopf.
21. Spitz, H. I., & Spitz, S. T. (2017). Family and couple's therapy. In B. J. Sadock, V. A. Sadock, & P. Ruiz (Eds.), *Comprehensive Textbook of Psychiatry* (10th ed., Vol. 2, pp. 2748–2760). Lippincott, Williams & Wilkins/Wolters Kluwer.
22. Sugarman, L. (1986). *Life-Span Development: Concepts, Theories and Interventions*. Methuen.
23. Sullivan, H. S. (1953). *The Interpersonal Theory of Psychiatry*. Norton.
24. Szasz, T. (1961). *The Myth of Mental Illness*. Hoeber-Harper.
25. Yalom, I. D., & Leszcz, M. (2005). *The Theory and Practice of Group Psychotherapy* (5th ed.). Basic Books.

Chapter

THERAPEUTIC RELATIONSHIPS AND COMMUNICATION

3

Contents

Introduction

Developing therapeutic relationships with clients is a critical skill that any nurse should strive to master. The therapeutic relationship is essential to the success of interventions with clients who require psychiatric care, even though it is important in all nursing specialties. This is because the therapeutic relationship and the communication within it serve as the foundation for treatment and success. The essential elements of building appropriate therapeutic nurse-client relationships are examined in this chapter, including self-awareness, acceptance, positive regard, genuine interest, trust, and therapeutic use of self. It looks at the things that need to get done at each stage of the nurse-client relationship and the methods a nurse can employ to make that happen. It also covers the four therapeutic roles that nurses can play: advocate, teacher, caregiver, and parent substitute. Information is exchanged between individuals through communication. Both verbal and nonverbal messages are simultaneously sent and received through the use of words and the behaviors that go along with them (Wasajja, 2018). The words a person uses to speak to one or more listeners are known as verbal communication. Words serve as symbols for the things and ideas under discussion. These symbols are given order and meaning when words are arranged into understandable phrases and sentences for both the speaker and the listener. The actual words that someone speaks are their content when communicating verbally. Context is the setting in which communication takes place' it can be the physical, social, emotional, or cultural surroundings as well as the passage of time. The situation or circumstances that elucidate the meaning of the message's content are included in the context.

The behavior that goes along with spoken words, such as body language, eye contact, facial expressions, tone of voice, hesitancy and rapidity in speech, grunts and groans, and proximity to the audience, is known as nonverbal communication. A speaker's mostly unconscious thoughts, feelings, needs, and values can be inferred from their nonverbal cues. The term "process" refers to all nonverbal cues used by the speaker to provide context and meaning. In order to determine whether or not they agree with the speaker's verbal content, listeners must analyze the speaker's nonverbal cues and pay attention to the sounds and behaviors that emphasize words. When content and process align, a coherent message is communicated. A client might say, "I know I haven't been myself." as an example. I require assistance. She speaks in a real and sincere tone, with a dejected expression on her face. The procedure verifies the veracity of the content. However, the speaker is sending out an inconsistent message when the content and the process are at odds—that is, when what the speaker says and does not agree. The message is inconsistent, for instance, if the client says, "I'm here to get help," but exhibits incongruent body language, clenched fists, an agitated and frowning facial expression, and snarls the words through clenched teeth. The method or seen conduct refutes the speaker's claims (content).

A message conveyed nonverbally is more accurate than one conveyed verbally. With a slumped posture, a resigned voice tone, downcast eyes, and a shameful facial expression, the statement "I'm sorry I yelled and screamed at you" is easily believable because the process and the content match. The same sentence is rendered invalid by a loud voice, furrowed brows, penetrating gaze, an indignant facial expression, hands on hips, and furious body language (incongruent message). "I'm apologizing because I think I have to," is the message that is being sent. Not that I'm sorry. "

Orientation and Directional Terms

Term	Definition	Illustration
Caregiver	Caregiver is a paid or unpaid person who helps an individual with activities of daily living. Caregivers who are members of a care recipient's family or social network, and who may have no specific professional training, are often described as informal caregivers.	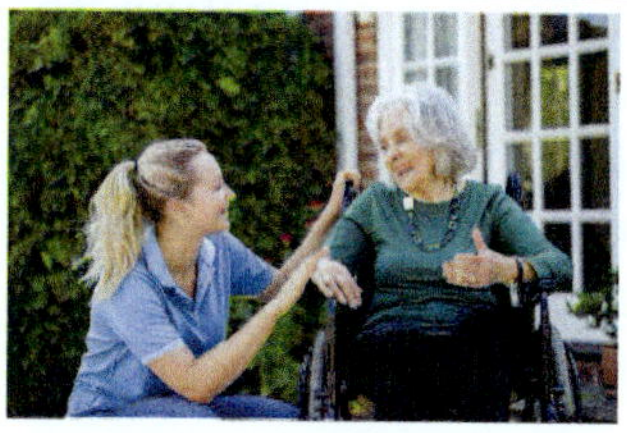
Facial expressions	Facial expressions are configurations of different micromotor (small muscle) movements in the face that are used to infer a person's discrete emotional state	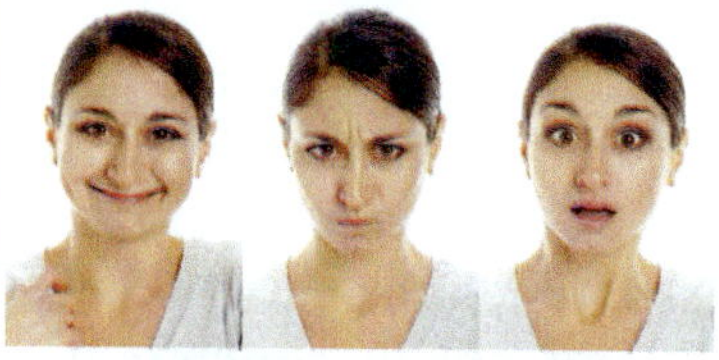
Nurse-client relationship	A relationship that establishes trust and rapport with a specific purpose of facilitating therapeutic communication and engaging the client in decision-making regarding their plan of care.	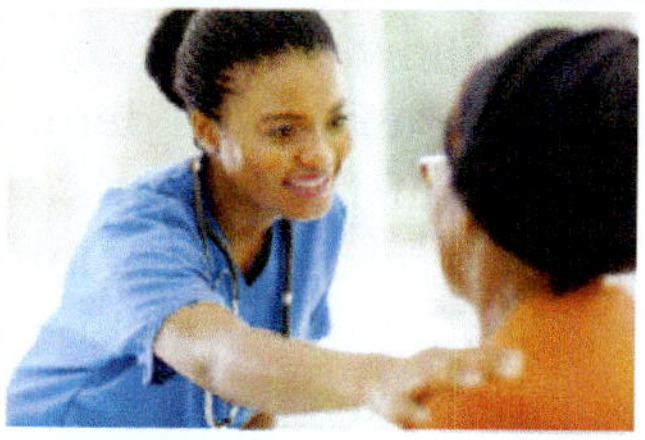
Therapeutic relationship	A therapeutic relationship is a connection between a therapist and a client that is built on trust, mutual respect, and a sense of hope. It provides a safe space for the client to express themselves freely without judgment and allows for collaboration in the therapeutic process.	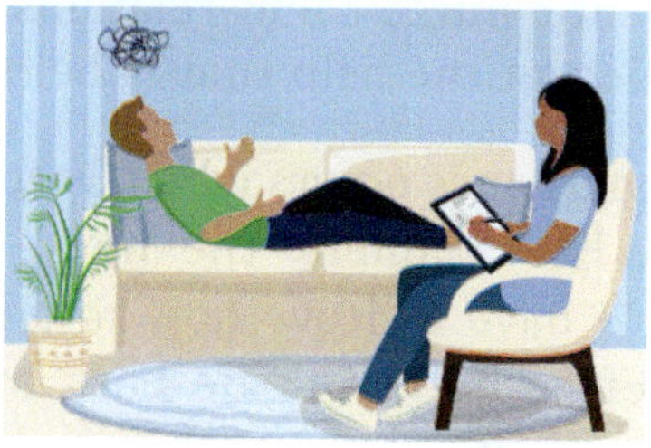
Self-disclosure	Self-disclosure involves sharing personal information – such as your thoughts, dreams, fears, goals, preferences, and experiences. It's an important way to strengthen relationships and build trust.	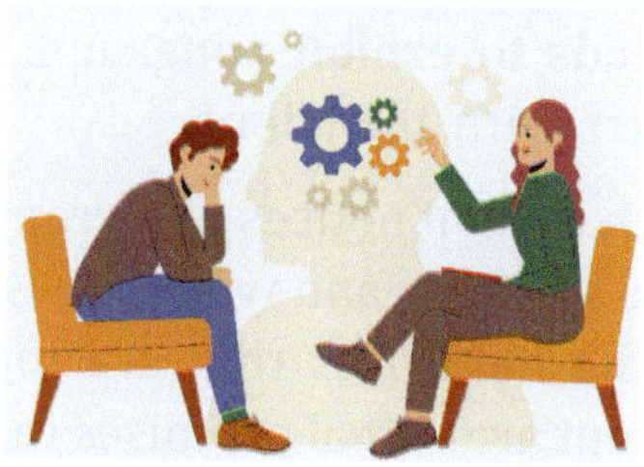

3.1. Components of a Therapeutic Relationship

The nurse has an obligation to cultivate the many elements that can improve the nurse-client relationship. These elements improve relationships and encourage communication in every facet of the nurse's life.

3.1.1. Trust

Trust is essential in the nurse-client relationship. When a client has faith in the nurse and perceives the nurse as trustworthy and dependable, trust is fostered. When the patient feels that the nurse will act and speak consistently and can be counted on to follow through on commitments, trust is built. The nurse can demonstrate many traits to help gain the client's trust, such as concern, interest, comprehension, consistency, honesty, honoring commitments, and attentive listening. Building trust through a compassionate therapeutic nurse-client relationship helps the client accept the help that is being provided.

Congruence occurs when words and actions match. For example, the nurse says to the client, "I have to leave now to go to a clinical conference, but I will be back at 2 PM," and indeed returns at 2 PM to see the client. The nurse needs to exhibit congruent behaviors to build trust with the client.

When a client notices a discrepancy between the nurse's actions and words, trust is damaged. Among the behaviors that are inconsistent or incongruent are verbal promises that are broken. For instance, the nurse promises the client that they will meet every Tuesday at 10 AM, but the nurse cancels their appointment due to a conflict with the conference schedule the following week. When a nurse speaks in a way that is inconsistent with his or her body language, that is another instance of incongruent behavior. An irate patient, for instance, approaches a nurse and claims that she doesn't like her. "Of course, I like you, Nancy! I am here to help you," says the nurse in response. However, the nurse turns away from Nancy and peers over her shoulder as she utters these words, indicating that the nonverbal and verbal parts of the message are not consistent.

Trust is built in the nurse–client relationship when the nurse exhibits the following behaviors:

- Caring;
- Openness;
- Objectivity;
- Respect;
- Interest;
- Understanding;
- Consistency;
- Treating the client as a human being;
- Suggesting without telling;
- Approachability;
- Listening;
- Keeping promises;
- Honesty.

3.1.2. Genuine Interest

The client feels the nurse is a real person who genuinely cares about them when the nurse is confident in herself, aware of her strengths and weaknesses, and laser-focused. When someone is acting dishonestly or artificially, such as asking a question and then not waiting for an answer, talking over them, or telling them everything will be okay, a client with mental illness can tell. The nurse should behave consistently and be forthright and honest. On occasion, though, a straightforward and honest response is not the most appropriate one from a professional standpoint. In these situations, the nurse might decide to share with the client a personal story that relates to what the client is currently worried about. However, the nurse must be selective when sharing personal experiences. These instances ought to come from the nurse's prior experiences rather than from a recent, still-painful incident or a problem the nurse is currently attempting to solve. The most beneficial self-disclosure examples for the client are those that are representative of ordinary, everyday situations and stay away from morally dubious subjects. The nurse might relate, for instance, how aggrieved she was by a colleague's tardiness or how concerned she was when a child failed an exam at school. Sharing intimate details of one's life, like a divorce or a partner's infidelity, is rarely beneficial. Sometimes self-disclosure is beneficial, but the nurse shouldn't let the client's problems take precedence over their own.

3.1.3. Empathy

The ability of a nurse to understand a client's meanings and feelings and convey that understanding to the client is known as empathy. It's regarded as one of the most important abilities a nurse should have to deliver compassionate, high-quality care. The nurse's ability to place oneself in the client's position does not imply that the nurse has shared the client's experiences exactly. However, the nurse can imagine the client's feelings about the experience by listening to them and gauging how important the situation is to them. When empathy arises, the nurse and the client both offer a "gift of self"—the nurse by listening intently enough to comprehend, and the client by feeling comfortable enough to share feelings. Empathy has been demonstrated to have a positive impact on client outcomes. When a nurse demonstrates empathy, patients typically feel more accepted of themselves and understood.

Several therapeutic communication techniques, such as reflection, restatement, and clarification, help the nurse send empathetic messages to the client. For example, a client says,

- "I'm so confused! My son just visited and wants to know where the safety deposit box key is'"
- Using reflection, the nurse responds;
- "You're confused because your son asked for the safety deposit key?"
- The nurse, using clarification, responds,l
- "Are you confused about the purpose of your son's visit?"

From these empathetic moments, a bond can be established to serve as the foundation for the nurse–client relationship.

The distinction between empathy and sympathy—two different emotions that one expresses concern or compassion for another—must be made by the nurse. The nurse may prevent the client from expressing their feelings by projecting their own worries onto them when they show sympathy. In the aforementioned scenario, the compassionate nurse would have replied, "I understand how perplexing sons can be.". I know how awful it feels to be confused, and my son is the same way with me. "The relationship may be impacted by the nurse's melancholy or even pity, which could make it more difficult for the nurse to concentrate on the needs of the client. The focus of sympathy frequently moves to the nurse's emotions, making it more difficult for the nurse to see the client's needs from an objective standpoint.

3.1.4. Acceptance

A nurse who remains composed and does not react adversely to a client's tantrums, rage, or acting out communicates acceptance to the client. Acceptance is not passing judgment on someone based on their behavior. This indicates that the individual is deemed worthy rather than that improper behavior is accepted. Setting rules for behavior in the nurse-client relationship is the responsibility of the nurse. The nurse lets the client feel whole while making it clear that certain behaviors are inappropriate by being firm and clear without becoming angry or passing judgment. As an illustration, a client wraps his arm around the nurse's waist. An appropriate response would be for the nurse to remove his hand and say,

- "John, do not place your hand on me. We are working on your relationship with your girlfriend and that does not require you to touch me. Now, let's continue."
- An inappropriate response would be,
- "John, stop that! What's gotten into you? I am leaving, and maybe I'll return tomorrow."

Refusing to return and walking away punishes the client without providing a clear solution for their inappropriate behavior.

3.1.5. Positive Regard

Regardless of the client's behavior, background, or way of life, the nurse can respect them if they see them as special, deserving human beings. Positive regard is a term used to describe this unconditional, nonjudgmental attitude that suggests respect. The nurse can show the client respect and positive regard by calling them by name, spending time with them, and listening to and talking to them honestly. When planning care, the nurse also demonstrates positive regard by taking the client's preferences and ideas into account. By doing this, the nurse is demonstrating to the client that they think the client can positively and meaningfully contribute to their own care plan. The nurse uses verbal and nonverbal communication techniques to show the client that they are being attended to fully, a practice known as presence or attending. Nonverbal cues like leaning in toward the client, keeping eye contact, being at ease, keeping your arms at your sides, and projecting an interested but impartial demeanor all contribute to a presence-filled environment.

When a nurse verbally attends, they refrain from passing judgment on the client's behavior. For instance, the client might say, "I screamed and yelled at my mother for an hour because I was so mad.". "Well, that didn't help, did it?" or "I can't believe you did that" are examples of value judgments the nurse may convey to the client, suggesting that they were "bad" or "wrong.". "What happened then?" or "You must have been really upset." would be better questions to ask. The nurse stays focused on the client and refrains from offering criticism or assigning values to the client's actions.

3.1.6. Self-Awareness and Therapeutic Use of Self

The nurse needs to know themselves before they can start to understand their clients. The process of becoming conscious of one's own values, beliefs, thoughts, feelings, attitudes, motives, biases, strengths, and limitations as well as how these attributes impact other people is known as self-awareness. It enables the nurse to watch, listen, and comprehend the nuanced reactions and responses of the clients during interactions with them. Values are impersonal benchmarks that define a person's sense of good and wrong as well as a set of rules for behavior. Hard work, sincerity, honesty, cleanliness, and orderliness are examples of sample values. The values clarification process can be useful in gaining understanding of oneself and one's personal values.

There are three steps in the values clarification process: acting, choosing, and pricing. When someone chooses, they freely weigh a variety of options and select the value that feels right to them. Prizing is the act of taking into account, valuing, and openly associating something with oneself. When someone acts, they are putting the values into practice. One student, for instance, who keeps things tidy and orderly, has been put to live with another student who strews food and clothes all over the place. The orderly student is initially perplexed as to why she feels uneasy around her roommate and is reluctant to go back to the room. Upon closer inspection, she discovers that their perspectives on how to use personal space differ (choosing). She then talks to her adviser and friends (prizing) about her conflict and decisions. In the end, she chooses to work out a compromise (acting) with her roommate.

Beliefs are convictions held to be true. Some examples of beliefs are: "Everyone over the age of sixty can't hear," "A sunny day is always a good day," and "Peas should be planted on St. Saint Patrick's Day. There are some beliefs that are supported by objective data. For instance, proponents of evolution have acknowledged the data supporting their theory of the origins of life. Some beliefs are illogical and can endure even in the face of contradicting empirical evidence or a lack of evidence to support them. For instance, a lot of people hold unfounded stereotypes about cultures other than their own that they acquired purely from the remarks of others or out of a fear of the unknown, without any supporting data.

General sentiments or a framework for organizing one's knowledge of the outside world are known as attitudes. Views of the world and people are influenced by a variety of attitudes, including positive, negative, pessimistic, optimistic, and hopeful. Choosing to see the bright side of an event, a remark, or a judgment is a sign of having a positive mental attitude. For instance, the person at the front of a busy grocery line pays with change and counts it out slowly. A positive-attitude line waiter would be appreciative of the additional minutes and start using them to unwind and practice deep breathing. A pessimistic outlook affects one's perception of the outside world and other people. For instance, someone who has encountered a rude server once could grow to despise wait staff in general. A person with such a bad attitude could act rudely and unpleasant toward every server they come across.

As the nurse acquires knowledge and experience, he or she should periodically review and modify beliefs and attitudes. Constant self-awareness enables the nurse to accept other people's potentially different values, attitudes, and beliefs. A person may harbor prejudice or bias toward a group of people due to preconceived notions or stereotypical images of that group if they fail to evaluate their own attitudes and beliefs. Being ethnocentric about one's own culture—thinking it to be better than others—occurs frequently, especially in those cases where the individual has never been exposed to any other culture. An illustration of a value clarification exercise that can help nurses become more conscious of their own attitudes and ideas regarding other cultures.

3.1.6.1. Therapeutic Use of Self

The nurse can use elements of his or her personality, experiences, values, feelings, intelligence, needs, coping mechanisms, and perceptions to build relationships with clients by becoming more self-aware and starting to understand attitudes. We refer to this as therapeutic use of self. To build therapeutic relationships with patients and support their growth, transformation, and healing, nurses use themselves as a therapeutic tool. To support their clients' development and prevent restricting their options to those that nurses value, nurses need to have a clear understanding of themselves, according to Peplau (1952), who first described this therapeutic use of self in the nurse-client relationship.

The conscious and unconscious reactions that the nurse's life experiences, education, spirituality, and cultural values shape her actions. Because they are accustomed to something, nurses—like everyone else—tend to employ a lot of automatic reactions or behaviors. They must look at these socially acceptable modes of reacting or acting and assess whether or not they support the therapeutic alliance.

The Johari window (Luft, 1970) is a tool that can be used to gain a better understanding of oneself. It generates a "word portrait" of an individual in four areas and shows how well that individual knows themselves and interacts with others.

The four areas evaluated are as follows:

- **Quadrant 1:** Open/public—self-qualities one knows about oneself and others also know;
- **Quadrant 2:** Blind/unaware—self-qualities known only to others;
- **Quadrant 3:** Hidden/private—self-qualities known only to oneself;
- **Quadrant 4:** Unknown—an empty quadrant to symbolize qualities as yet undiscovered by oneself or others.

The nurse must first evaluate his or her own qualities by making a list of them, including values, attitudes, feelings, strengths, behaviors, accomplishments, needs, desires, and thoughts, before establishing a Johari window. The second step involves interviewing people to learn about their opinions of the nurse and asking them to list any positive or negative traits they see in her. For this exercise to be beneficial, the opinions expressed must be truthful, and those who list flaws should not face repercussions. Comparing lists and placing attributes in the appropriate quadrant is the third step.

A nurse who shares little personal information with others is indicated by a smaller quadrant 1' if the list in quadrant 1 is the longest, it suggests that the nurse is receptive to others. The individual shows little insight if both quadrants 1 and 3 are small. Any modifications made to one quadrant have an equal impact on the other quadrants. Working to move traits from quadrants 2, 3, and 4 into quadrant 1 (qualities known to self and others) is the aim. This shows that the nurse is becoming more conscious of and aware of herself.

3.1.6.2. Patterns of Knowing

Preconceptions, or the ways one person expects another to act or speak, have been identified by nurse theorist Hildegard Peplau (1952) as a barrier to the development of an authentic relationship. People frequently are unable to get to know one another because of preconceptions. It could be difficult for a nurse to establish a therapeutic relationship with a client if they have preconceived notions or conflicting personal beliefs and values. An illustration of preconceptions that obstruct a therapeutic relationship is Mr. Dot Lopez, a client, who refuses to have Samuel, a male nurse, take care of him because he believes that all male nurses are homosexual. Samuel is relieved that Mr. Lopez has declined to collaborate with him because he harbors the preconceived stereotype that all Hispanic men are violent. Erroneous assumptions are preventing both men from working together on some crucial projects. Nursing knowledge can be categorized into four categories according to Carper (1978): aesthetic knowing, which comes from nursing art, personal knowing, which comes from life experiences, ethical knowing, which comes from nursing moral knowledge, and empirical knowing, which comes from the science of nursing. The nurse can clearly observe and comprehend each client interaction by using these patterns. Being aware of the sources of knowledge and how it influences behavior aids in the nurse's self-awareness. To facilitate a truly authentic encounter, Munhall (1993) added another pattern that she dubbed unknowing: the nurse admitting that they do not know the client or the client's subjective world. When a nurse is ignorant, they are receptive to the client's opinions and do not try to force their own beliefs or values on them. The nurse must work on cultivating this openness and acceptance toward the client because in psychiatric nursing, the nurse's negative preconceptions can negatively impact the therapeutic relationship (Table 3.1).

Table 3.1. *Carper's Patterns of Nursing Knowledge*

Pattern	Example
Empirical knowing (obtained from the science of nursing)	The client with panic disorder begins to have an attack. Panic attacks will raise pulse rate.
Personal knowing (obtained from life experience)	The client's face shows the panic.
Ethical knowing (obtained from the moral knowledge of nursing)	Although the nurse's shift has ended, he or she remains with the client.
Aesthetic knowing (obtained from the art of nursing)	Although the client shows outward signals now, the nurse has sensed previously the client's jumpiness and subtle differences in the client's demeanor and behavior.

Source: Adapted from Carper, B. (1978). Fundamental patterns of knowing in nursing. Advances in Nursing Sciences, 1(1), 13–23.

3.2. Types of Relationships

Every relationship is different due to the different ways that the circumstances and traits of the individuals involved can be combined. All relationships fall into one of three main categories, even though each one is unique: social, intimate, or therapeutic.

3.2.1. Social Relationship

The main goals of establishing a social relationship are friendship, socialization, companionship, or task completion. Although it can be superficial, communication satisfies people's basic need for interaction by primarily focusing on the sharing of thoughts, emotions, and experiences. It's common to give advice. Roles can change in social situations. The results of this type of relationship are seldom evaluated. A social interaction occurs when a nurse welcomes a patient, strikes up a conversation about the weather, a sporting event, or just strikes up a conversation. This is acceptable in the nursing profession, but limited social interaction is necessary for the nurse-client relationship to achieve the established goals. Serious work that advances the client will not be done if the relationship turns more social than therapeutic.

3.2.2. Intimate Relationship

Two individuals who are emotionally devoted to one another are necessary for a successful intimate relationship. Both parties are focused on meeting their own needs as well as assisting one another in doing the same. Together with sharing common objectives, the relationship may entail emotional or sexual intimacy. The interaction may or may not be evaluated continuously. The nurse-client relationship is not the place for an intimate relationship.

3.2.3. Therapeutic Relationship

The focus of the therapeutic relationship is solely on the needs, experiences, feelings, and ideas of the client, which sets it apart from social or intimate relationships in many ways. The client and the nurse agree on the areas that need attention and how best to assess the results. To interact with the client, the nurse makes use of her interpersonal strengths, communication skills, and comprehension of human behavior. The boundaries of the therapeutic alliance are well defined' the client's needs, not the nurse's, are the primary focus. The client's likeability or gratitude should not be a source of concern for the nurse. A nurse who exhibits this level of concern is likely attending to a personal need to be liked or needed. The nurse must be careful not to let the therapeutic alliance devolve into a more social one and must maintain a constant focus on the client's needs rather than their own.

The therapeutic alliance may be enhanced or hampered by the nurse's degree of self-awareness. For instance, the relationship is more likely to remain social if the nurse feels uneasy around the client because superficiality is safer. Knowing what worries the nurse has can help him or her talk about them with the instructor, which can lead to a more therapeutic relationship.

3.3. Establishing the Therapeutic Relationship

Nurses who are self-aware and confident in themselves are prepared to build healthy therapeutic relationships with patients. Over the course of a lifetime, personal growth occurs, so the nurse cannot claim to have perfect self-knowledge. However, it's a good idea to be aware of one's strengths and limitations at any given time.

3.3.1. Phases

Peplau dedicated thirty-five years of study and writing to the examination of the phases and interpersonal processes involved in the nurse-client relationship. Her research offers a framework that the nursing field can use to track and analyze improvements in interpersonal relationships. Orientation, working, and resolution or termination are the three stages of the Peplau (1952) model. These phases overlap and interact with one another in real life, making them less distinct (Table 3.2).

Table 3.2. *Phases of the Nurse–Client Relationship*

	Working		
Orientation	**Identification**	**Exploitation**	**Termination**
Client			
• Seeks assistance • Conveys needs • Asks questions • Shares preconceptions and expectations of nurse based on past experience	• Participates in identifying problems • Begins to be aware of time • Responds to help • Identifies with nurse • Recognizes nurse as a person • Explores feelings • Fluctuates dependence, independence, and interdependence in relationship with nurse • Increases focal attention • Changes appearance (for better or worse) • Understands continuity between sessions (process and content) • Testing maneuvers decrease	• Makes full use of services • Identifies new goals • Attempts to attain new goals • Rapid shifts in behavior: dependent and independent • Exploitative behavior • Self-directing • Develops skill in interpersonal relationships and problem-solving • Displays changes in manner of communication (more open, flexible)	• Abandons old needs • Aspires to new goals • Becomes independent of helping person • Applies new problem-solving skills • Maintains changes in style of communication and interaction • Shows positive changes in view of self • Integrates illness • Exhibits ability to stand alone
Nurse			
• Responds to client • Gives parameters of meetings • Explains roles • Gathers data • Helps client identify problem • Helps client plan use of community resources and services • Reduces anxiety and tension • Practices active listening • Focuses client's energies • Clarifies preconceptions and expectations of nurse	• Maintains separate identity • Exhibits ability to edit speech or control focal attention • Shows unconditional acceptance • Helps express needs and feelings • Assesses and adjusts to needs • Provides information • Provides experiences that diminish feelings of helplessness • Does not allow anxiety to overwhelm client • Helps client focus on cues • Helps client develop responses to cues • Uses word stimuli	• Continues assessment • Meets needs as they emerge • Understands reason for shifts in behavior • Initiates rehabilitative plans • Reduces anxiety • Identifies positive factors • Helps plan for total needs • Facilitates forward movement of personality • Deals with therapeutic impasse	• Sustains relationship as long as client feels necessary • Promotes family interaction to assist with goal planning • Teaches preventive measures • Uses community agencies • Teaches self-care • Terminates nurse–client relationship

Source: Adapted from Forchuck, C., & Brown, B. (1989). Establishing a nurse-client relationship. Journal of Psychosocial Nursing, 27(2), 30–34.

3.3.2. Orientation

When the nurse and client first meet and the client starts identifying issues to look into, the orientation phase comes to an end. In the orientation phase, the nurse defines roles, defines the goal of the meeting and its parameters, pinpoints the client's issues, and makes clear expectations. The nurse has important work to do before seeing the client. The nurse gathers the necessary paperwork, reads the client's background information, learns about any medications the client is taking, and sets up a calm, comfortable, and private environment. It's time for you to evaluate yourself. When assisting this client, the nurse should take into account both his or her own strengths and weaknesses. Does the client's history of domestic violence indicate any areas where the nurse should be concerned? For instance, if the client is a spouse batterer and the nurse's father was a domestic abuser, the situation may indicate difficulties. Preconceptions about the client must be examined by the nurse to make sure that he or she can set them aside and get to know the person. How does it make him or her feel? What memories does it prompt, and can he or she work with the client without these memories interfering? The nurse must approach every client impartially and without bias. The nurse should talk with a mentor about any possible trouble spots.

Table 3.3. *Communication during the Phases of the Nurse–Client Relationship*

Phase of Relationship	Sample Conversation	Communication Skill
Orientation	*Nurse:* "Hello, Mr. O'Hare. I am Sally Fourth, a nursing student from Orange County Community College. I will be coming to the hospital for the next six Mondays. I would like to meet with you each time I am here to help support you as you work on your treatment goals."	Establishing trust; placing boundaries on the relationship and first mention of termination in 6 weeks
Orientation	*Nurse:* "Mr. O'Hare, we will meet every Monday from June 1 to July 15 at 11 AM in conference room 2. We can use that time to work on your feelings of loss since the death of your twin sister."	Establishing specifics of the relationship time, date, place, and duration of meetings (can be written as a formal contract or stated as an informal contract)
Orientation	*Nurse:* "Mr. O'Hare, it is important that I tell you I will be sharing some of what we talk about with my instructor, peers, and staff at clinical conference. I will not be sharing any information with your wife or children without your permission. If I feel a piece of information may be helpful, I will ask you first if I may share it with your wife."	Establishing confidentiality
Working	*Client:* "Nurse, I miss my sister Eileen so much." *Nurse:* "Mr. O'Hare, how long have you been without your sister?"	Gathering data
Working	*Client:* "Without my twin, I am not half the person I was." *Nurse:* "Mr. O'Hare, let's look at the strengths you have."	Promoting self-esteem
Working	*Client:* "Oh, why talk about me? I'm nothing without my twin." *Nurse:* "Mr. O'Hare, you are a person in your own right. I believe working together we can identify strengths you have. Will you try with me?"	Overcoming resistance
Termination	*Nurse:* "Well, Mr. O'Hare, as you know I only have 1 week left to meet with you." *Client:* "I am going to miss you. I feel better when you are here." *Nurse:* "I will miss you also, Mr. O'Hare."	Sharing of the termination experience with the client demonstrates the partnership and the caring of the relationship

Source: https://tms.iau.ir/file/download/download/1660127163-psychiatric-mental-health-nursing-8th-edition-2020-.pdf.

The nurse starts to establish trust with the client during the orientation phase. Creating a therapeutic atmosphere that encourages trust and understanding is the nurse's job. At this point, the nurse should disclose any pertinent information about themselves, such as their name, reason for being on the unit, and degree of education. For instance, "Hello, James". Ms. Ames here, and I'll be your nurse for the ensuing six Tuesdays. I attend the University of Mississippi as a senior nursing student." (Table 3.3).

It is imperative that the nurse pays close attention to the client's history, perceptions, and misconceptions. He or she must exude compassion and comprehension. Relationships that have a good start have a higher chance of succeeding and reaching their objectives.

If the client's past interactions with nurses were disappointing, they might be wary during their initial meeting. The client may act out, talk incoherently, or exaggerate incidents as a ruse to avoid talking about the true issues. It might require multiple sessions for the client to develop confidence in the nurse's ability to be trusted.

3.3.2.1. Nurse–Client Contracts

The nurse must reiterate the roles that both the client and the nurse have, even though many clients have previous experiences in the mental health system. These duties should initially be agreed upon by the client and the nurse in a verbal or informal contract. A formal or written contract might be required in some situations. A couple of these situations include when a written contract was previously required with the client or when the client "forgets" the verbal agreement.

The contract should state the following:

- Time, place, and length of sessions;
- When sessions will terminate;
- Who will be involved in the treatment plan (family members or health team members);
- Client responsibilities (arrive on time and end on time);
- Nurse's responsibilities (arrive on time, end on time, maintain confidentiality at all times, evaluate progress with client, and document sessions).

3.3.2.2. Confidentiality

Respecting the client's right to privacy regarding any information pertaining to their physical and mental health as well as any associated care is what is meant by confidentiality. It entails restricting access to the information a client discloses to those who are directly involved in their care. Third parties are only permitted access to this information under very specific circumstances' in many states, for instance, staff members are required by law to report suspicions of elder and child abuse.

Adult clients have the option to access clinical information and choose which family members, if any, will be involved in their care. The individuals closest to the client and in charge of their care should ideally be involved. However, the client has to choose who gets to be involved. Boundaries need to be clear for the client to feel comfortable. Regarding who will have access to client assessment data and progress evaluations, the nurse must be very clear. He or she should explain to the client that the mental health team shares pertinent information amongst itself to deliver consistent care and that family members will only be included with the client's consent. If the client has a guardian appointed, that person has the authority to examine client records and decide on treatments that are best for the client. A child's parent or designated guardian has access to information and can decide what course of treatment to follow in consultation with the medical team. The nurse must be alert if a client asks him or her to keep a secret because this information may relate to the client's harming him or herself or others. The nurse should not pledge to keep information private. The nurse may be compromising the client's trust if they have promised not to disclose before receiving the message. Most of the time, the client still brings up concerns even when the nurse declines to agree to keep information private. The following is an example of a good response to a client who is suicidal but requests secrecy:

- **Client:** "I am going to jump off the 14th floor of my apartment building tonight, but please don't tell anyone."
- **Nurse:** "I cannot keep such a promise, especially if it involves your safety. I sense you are feeling frightened. The staff and I will help you stay safe."

The Tarasoff vs. Should a client make a homicidal threat, the Regents of the University of California decision from 1976 releases professionals from privileged communication with their clients. The nurse must inform the police and the intended victims of this threat, per the decision. In this case, the nurse has a duty to notify the attending physician and nursing supervisor of the potential for homicide so that the intended victim and the police are informed.

The client's issues are recorded by the nurse using scheduled interventions. The patient must be aware that the nurse will gather information about them to plan their medical care, including prescriptions, and to safeguard their civil rights in addition to aiding in diagnosis. The client must understand the boundaries of confidentiality in nurse-client interactions, as well as how the nurse will utilize and distribute this information to other healthcare professionals.

3 .3.2.3. Self-Disclosure

Self-disclosure is the act of sharing with clients private details about oneself, including ideas, feelings, and biographical details. It was customary for nurses to disclose only their name and a general description of where they reside, like "I live in Ocean County.". But these days, it's thought that a little deliberate, well-thought-out self-disclosure can enhance the relationship between the nurse and the patient. Through self-disclosure, the nurse can educate clients, show support, and reassure them that anxiety is common and that many people struggle with stress and other issues in their lives.

Self-disclosure could make the client feel more at ease and open to sharing ideas and emotions, or it could give the client more understanding of their circumstances. The nurse must take cultural considerations into account when using self-disclosure. Certain clients might feel uncomfortable with self-disclosure because they think it's too personal or improper. It is important to plan ahead and carefully consider any potential harm or inappropriateness before disclosing personal information to a client. Self-disclosing personal information on the spur of the moment can backfire. For instance, the nurse might say, "My parents got divorced when I was 12, and it was a horrible time for me," while working with a client whose parents are divorcing. The client has been made to feel as though this will be a terrible experience by the nurse, who has taken the focus off of them. Even if the nurse intended to convey empathy, the outcome might be completely the opposite.

3.3.2.4. Working

Typically, the nurse-client relationship's working phase is split into two smaller phases. The client determines the problems or concerns that are causing them during the problem identification process. When a client is being exploited, the nurse helps them explore their emotions and reactions, improve their coping mechanisms, and cultivate a more positive view of themselves. This promotes behavior modification and the growth of independence. It should be noted that Peplau used the word "exploitation" very differently than it is used today, which refers to unfairly using or taking advantage of a person or circumstance. Because of this, it would be more accurate to think of this phase as a deep investigation and development of previously discussed themes with the client. The nurse and the client are now able to examine the issues and work on them within the safety of the relationship because of the trust that has been built between them. When the client discloses experiences, problems, behaviors, or issues, the nurse must be trusted not to reject them or become upset.

The patient may occasionally put the nurse to the test by making up wild tales or acting out actions. The nurse is put to the test when it comes to maintaining focus and avoiding distraction or reaction. The client will frequently use testing behaviors to sidestep the topic when they feel uncomfortable because they are approaching the truth too closely. In response, the nurse might say something like, "It appears that we have put you in an uncomfortable situation. "Would you like to let it go for now?" pulls the focus away from the testing behavior and onto the current problem.

The nurse needs to keep in mind that the client is the one who looks at and investigates problematic relationships and situations. The nurse should let the client make their own decisions about situations and refrain from passing judgment or offering advice. The client can be assisted by the nurse in identifying behavioral patterns and whether the anticipated response materializes or not. For instance, a depressed client confides in the nurse about her children's lack of concern for her. The client can investigate her communication style with her kids with the nurse's help and direction. She might find that her communication style consists of criticism and complaint. The nurse can then work with the client to investigate future communication strategies that will work better.

The specific tasks of the working phase include the following:

- Maintaining the relationship;
- Gathering more data;
- Exploring perceptions of reality;
- Developing positive coping mechanisms;
- Promoting a positive self-concept;
- Encouraging verbalization of feelings;
- Facilitating behavior change;
- Working through resistance;
- Evaluating progress and redefining goals as appropriate;
- Providing opportunities for the client to practice new behaviors;
- Promoting independence.

It is common for the client to unintentionally transfer feelings for significant others to the nurse during their work together. We refer to this as transference. For instance, the client may react negatively and resist the nurse, who is also seen as an authority, if they have had bad experiences with other authority figures like parents, teachers, or principals. Countertransference is the term for what happens when a nurse reacts to a patient based on their own unconscious needs and conflicts. For instance, the nurse may become enraged with a client who refuses to listen to her advice if she is the youngest in her family and frequently felt that no one paid attention to her when she was younger. Once more, self-awareness is crucial for the nurse to recognize potential instances of transference and countertransference. Knowing these "hot spots" will help the nurse respond appropriately and prevent relationship problems caused by unresolved issues from arising in the future.

3.3.2.5. Termination

The nurse-client relationship ends with the termination or resolution phase. It starts when the issues are fixed and finishes when the partnership is dissolved. When a relationship ends, both the nurse and the client typically feel something is lost' in the case of the client, this could be especially true. Clients frequently act irate or act as though the issue has not been resolved in an attempt to avoid being fired. The nurse can validate the client's feelings of anger and reassure them that this reaction is typical when a relationship is ending. The nurse should not assume that the sessions were ineffective if the client attempts to revisit and discuss previously settled issues. Rather, the nurse should recognize the client's stalling strategies and redirect the client's attention to recently acquired behaviors and skills to address the issue. While it is acceptable to tell the client that the nurse enjoyed their time together and will think of them, it is not appropriate for the nurse to consent to see the client for purposes other than therapy.

3.4. Avoiding Behaviors that Diminish the Therapeutic Relationship

Because of their position in the nursing profession, the nurse has authority over the client. If there is an excessive amount of familiarity, an intimate relationship, or a breach of confidentiality, that power may be abused.

3.4.1. Inappropriate Boundaries

All employees run the risk of permitting a therapeutic alliance to develop into an unsuitable one, regardless of experience level. Being conscious of one's own emotions and the impact one has on others is crucial for nurses. This allows them to help uphold the boundaries of their professional relationships. For optimal therapeutic results, the nurse must uphold professional boundaries. It is the nurse's duty to establish the parameters of the relationship precisely during the orientation stage and to make sure those parameters are upheld during the partnership. Although the nurse should be kind and sympathetic, she shouldn't make an effort to become friends with the client. The conversation tends to remain surface-level when social interactions persist after the initial few minutes of a meeting. This neglect of the issues that have been scheduled for discussion weakens the working relationship.

If the nurse feels that "there is no way I would ever do anything nontherapeutic," there is a significant chance that they will cross boundaries. Boundary violations frequently start out innocently or even with good intentions, like when a nurse shares personal relationship issues with a client in the hopes that it will benefit them. Personal information cannot be taken back once it has been disclosed. It is impossible to repair the damage done to the therapeutic alliance. It is the responsibility of the nurse to uphold professional boundaries whether they are attracted to a client or the other way around. Giving a client one's home address or phone number, or accepting gifts, would be viewed as unethical behavior. Nurses have to constantly evaluate themselves, make sure their emotions are under control, and concentrate on the needs and interests of their clients. Using Table 3.4 Nursing Boundary Index, nurses can evaluate their conduct.

Table 3.4. *Nursing Boundary Index*

Please rate yourself according to the frequency that the following statements reflect your behavior, thoughts, or feelings within the past 2 years while providing patient care.

1.	Have you ever received any feedback about your behavior for being overly intrusive with patients or their families?	Never Rarely Sometimes Often
2.	Do you ever have difficulty setting limits with patients?	Never Rarely Sometimes Often
3.	Do you arrive early or stay late to be with your patient for a longer period of time?	Never Rarely Sometimes Often
4.	Do you ever find yourself relating to patients or peers as you might to a family member?	Never Rarely Sometimes Often
5.	Have you ever acted on sexual feelings you have for a patient?	Never Rarely Sometimes Often
6.	Do you feel that you are the only one who understands the patient?	Never Rarely Sometimes Often
7.	Have you ever received feedback that you get "too involved" with patients or families?	Never Rarely Sometimes Often
8.	Do you derive conscious satisfaction from patients' praise, appreciation, or affection?	Never Rarely Sometimes Often
9.	Do you ever feel that other staff members are too critical of "your" patient?	Never Rarely Sometimes Often
10.	Do you ever feel that other staff members are jealous of your relationship with a patient?	Never Rarely Sometimes Often
11.	Have you ever tried to "match-make" a patient with one of your friends?	Never Rarely Sometimes Often
12.	Do you find it difficult to handle patients' unreasonable requests for assistance, verbal abuse, or sexual language?	Never Rarely Sometimes Often

Any item that is responded to with a "sometimes" or "often" should alert the nurse to a possible area of vulnerability. If the item is responded to with a "rarely," the nurse should determine whether it was an isolated event or a possible pattern of behavior.

Source: https://tms.iau.ir/file/download/download/1660127163-psychiatric-mental-health-nursing-8th-edition-2020-.pdf.

3.4.2. Feelings of Sympathy and Encouraging Client Dependency

It is imperative for the nurse to avoid allowing empathy to morph into sympathy for the patient. In contrast to using empathy therapeutically, a nurse who feels sorry for a client frequently makes an effort to appease them in an attempt to make up for it. The nurse's behavior becomes easier for the client to control when it stems from sympathy. This inhibits the client's ability to grow, discourages the client from investigating their issues, ideas, and feelings, and frequently results in client dependency. The patient may become more dependent on the nurse for support or assistance, or they may regress and behave as though they are incapable of performing previously completed tasks. These may indicate that the nurse has been providing the client with "overdoing" care, which could be contributing to the client's dependency. It is common for clients to put the nurse to the test to see how much she will do. The client has grown too reliant if they only cooperate when the nurse is present and do not behave as agreed upon when the nurse is not around. In each of these situations, the nurse should evaluate their professional conduct and put the client's needs and therapeutic objectives back in the forefront.

3.4.3. Nonacceptance and Avoidance

If the nurse finds the client's behavior objectionable or repulsive and lets those feelings show by avoiding the client, responding angrily verbally, expressing annoyance with facial expressions, or turning away from the client, the nurse-client relationship may be in danger. Before starting a relationship, the nurse should be aware of the client's behavior and background' if the nurse thinks there might be a conflict, he or she needs to discuss this possibility with a colleague. The nurse must also look into any prejudice that might paint the client in a negative light if they are aware of it. Occasionally, through discussing and facing these emotions, the nurse can accept the patient and prevent bias from undermining the relationship. However, the nurse ought to think about asking for a different assignment if they are unable to overcome such unpleasant emotions. Regardless of the client's past, the nurse has an obligation to accept and show positive regard for each individual. The nurse has to keep growing in self-awareness and to face and overcome any biases that might jeopardize the nurse-client bond.

Possible Warnings or Signals of Abuse of the Nurse–Client Relationship:

- Secrets' reluctance to talk to others about the work being done with clients;
- Sudden increase in phone calls between nurse and client or calls outside clinical hours;
- The nurse making more exceptions for the client than normal;
- Inappropriate gift-giving between client and nurse;
- Loaning, trading, or selling goods or possessions;
- Nurse disclosure of personal issues or information;
- Inappropriate touching, comforting, or physical contact;
- Overdoing, overprotecting, or overidentifying with the client;
- Change in nurse's body language, dress, or appearance (with no other satisfactory explanation);
- Extended one-on-one sessions or home visits;
- Spending off-duty time with the client;
- Thinking about the client frequently when away from work;
- Becoming defensive if another person questions the nurse's care of the client;
- Ignoring agency policies.

3.5. Roles of the Nurse in a Therapeutic Relationship

Psychiatric nurses use a variety of roles to give clients the necessary care, just like they would in any other nursing setting. The nurse is aware of how critical it is to adopt the proper role for the work that they are performing with the client.

3.5.1. Teacher

The majority of client care facets inherently involve the teacher role. In the working stage of the nurse-client relationship, the nurse might impart to the client fresh coping and problem-solving techniques. He or she might give the client instructions regarding the prescribed dosage and neighborhood resources. Nurses need to be aware of the boundaries of their knowledge base and feel secure in their expertise in order to be an effective teacher. The nurse should be knowledgeable about the community, online resources, and healthcare setting resources that can help clients find the information they need. When and where to refer clients for additional information, the nurse must be forthright about the information that they can offer. Client trust is increased by this conduct and candor.

3.5.2. Caregiver

In mental health settings, establishing a therapeutic relationship with the client to foster trust, explore feelings, help the client solve problems, and support their psychosocial needs is the main caregiving role. If the client also needs physical nursing care, the nurse might have to explain to them why touch is necessary while providing that care. The therapeutic relationship may suffer if some clients mistake physical care for intimacy and sexual desire. The nurse must take into account the parameters and boundaries of the relationship as well as reiterate the objectives that were decided upon at the outset of the partnership.

3.5.3. Advocate

As the client's advocate, the nurse provides information and then stands by them no matter what choice they make. Because of the nature of the client's illness, advocacy in psychiatric-mental health nursing differs slightly from that in medical-surgical settings. For instance, a nurse cannot condone a client's choice to harm themselves or another individual. Acting on a client's behalf when they are unable to do so is known as advocacy. This entails protecting oneself from mistreatment and exploitation by a healthcare provider or other authority figure, encouraging informed consent, avoiding pointless tests and procedures, gaining access to necessary services and benefits, and guaranteeing one's privacy and dignity. The nurse has just acted as the client's advocate, for instance, if the doctor starts to examine the patient without closing the drapes and the nurse intervenes to properly drape the patient and close the curtains. Advocacy comes with risks. In the preceding instance, the doctor might have said something to the nurse out of embarrassment and rage. The nurse must not allow intimidation to divert him or her from maintaining focus on the propriety of their actions.

Being aware of other medical professionals is another requirement of the advocate role for nurses. Staff members can occasionally be reluctant to intervene or see what is going on when a colleague crosses the line in a professional relationship. When they witness boundary violations, nurses need to speak with the coworker or a supervisor before taking any further action. The legal obligation of nurses to report boundary violations and unethical behavior by other healthcare providers is outlined in state nurse practice acts.

The role of the nurse as an advocate is up for discussion. Sometimes, as when a nurse supports a suicidal client's involuntary hospitalization, they fail to uphold the client's autonomy or right to self-determination. In these situations, the client's wishes are directly at odds with acting in their best interest, which is to keep them safe. This is seen by some critics as paternalism and a meddling in the actual function of advocacy. Furthermore, they believe that advocacy is not just a nursing-specific role, but also one that applies to the fields of medicine, social work, and other healthcare providers.

3.5.4. Parent Surrogate

A nurse may be inclined to adopt a parental role when a client behaves in a childlike manner or when the nurse is asked to perform personal care tasks like feeding or bathing. This can be shown in the nurse's word choice and nonverbal cues. The nurse might start to come across as authoritative and have the mindset of "I know what's best for you.". The client usually reacts by becoming more obstinate and childlike. Both parties are unaware that their communication style has shifted from adult-to-adult to parent-child. In these situations, it is simple for the client to see the nurse as a parent surrogate. In these kinds of circumstances, the nurse needs to be precise and strong, setting boundaries or restating existing ones. While setting boundaries, the nurse can continue to nurture the client by maintaining an approachable, laid-back, and nonjudgmental demeanor. It is the nurse's responsibility to make sure the relationship stays therapeutic and does not turn personal or social.

Methods to Avoid Inappropriate Relationships between Nurses and Clients:

- Realize that all staff members, whether male or female, junior or senior, or from any discipline, are at risk for overinvolvement and loss of boundaries.
- Assume that boundary violations will occur. Supervisors should recognize potential "problem" clients and regularly raise the issue of sexual feelings or boundary loss with staff members.
- Provide opportunities for staff members to discuss their dilemmas and effective ways of dealing with them.
- Develop orientation programs to include how to set limits, how to recognize clues that the relationship is losing boundaries, what the institution expects of the professional, clearly defined consequences, case studies, how to develop skills to maintain boundaries, and recommended reading.
- Provide resources for confidential and nonjudgmental assistance.
- Hold regular meetings to discuss inappropriate relationships and feelings toward clients.
- Provide senior staff to lead groups and model effective therapeutic interventions with difficult clients.
- Use clinical vignettes for training.
- Use situations that reflect not only sexual dilemmas but also other boundary violations, including problems with abuse of authority and power.

3.6. Therapeutic Communication

Therapeutic communication is an interpersonal exchange in which the nurse attends to the client's individual needs to facilitate an efficient information sharing process. The nurse can better comprehend and relate to the client's experience by using therapeutic communication techniques with skill. To effectively apply the nursing process and meet standards of care for their clients, all nurses must possess therapeutic communication skills.

Therapeutic communication can help nurses accomplish many goals:

- Establish a therapeutic nurse–client relationship.
- Identify the most important client concern at that moment (the client-centered goal).
- Assess the client's perception of the problem as it unfolds. This includes detailed actions (behaviors and messages) of the people involved and the client's thoughts and feelings about the situation, others, and self.
- Facilitate the client's expression of emotions.
- Teach the client and family the necessary self-care skills.
- Recognize the client's needs.
- Implement interventions designed to address the client's needs.
- Guide the client toward identifying a plan of action to a satisfying and socially acceptable resolution.

When working with clients, one of the most crucial things a nurse must do is establish a therapeutic relationship. The beginning, maintenance, and end of a therapeutic relationship are all facilitated by communication. Confidentiality, self-disclosure, and therapeutic use of self are all covered concerning the therapeutic relationship. To engage in therapeutic communication, the nurse must also take into account the following: use of touch, privacy and boundary respect, active listening, and observation.

3.6.1. Privacy and Respecting Boundaries

In therapeutic communication, privacy is preferred but not always feasible. If the nurse thinks that the conference room is a suitable location for the interview, then it is the best choice. Depending on the physical arrangement of the setting, the nurse may also speak with the client at the end of the hall or in a private corner of the day room or lobby. If engaging with the client in their room is therapeutic, the nurse must assess this. For instance, it is not the ideal environment for the client's room if they have trouble setting limits or if they have been making sexual remarks. One would prefer a more formal setting.

The study of communication distance zones between individuals is known as proxemics. When speaking with someone they know, as opposed to a stranger, people are more at ease over shorter distances (McCall, 2017).

People from the United States, Canada, and many Eastern European nations generally observe four distance zones:

- **Intimate Zone (0–18 in between people):** This amount of space is comfortable for parents with young children, people who mutually desire personal contact, or people whispering. Invasion of this intimate zone by anyone else is threatening and produces anxiety.
- **Personal Zone (18–36 in):** This distance is comfortable between family and friends who are talking.
- **Social Zone (4–12 ft):** This distance is acceptable for communication in social, work, and business settings.
- **Public Zone (12–25 ft):** This is an acceptable distance between a speaker and an audience, small

groups, and other informal functions (Hall, 1963).

When conversing, some individuals from diverse cultural backgrounds—such as those from the Mediterranean, East Indian, Asian, and Middle Eastern backgrounds—feel more at ease when there is less than 4 to 12 feet between them. When speaking with clients from these cultures, the European American or African American nurse might feel awkward if they stand close together. Clients from these backgrounds, on the other hand, might view the nurse as distant and uncaring (Andrews and Boyle, 2015).

When one person enters the other's personal or intimate space, the client and the nurse may feel threatened and become tense, agitated, fidgety, or even try to flee. The nurse should always get the client's consent before entering the intimate or personal area. When taking a client's blood pressure during an assessment in a community setting, for instance, a nurse should say, "Mr. Smith, let me put this cuff around your arm and use my stethoscope to take your blood pressure. He or she should ask, "Is this acceptable to you?," using a yes-or-no format to ensure that the client knows exactly how to respond. Yes-or-no questions are appropriate in this situation.

The ideal distance for a therapeutic communication exchange between a nurse and a client is between three and six feet. Depending on how frequently the client has infringed on the nurse's personal space and the safety of the circumstance, the nurse should progressively impose boundaries if a client does so (0–18 in).

3.6.2. Touch

As intimacy increases, the need for distance decreases. Knapp (1980) identified five types of touch:

- **Functional**–professional touch is used in examinations or procedures such as when the nurse touches a client to assess skin turgor or a massage therapist performs a massage.
- **Social**–polite touch is used in greeting, such as a handshake and the "air kisses" some people use to greet acquaintances, or when a gentle hand guides someone in the correct direction.
- **Friendship**–warmth touch involves a hug in greeting, an arm thrown around the shoulder of a good friend, or the backslapping some people use to greet friends and relatives.
- **Love**–intimacy touch involves tight hugs and kisses between lovers or close relatives.
- **Sexual**–arousal touch is used by lovers.

When touching a client is appropriate and welcomed, it can be consoling and encouraging. When observing a client, the nurse should look for signs that indicate whether or not touch is appropriate. It is appropriate and therapeutic, for instance, to hold the hand of a distraught mother whose child is ill. However, the mother indicates to the nurse that she finds it awkward to be touched if she pulls her hand away. The client may be questioned by the nurse about touching (for example. "May I please give you a squeeze?").

Based on the client's requirements, history, and preferences, the nurse must assess how touch is used. Touch may be comforting to the nurse, but it may not be to the client. Similarly, a patient may utilize physical contact excessively, in which case the nurse must establish suitable limits.

Touch is an infringement of private and intimate space, although it can be consoling and healing. Some mentally ill clients find it difficult to comprehend the idea of personal boundaries or to discern when it is appropriate or inappropriate to touch someone. Individuals who have experienced abuse in the past have often been touched in painful ways by others, usually without their permission. When touch hurts them, they might be reluctant or even unable to express it to others. As such, there are policies prohibiting clients from touching staff members or one another in the majority of psychiatric inpatient, outpatient, and ambulatory care units. Employees should set an example for their clients by not entering their personal or intimate spaces unless it's necessary to provide nursing care. Before beginning any nursing care procedure involving physical contact with a client, a staff member must verbally prepare the client. When a clients experience touch, they may see it as a threat and try to defend themselves by hitting the staff member.

3.6.3. Active Listening and Observation

The nurse needs to use both active listening and active observation to receive the sender's simultaneous messages. Refusing to engage in other internal mental tasks while actively listening entails focusing solely on what the client is saying. Active observation entails observing the nonverbal cues used by the speaker while they are speaking.

Peplau (1952) initiated the therapeutic interaction with observation. The nurse watches the client's actions and assists them in providing thorough explanations of those actions. The nurse records these particulars as well. The nurse evaluates the information gathered, ascertains the underlying needs related to the behavior, and connects the points (creates connections between different parts of the conversation) to assist the client in gaining an understanding of his or her interpersonal skills. When learning the skill of therapeutic communication, students frequently mistakenly believe that they need to have questions prepared for the client as soon as they conclude speaking. As a result, they are not really listening to what the client is saying because they are always considering the next question. This could lead to a vague, superficial, and frustrating conversation for both parties, as the nurse may not comprehend the client's concerns. A cursory conversation can lead to the nurse complaining that the patient isn't taking responsibility for their own recovery, isn't cooperating, or is repeating things. However, if a nurse asks the same question over and over again without paying attention to the client's responses, it may lead to superficiality. Rather than working from the client's actual circumstances, the nurse makes assumptions based on a lack of information.

It is nearly impossible for a nurse to remain impartial while hearing a client's story. The way a person interprets a message is frequently influenced by their life experiences, background knowledge, values, and prejudices. To get the full story from the client's perspective, dispel presumptions, and foster empathy with the client, the nurse must ask targeted questions during therapeutic communication. Being empathetic means having the capacity to temporarily put oneself in another person's shoes. To foster empathy, nurses should try to get as much information as they can directly from clients about a problem to avoid adding their own perspectives and experiences. To fully comprehend the client's perspective of an event or problem, the nurse asks as many questions as necessary.

Active listening and observation help the nurse:

- Recognize the issue that is most important to the client at this time;
- Know what further questions to ask the client;
- Use additional therapeutic communication techniques to guide the client to describe his or her perceptions fully;
- Understand the client's perceptions of the issue instead of jumping to conclusions;
- Interpret and respond to the message objectively.

3.7. Verbal Communication Skills

3.7.1. Using Concrete Messages

To ensure that the client understands what is being said, the nurse should speak to them in as clear a manner as possible. Concrete messages are crucial for accurate information exchange because anxious people lose cognitive processing skills—the more anxious they are, the less able they are to process concepts. Concrete questions are simple, straightforward, and easy to understand. For example, "What health symptoms caused you to come to the hospital today?" or "When was the last time you took your antidepressant medications?" are examples of statements that are explicit and require no interpretation. They get more precise answers and save you from having to ask the same questions over and over again, which breaks up the therapeutic exchange.

Conversely, abstract messages are characterized by ambiguous word patterns and frequently contain difficult-to-understand figures of speech. They necessitate that the listener decipher the speaker's intentions. When a nurse inquires about a patient's reason for admission to the unit, for instance, "How did you get here?" the message is abstract because the terms "how" and "here" are ambiguous. Unsure of their location, a nervous client may ask, "Where am I?" or interpret this as a query regarding how they were transported to the hospital, saying, "The ambulance brought me.". Clients with anxiety, language barriers, cognitive impairments, or mental disorders frequently understand information at a concrete level and struggle to respond to abstract questions. The nurse must ensure that all queries and remarks are precise and unambiguous.

3.7.2. Using Therapeutic Communication Techniques

When interacting with clients, the nurse can employ a variety of therapeutic communication strategies. The goal of the conversation and the client's capacity for verbal communication determine which technique is used. In general, the nurse uses methods that help the client and nurse interact and communicate more effectively. Table 3.5 enumerates these methods and provides illustrations. The client is encouraged to talk about their feelings or concerns in greater detail by using techniques like exploring, focusing, restating, and reflecting. Other strategies aid in clarification or focus of the spoken word. The nurse may use strategies like presenting reality or making an observation to provide the client with feedback.

Table 3.5. *Therapeutic Communication Techniques*

Therapeutic Communication Technique	Examples	Rationale
Accepting—indicating reception	"Yes." "I follow what you said." Nodding	An accepting response indicates the nurse has heard and followed the train of thought. It does not indicate agreement but is nonjudgmental. Facial expression, tone of voice, and so forth also must convey acceptance or the words lose their meaning.
Broad openings—allowing the client to take the initiative in introducing the topic	"Is there something you'd like to talk about?" "Where would you like to begin?"	Broad openings make it explicit that the client has the lead in the interaction. For the client who is hesitant about talking, broad openings may stimulate him or her to take the initiative.
Consensual validation—searching for mutual understanding, for accord in the meaning of the words	"Tell me whether my understanding of it agrees with yours." "Are you using this word to convey that…?"	For verbal communication to be meaningful, it is essential that the words being used have the same meaning for both or all participants. Sometimes, words, phrases, or slang terms have different meanings to different people and can be easily misunderstood.
Encouraging comparison—asking that similarities and differences be noted	"Was it something like…?" "Have you had similar experiences?"	Comparing ideas, experiences, or relationships brings out many recurring themes. The client benefits from making these comparisons because he or she might recall past coping strategies that were effective or remember that he or she has survived a similar situation.
Encouraging description of perceptions—asking the client to verbalize what he or she perceives	"Tell me when you feel anxious." "What is happening?" "What does the voice seem to be saying?"	To understand the client, the nurse must see things from his or her perspective. Encouraging the client to fully describe ideas may relieve the tension the client is feeling, and he or she might be less likely to take action on ideas that are harmful or frightening.
Encouraging expression—asking the client to appraise the quality of his or her experiences	"What are your feelings in regard to…?" "Does this contribute to your distress?"	The nurse asks the client to consider people and events in light of his or her own values. Doing so encourages the client to make his or her own appraisal rather than to accept the opinion of others.

Exploring—delving further into a subject or an idea	"Tell me more about that." "Would you describe it more fully?" "What kind of work?"	When clients deal with topics superficially, exploring can help them examine the issue more fully. Any problem or concern can be better understood if explored in depth. If the client expresses an unwillingness to explore a subject, however, the nurse must respect his or her wishes.
Focusing—concentrating on a single point	"This point seems worth looking at more closely." "Of all the concerns you've mentioned, which is most troublesome?"	The nurse encourages the client to concentrate his or her energies on a single point, which may prevent a multitude of factors or problems from overwhelming the client. It is also a useful technique when a client jumps from one topic to another.
Formulating a plan of action—asking the client to consider kinds of behavior likely to be appropriate in future situations	"What could you do to let your anger out harmlessly?" "Next time this comes up, what might you do to handle it?"	It may be helpful for the client to plan in advance what he or she might do in future similar situations. Making definite plans increases the likelihood that the client will cope more effectively in a similar situation.
General leads—giving encouragement to continue	"Go on." "And then?" "Tell me about it."	General leads indicate that the nurse is listening and following what the client is saying without taking away the initiative for the interaction. They also encourage the client to continue if he or she is hesitant or uncomfortable about the topic.
Giving information—making available the facts that the client needs	"My name is …" "Visiting hours are …" "My purpose in being here is …"	Informing the client of facts increases his or her knowledge about a topic or lets the client know what to expect. The nurse is functioning as a resource person. Giving information also builds trust with the client.
Giving recognition—acknowledging, indicating awareness	"Good morning, Mr. S …" "You've finished your list of things to do." "I notice that you've combed your hair." "You appear	Greeting the client by name, indicating awareness of change, or noting efforts the client has made all show that the nurse recognizes the client as a person, as an individual. Such recognition does not carry the notion of value, that is, of being "good" or "bad."

	tense.”	
Making observations—verbalizing what the nurse perceives	“Are you uncomfortable when…?” “I notice that you’re biting your lip.”	Sometimes clients cannot verbalize or make themselves understood. Or the client may not be ready to talk.
Offering self—making oneself available	“I’ll sit with you awhile.” “I’ll stay here with you.” “I’m interested in what you think.”	The nurse can offer his or her presence, interest, and desire to understand. It is important that this offer is unconditional; that is, the client does not have to respond verbally to get the nurse’s attention.
Placing event in time or sequence—clarifying the relationship of events in time	“What seemed to lead up to…?” “Was this before or after…?” “When did this happen?”	Putting events in proper sequence helps both the nurse and the client to see them in perspective. The client may gain insight into cause-and-effect behavior and consequences or the client may be able to see that perhaps some things are not related. The nurse may gain information about recurrent patterns or themes in the client’s behavior or relationships.
Presenting reality—offering for consideration that which is real	“I see no one else in the room.” “That sound was a car backfiring.” “Your mother is not here; I am a nurse.”	When it is obvious that the client is misinterpreting reality, the nurse can indicate what is real. The nurse does this by calmly and quietly expressing his or her perceptions or the facts, not by way of arguing with the client or belittling his or her experience. The intent is to indicate an alternative line of thought for the client to consider, not to “convince” the client that he or she is wrong.
Reflecting—directing client actions, thoughts, and feelings back to client	*Client:* “Do you think I should tell the doctor…?” *Nurse:* “Do you think you should?” *Client:* “My brother spends all my money and then has nerve to ask for more.” *Nurse:* “This causes you to feel angry?” *Client:* “I can’t sleep. I stay	Reflection encourages the client to recognize and accept his or her own feelings. The nurse indicates that the client’s point of view has value and that the client has the right to have opinions, make decisions, and think independently.

Restating—repeating the main idea expressed	awake all night." *Nurse:* "You have difficulty sleeping." *Client:* "I'm really mad, I'm really upset." *Nurse:* "You're really mad and upset."	The nurse repeats what the client has said in approximately or nearly the same words the client has used. This restatement lets the client know that he or she communicated the idea effectively. This encourages the client to continue. Or if the client has been misunderstood, he or she can clarify his or her thoughts.
Seeking information—seeking to make clear that which is not meaningful or that which is vague	"I'm not sure that I follow." "Have I heard you correctly?"	The nurse should seek clarification throughout interactions with clients. Doing so can help the nurse to avoid making assumptions that understanding has occurred when it has not. It helps the client articulate thoughts, feelings, and ideas more clearly.
Silence—absence of verbal communication, which provides time for the client to put thoughts or feelings into words, to regain composure, or to continue talking	Nurse says nothing but continues to maintain eye contact and conveys interest.	Silence often encourages the client to verbalize, provided that it is interested and expectant. Silence gives the client time to organize thoughts, direct the topic of interaction, or focus on issues that are most important. Much nonverbal behavior takes place during silence, and the nurse needs to be aware of the client and his or her own nonverbal behavior.
Suggesting collaboration—offering to share, to strive, and to work with the client for his or her benefit	"Perhaps you and I can discuss and discover the triggers for your anxiety." "Let's go to your room, and I'll help you find what you're looking for."	The nurse seeks to offer a relationship in which the client can identify problems in living with others, grow emotionally, and improve the ability to form satisfactory relationships. The nurse offers to do things with, rather than for, the client.
Summarizing—organizing and summing up that which has gone before	"Have I got this straight?" "You've said that…." "During the past hour, you and I have discussed…."	Summarization seeks to bring out the important points of the discussion and seeks to increase the awareness and understanding of both participants. It omits the irrelevant and organizes the pertinent aspects of the interaction. It allows both client and nurse to depart with the same ideas and provides a sense of closure at the completion of each discussion.

Translating into feelings—seeking to verbalize client's feelings that he or she expresses only indirectly	*Client:* "I'm dead." *Nurse:* "Are you suggesting that you feel lifeless?" *Client:* "I'm way out in the ocean." *Nurse:* "You seem to feel lonely or deserted."	Often what the client says, when taken literally, seems meaningless or far removed from reality. To understand, the nurse must concentrate on what the client might be feeling to express him or herself this way.
Verbalizing the implied—voicing what the client has hinted at or suggested	*Client:* "I can't talk to you or anyone. It's a waste of time." *Nurse:* "Do you feel that no one understands?"	Putting into words what the client has implied or said indirectly tends to make the discussion less obscure. The nurse should be as direct as possible without being unfeelingly blunt or obtuse. The client may have difficulty communicating directly. The nurse should take care to express only what is fairly obvious; otherwise, the nurse may be jumping to conclusions or interpreting the client's communication.
Voicing doubt—expressing uncertainty about the reality of the client's perceptions	"Isn't that unusual?" "Really?" "That's hard to believe."	Another means of responding to distortions of reality is to express doubt. Such expression permits the client to become aware that others do not necessarily perceive events in the same way or draw the same conclusions. This does not mean the client will alter his or her point of view, but at least the nurse will encourage the client to reconsider or reevaluate what has happened. The nurse neither agreed nor disagreed; however, he or she has not let the misperceptions and distortions pass without comment.

Source: Adapted from Hays, J. S., & Larson, K. (1963). Interactions with patients. New York, NY: Macmillan Press.

3.7.3. Avoiding Nontherapeutic Communication

In contrast, nurses should refrain from using a lot of nontherapeutic methods. These answers sever the connection and make it more challenging for it to continue. Though they might be meant to reassure the client, responses like "everything will work out" or "maybe tomorrow will be a better day" could actually get in the way of communication. When a nurse asks a client "why," it could be interpreted as criticism and suggest that the client thinks poorly of the nurse. Numerous of these reactions are typical in social situations. As a result, the nurse needs to practice refraining from saying things like this (Table 3.6).

Table 3.6. *Nontherapeutic Communication Techniques*

Techniques	Examples	Rationale
Advising—telling the client what to do	"I think you should …" "Why don't you …"	Giving advice implies that only the nurse knows what is best for the client.
Agreeing—indicating accord with the client	"That's right." "I agree."	Approval indicates the client is "right" rather than "wrong." This gives the client the impression that he or she is "right" because of agreement with the nurse. Opinions and conclusions should be exclusively the client's. When the nurse agrees with the client, there is no opportunity for the client to change his or her mind without being "wrong."
Belittling feelings expressed—misjudging the degree of the client's discomfort	*Client:* "I have nothing to live for … I wish I was dead." *Nurse:* "Everybody gets down in the dumps," or "I've felt that way myself."	When the nurse tries to equate the intense and overwhelming feelings the client has expressed to "everybody" or to the nurse's own feelings, the nurse implies that the discomfort is temporary, mild, self-limiting, or not that important. The client is focused on his or her own worries and feelings; hearing the problems or feelings of others is not helpful.
Challenging—demanding proof from the client	"But how can you be president of the United States?" "If you're dead, why is your heart beating?"	Often, the nurse believes that if he or she can challenge the client to prove unrealistic ideas, the client will realize there is no "proof" and then will recognize reality. Actually, challenging causes the client to defend the delusions or misperceptions more strongly than before.
	"This hospital has a fine	Defending what the client has criticized implies that he

Defending—attempting to protect someone or something from verbal attack	reputation." "I'm sure your doctor has your best interests in mind."	or she has no right to express impressions, opinions, or feelings. Telling the client that his or her criticism is unjust or unfounded does not change the client's feelings but only serves to block further communication.
Disagreeing—opposing the client's ideas	"That's wrong." "I definitely disagree with …" "I don't believe that."	Disagreeing implies the client is "wrong." Consequently, the client feels defensive about his or her point of view or ideas.
Disapproving—denouncing the client's behavior or ideas	"That's bad." "I'd rather you wouldn't …"	Disapproval implies that the nurse has the right to pass judgment on the client's thoughts or actions. It further implies that the client is expected to please the nurse.
Giving approval—sanctioning the client's behavior or ideas	"That's good." "I'm glad that …"	Saying what the client thinks or feels is "good" implies that the opposite is "bad." Approval, then, tends to limit the client's freedom to think, speak, or act in a certain way. This can lead to the client's acting in a particular way just to please the nurse.
Giving literal responses—responding to a figurative comment as though it were a statement of fact	*Client:* "They're looking in my head with a television camera." *Nurse:* "Try not to watch television" or "What channel?"	Often, the client is at a loss to describe his or her feelings, so such comments are the best he or she can do. Usually, it is helpful for the nurse to focus on the client's feelings in response to such statements.
Indicating the existence of an external source—attributing the source of thoughts, feelings, and behaviors to others or to outside influences	"What makes you say that?" "What made you do that?" "Who told you that you were a prophet?"	The nurse can ask, "What happened?" or "What events led you to draw such a conclusion?" However, to question, "What made you think that?" implies that the client was made or compelled to think in a certain way. Usually, the nurse does not intend to suggest that the source is external, but that is often what the client thinks.
Interpreting—asking to make conscious that which is unconscious; telling the client the meaning of his or her experience	"What you really mean is …" "Unconsciously you're saying …"	The client's thoughts and feelings are his or her own, not to be interpreted by the nurse for hidden meaning. Only the client can identify or confirm the presence of feelings.
Introducing an unrelated topic—	*Client:* "I'd like to die." *Nurse:* "Did you	The nurse takes the initiative for the interaction away from the client. This usually happens because the nurse is uncomfortable, doesn't know how to respond, or has a topic he or she would rather discuss. The client's thoughts and feelings are his or her own, not

	last evening?"	to be interpreted by the nurse for hidden meaning. Only the client can identify or confirm the presence of feelings.
Making stereotyped comments—offering meaningless clichés or trite comments	"It's for your own good." "Keep your chin up." "Just have a positive attitude and you'll be better in no time."	Social conversation contains many clichés and much meaningless chit-chat. Such comments are of no value in the nurse–client relationship. Any automatic responses lack the nurse's consideration or thoughtfulness.
Probing—persistent questioning of the client	"Now tell me about this problem. You know I have to find out." "Tell me your psychiatric history."	Probing tends to make the client feel used or invaded. Clients have the right not to talk about issues or concerns if they choose. Pushing and probing by the nurse will not encourage the client to talk.
Reassuring—indicating there is no reason for anxiety or other feelings of discomfort	"I wouldn't worry about that." "Everything will be alright." "You're coming along just fine."	Attempts to dispel the client's anxiety by implying that there is not sufficient reason for concern completely devalue the client's feelings. Vague reassurances without accompanying facts are meaningless to the client.
Rejecting—refusing to consider or showing contempt for the client's ideas or behaviors	"Let's not discuss …" "I don't want to hear about …"	When the nurse rejects any topic, he or she closes it off from exploration. In turn, the client may feel personally rejected along with his or her ideas.
Requesting an explanation—asking the client to provide reasons for thoughts, feelings, behaviors, and events	"Why do you think that?" "Why do you feel that way?"	There is a difference between asking the client to describe what is occurring or has taken place and asking him or her to explain why. Usually, a "why" question is intimidating. In addition, the client is unlikely to know "why" and may become defensive trying to explain him or herself.
Testing—appraising the client's degree of insight	"Do you know what kind of hospital this is?" "Do you still have the idea that…?"	These types of questions force the client to try to recognize his or her problems. The client's acknowledgment that he or she doesn't know these things may meet the nurse's needs but is not helpful for the client.
	Client: "I'm nothing." *Nurse:* "Of course you're	
Using denial—refusing to admit that a problem exists	course you're something—everybody's something." *Client:* "I'm dead." *Nurse:* "Don't be silly."	The nurse denies the client's feelings or the seriousness of the situation by dismissing his or her comments without attempting to discover the feelings or meaning behind them.

Source: Adapted from Hays, J. S., & Larson, K. (1963). Interactions with patients. New York, NY: Macmillan Press.

3.7.4. Interpreting Signals or Cues

The nurse listens and watches intently for cues that indicate what the client is trying to say. Cues are nonverbal or spoken signals that indicate important terms or concerns to the client. They can be overt or covert. Active listening has the benefit of helping one find cues. Cues may be submerged in a client's words or revealed through actions taken during dialogue. Cue words that the client uses can often tell the nurse what questions to ask next or how to react to the client. These cue words or concepts serve as the foundation for the nurse's responses.

Understanding this can relieve pressure on students who are worried and anxious about what question to ask next. The following example illustrates questions the nurse might ask when responding to a client's cue:

- **Client:** "I had a boyfriend when I was younger."
- **Nurse:** "You had a boyfriend?" (reflecting) "Tell me about you and your boyfriend." (encouraging description) "How old were you when you had this boyfriend?" (placing events in time or sequence)

If a client has difficulty attending to a conversation and drifts into a rambling discussion or a flight of ideas, the nurse listens carefully for a theme or a topic around which the client composes his or her words. Using the theme, the nurse can assess the nonverbal behaviors that accompany the client's words and build responses based on these cues. In the following examples, certain cues help the nurse formulate further communication based on themes.

- Theme of Sadness:
  - **Client:** "Oh, hi, nurse." (face is sad' eyes look teary' voice is low, with little inflection)
  - **Nurse:** "You seem sad today, Mrs. Venezia."
  - **Client:** "Yes, it is the anniversary of my husband's death."
  - **Nurse:** "How long ago did your husband die?" (or the nurse can use the other cue)
  - **Nurse:** "Tell me about your husband's death, Mrs. Venezia."
- Theme of Loss of Control:
  - **Client:** "I had a fender bender this morning. I'm OK. I lost my wallet, and I have to go to the bank to cover a check I wrote last night. I can't get in contact with my husband at work. I don't know where to start."
  - **Nurse:** "I sense you feel out of control." (translating into feelings)

To let the listener know what they mean, clients can employ a variety of word patterns. Clear, direct declarations of intent, like "I want to die," are known as overt cues. It is evident from the message that the client is considering self-harm or suicide. Uncertain or oblique signals that require interpretation and investigation are known as covert cues. An example of one would be a client stating, "Nothing can help me". The client seems to be expressing that they feel so helpless and hopeless that they intend to take their own lives, but the nurse is not sure. To protect the client and to understand their intentions, the nurse can investigate this hidden cue. When questioned directly, the majority of suicidal individuals often confess their plan and exhibit ambivalence about whether to live or die. The nurse uses a yes-or-no question to get a clear response when they suspect suicide or self-harm.

- Theme of Hopelessness and Suicidal Ideation:
  - **Client:** "Life is hard. I want it to be done. There is no rest. Sleep, sleep is good ... forever."
  - **Nurse:** "I hear you saying things seem hopeless. I wonder if you are planning to kill yourself." (verbalizing the implied)

Other word patterns that need further clarification for meaning include metaphors, proverbs, and clichés. When a client uses these figures of speech, the nurse must follow up with questions to clarify what the client is trying to say.

- A metaphor is a phrase that describes an object or a situation by comparing it with something else familiar.
  - **Client:** "My son's bedroom looks like a bomb went off."
  - **Nurse:** "You're saying your son is not very neat." (verbalizing the implied)
  - **Client:** "My mind is like mashed potatoes."
  - **Nurse:** "I sense you find it difficult to put thoughts together." (translating into feelings)
- Proverbs are old accepted sayings with generally accepted meanings.
  - **Client:** "People who live in glass houses shouldn't throw stones."
  - **Nurse:** "Who do you believe is criticizing you but actually has similar problems?" (encouraging description of perception)

A cliché is an overused expression that typically perpetuates a stereotype. For instance, if a client remarks, "She has more guts than brains," it implies that the speaker doesn't think the woman in question is intelligent, doesn't act before considering her options, or lacks common sense. "Give me an example of how you see her as having more guts than brains," the nurse can focus on getting to the heart of the matter and understand the client's meaning.

3.8. Nonverbal Communication Skills

The actions someone takes while speaking is known as nonverbal communication. It encompasses body language, boundaries, time, space, and facial expressions as well as eye contact. If anything, nonverbal communication is even more crucial than verbal communication. It is estimated that two-thirds of meaning are communicated nonverbally and one-third is transmitted through words. While nonverbal communication reveals the speaker's true meaning, verbal communication may express what the speaker thinks the listener wants to hear. The unconscious mind expresses feelings about the spoken content, the circumstance, the setting, and the relationship between the speaker and the listener through nonverbal communication. When there is a discrepancy between the two, nonverbal communication is frequently more accurate than verbal communication. Individuals are more likely to be able to control their nonverbal communication than their verbal communication. Meaning is communicated through both verbal and nonverbal cues. Some people emphasize what they are saying with hand gestures. A nod can signify agreement, but a puzzled expression can be read as confusion. Verifying the meaning of nonverbal cues is crucial because misconceptions or presumptions can result in miscommunication.

3.8.1. Facial Expression

The most obvious, intricate, and occasionally perplexing nonverbal cues come from a person's face. Words and facial expressions work together to convey meaning, revealing the speaker's inner monologue. Facial expressions can be categorized into expressive, impassive, and confusing:

- An expressive face portrays the person's moment-by-moment thoughts, feelings, and needs. These expressions may be evident even when the person does not want to reveal his or her emotions.
- An impassive face is frozen into an emotionless deadpan expression similar to a mask.
- A confusing facial expression is one that is the opposite of what the person wants to convey. A person who is verbally expressing sad or angry feelings while smiling is exhibiting a confusing facial expression.

The way one looks frequently influences how the other person responds. Facial expressions that are powerful and emotive can influence someone to believe what you're saying. For instance, a client can trick the nurse into staying longer than expected by acting bewildered and confused. The meaning of common facial expressions like happy, sad, embarrassed, and angry is usually universal, but the nurse should recognize the expression and get the client's confirmation before interpreting it' for example, "You're smiling, but I sense you are angry" (Wasajja, 2018).

Common nonverbal cues include frowns, smiles, puzzlement, relief, fear, surprise, and anger. Yawning, turning away from the speaker, and not meeting their eyes are telltale signs of boredom, dishonesty, or disinterest. The nurse detects nonverbal communication and verifies that it is consistent with the content to guarantee the accuracy of the information (Wasajja, 2018). As an illustration, consider "Mr. Jones, you scowled as you said, "Everything's fine today". I get the impression that things aren't really going well.

3.8.2. Body Language

Body language (e.g. body positions, gestures, and postures) is a type of nonverbal communication. Closed body language—crossed legs, folded arms across the chest, etc.—indicates that the person receiving the interaction may be threatened and may become defensive or unaccepting. Sitting facing the client with both feet on the ground, knees parallel, hands by the sides of the body, and legs either uncrossed or crossed only at the ankles is a better, more accommodative body position. This stance of acceptance, care, trust, and unconditional positive regard is demonstrated. The nurse faces the client, leans slightly in their direction, and makes nonthreatening eye contact as a sign of interest and acceptance. Hand gestures give the text additional meaning. The meaning of words can be reinforced or punctuated with a small lift of the hand from a chair's arm. With both hands raised and shoulders shrugged, the expression "I don't know" is frequently used. Some people act out or demonstrate what they are saying with a lot of hand gestures, while others use very few. It's crucial to consider how the nurse and client are positioned in relation to one another. While sitting behind a desk (creating a physical barrier) can increase the formality of the setting and may decrease the client's willingness to open up and communicate freely, sitting beside or across from the client can help them feel more at ease. But for some clients—like those who struggle to set limits—the nurse might want to establish a more formal environment.

3.8.3. Vocal Cues

Vocal cues are nonverbal cues that are transmitted in addition to the content. The sender's message is enhanced by changes in voice volume, tone, pitch, intensity, emphasis, speed, and pauses. Loudness, or volume, can convey a variety of emotions, including fear, happiness, rage, or deafness. One's tone can convey whether they are bored, agitated, or at ease. The pitch ranges from low and menacing to high and shrill. The strength, force, and power of the words—that is, their intensity—indicates the significance of the message. Accentuating words or phrases that draw attention to a topic or provide context is known as emphasizing it. The quantity of words spoken in a minute is called speed. Pauses enhance the message as well' they frequently add emphasis or emotion. Anxiety is frequently indicated by a message delivered quickly and in a high pitch. Circumstantiality is the use of superfluous words with drawn-out, boring descriptions. It might mean the client is not a good historian or is unsure of what is important. A person who answers slowly and hesitantly may be depressed, confused, struggling to find the right words to describe an experience, or thinking back on the past. Instead of assuming to know what the client is thinking or feeling, the nurse must validate these nonverbal cues (e.g., "Mr. Smith, you seem apprehensive. Is it your current state of mind?").

3.8.4. Eye Contact

The eyes reflect our emotions so much that they have been called the mirror of the soul. The eyes convey a range of emotions, including curiosity, humor, hatred, happiness, sadness, terror, warning, and pleading. When speaking, eye contact—looking directly into the other person's eyes—decreases while speaking, but it increases when listening and is used to assess the other person, the environment, and whose turn it is to speak (Wasajja, 2018). It's crucial that the nurse avoids "staring" at the client, even though maintaining good eye contact is usually preferred.

3.8.5. Silence

Long pauses or silences in conversation can mean a variety of things. It's possible that the client is depressed and finds it difficult to talk. Pauses can sometimes be an indication that the client is carefully thinking through the question before answering. The patient may occasionally appear to be "lost in his or her own thoughts" and not focus on the nurse. Even if it seems like a long time, it is crucial to give the client enough time to respond. If the nurse "jumps in" with another question or tries to phrase the question differently, it might confuse the client. Additionally, in certain cultures, verbal communication has a slower cadence with lots of pauses. If a nurse does not wait for the client's response, the client might think the nurse is impolite or impatient.

3.9. Understanding the Meaning of Communication

In social and therapeutic communication, messages frequently have multiple levels of meaning beyond the meaning conveyed through spoken words. The nurse has to make an effort to understand every nuance of the client's communication. A depressed client might say, for instance, "I'm so tired that I just can't go on.". The nurse may conclude that the client is suffering from the exhaustion that frequently accompanies depression if they simply take the words at face value. But, remarks like the one in the preceding example could indicate that the client wants to pass away. To ascertain whether the client is suicidal, the nurse will need to evaluate the client's statement in more detail.

Sometimes, clients find it easier to express their needs and feelings through acting out their feelings than it is to put their thoughts and feelings into words. People who, for instance, project an image of strength and dominance while manipulating and criticizing others may actually be insecure and have low self-esteem. Instead of expressing their genuine emotions through words, they behave as though they do. Jealousy and mistrust of others, as well as attempts to feel stronger and more important by controlling or criticizing others, are common manifestations of insecurity and low self-esteem.

Determining the meaning of a message accurately requires a thorough understanding of the communication context. Consider how two different situations—angry during a fight and learning that a friend is preparing a surprise party for them—make "I'm going to kill you!" mean different things. A nurse's ability to comprehend the situation's context increases informational value and lowers the likelihood of making assumptions.

The nurse must collect data from both verbal and nonverbal sources, validate findings with the client, and provide context clarification. When a client says, "I collapsed," for instance, she might be referring to a faint or weakness that required her to sit down. Alternatively, she might be saying that she went to bed because she was exhausted. The nurse could ask, "What do you mean collapsed?" (seeking clarification) or, "Describe where you were and what you were doing when you collapsed" to further explain these terms and put them in the context of the action. arranging things chronologically and logically. Contextual assessment considers who was present, what transpired, when it happened, how it developed, and the reasons behind the client's belief that it happened the way it did.

3.9.1. Understanding Spirituality

Spirituality is a person's personal belief system related to life, health, illness, death, and their connection to the universe. It is separate from organized religion, which involves specific beliefs about powerful forces that govern the universe and provide guidelines for living in harmony. Spiritual and religious beliefs are often shared and followed by others who practice similar rituals and rules in daily life. These beliefs can offer comfort, and hope, and influence a person's well-being and healthcare choices. As a nurse, it is important to understand and respect your own spiritual and religious beliefs. These beliefs are deeply personal and can vary greatly among individuals. It is crucial to remain impartial and accepting of a client's beliefs, without letting them impact the care provided. Nurses must assess the spiritual and religious needs of each client and avoid imposing their own beliefs on them. It is essential to ensure that clients are treated with respect and not marginalized for their differing beliefs and values.

The nurse has to be conscious of and respectful of the client's spiritual and religious beliefs as the therapeutic relationship progresses. Behaving judgmentally or ignoring someone will quickly erode their trust and may even end the relationship. For instance, while assisting a Native American patient, a nurse might notice that the patient is gazing up at the sky and conversing with "Grandmother Moon". The nurse might interpret the client's actions as inappropriate if she was unaware that the client believes that the sun, moon, earth, and trees are all spirits.

3.10. The Therapeutic Communication Session

3.10.1. Goals

The nurse uses all the therapeutic communication techniques and skills previously described to help achieve the following goals:

- Establish rapport with the client by being empathetic, genuine, caring, and unconditionally accepting of the client regardless of his or her behavior or beliefs.

- Actively listen to the client to identify the issues of concern and to formulate a client-centered goal for the interaction.
- Gain an in-depth understanding of the client's perception of the issue and foster empathy in the nurse–client relationship.
- Explore the client's thoughts and feelings.
- Facilitate the client's expression of thoughts and feelings.
- Guide the client in developing new skills in problem-solving.
- Promote the client's evaluation of solutions.

The time and environment for therapeutic communication, such as a thorough one-on-one conversation with a designated client, can frequently be planned by the nurse. The nurse will have a general idea of the topic—such as finding out what the client views as his or her main concern or following up on an interaction from a previous encounter—and will have time to consider where to meet and what to say. However, occasionally a client will ask to speak with the nurse directly, or the nurse may choose to approach a client who is crying and sitting by themselves. In these circumstances, the nurse may be aware that the goal will be to ascertain the client's current state of affairs.

It is appropriate to introduce oneself and create a relationship contract when meeting a client for the first time to initiate therapeutic communication. The client's preferred method of address may be inquired about by the nurse. A relationship contract outlines the care the nurse will provide, the times the nurse will visit the client and the terms the client must agree to. If the nurse and the client have never met before, they can strike up a conversation to help break the ice and get to know one another after the introduction and contract have been established. The nurse can then assist the client in identifying the main area of concern by asking a broad opening question. Asking open-ended questions at the start of a therapeutic communication session helps the client focus on the things that are important to them.

3.10.1.1. Nondirective Role

It's common for the client to identify the issue they wish to talk about when starting a therapeutic relationship—rather than the nurse. To determine the subject of concern, the nurse applies active listening techniques. Information on this topic is gathered with the client in mind, who specifies the goal. During this discussion, the nurse serves as a guide. The goal of the therapeutic conversation is to be accomplished within the allotted time.

The following are examples of client-centered goals:

- The client will discuss her concerns about her 16-year-old daughter who is having trouble in school.
- The client will describe the difficulty she has with the side effects of her medication.
- The client will share his distress about his son's drug abuse.
- The client will identify the greatest concerns she has about being a single parent.

In this kind of therapeutic communication, the nurse is taking on a non-directive role, gathering information and assisting the client in identifying and discussing the topic of concern through open-ended questions and broad openings. Most of the talking is done by the client. Throughout the interaction, the nurse supports the client in identifying problems and expressing their feelings. In certain therapeutic conversations, the client's main goal is to feel heard and to speak with an interested listener. Just talking about a traumatic experience can frequently free the client to express feelings and ideas that they have been suppressing. It functions as a means of releasing emotions and lessening the emotional burden without having to change the circumstances. At other times, the client might need to reflect and talk about enjoyable memories from the past. Reminiscing about past events, such as what was going on in the world when they were growing up, how they met and got married, and other life events, can be a great source of comfort for older adults.

3.10.1.2. Directive Role

The nurse takes on a directive role when a client is suicidal, going through a crisis, or losing their sense of reality. They ask straightforward yes-or-no questions and use problem-solving techniques to help the client come up with new coping strategies for handling current problems. In this instance, the client's safety is in jeopardy, so the nurse takes on a directive role. The nurse employs therapeutic communication to carry out numerous interventions in the client's care plan as their relationship develops. A thorough description of a problem or an incident can be obtained by the nurse by using active listening techniques, asking lots of open-ended questions, and expanding on the client's answers. This also helps the nurse comprehend the client's experience. Some clients require the assistance of the nurse to explain how an event transpired over time because they lack the necessary skill or patience. Clients frequently only tell stories from the start to the finish, omitting important details about their own actions. By employing strategies like clarification and placing an event in the proper order or time frame, the nurse can assist the client.

3.10.1.3. Asking for Clarification

Nurses frequently think that they ought to be able to comprehend their clients' words at all times. Uncertainty in the client's thoughts and communications makes this impractical at times. In the event of uncertainty, the nurse should always seek clarification rather than assuming that they understand. Accurate data collection depends critically on the nurse asking clarifying questions to make sure they understand what the client is trying to say. The nurse might need to go back to a previously discussed topic if additional details or clarification are needed. In certain cases, the nurse might also need to clarify information by asking questions. Subsequently, the nurse can employ the therapeutic method of consensual validation, which involves repeating the nurse's understanding of the event the client just described, to check if the client's perceptions match. Instead of working from assumptions, it's critical to go back and clarify.

3.10.1.4. Client's Avoidance of the Anxiety-Producing Topic

Occasionally, clients start talking about a non-essential topic because it doesn't seem as serious as the problem that is making them more anxious. While talking about a subject, the client appears to be distracted. The nurse can gain an understanding of what is happening by actively listening and noticing shifts in the intensity of the nonverbal process. Many options can help the nurse determine which topic is more important:

- Ask the client which issue is more important at this time.
- Go with the new topic because the client has given nonverbal messages that this is the issue that needs to be discussed.

- Reflect the client's behavior, signaling there is a more important issue to be discussed.
- Mentally file the other topic away for later exploration.
- Ignore the new topic because it seems that the client is trying to avoid the original topic.

3.10.2. Guiding the Client in Problem-Solving and Empowering the Client to Change

Several therapeutic contexts require problem-solving. It is not expected of the nurse to be an expert or to advise the client on how to resolve their issue. Instead, the nurse ought to assist the client in considering options and resolving issues. In many therapeutic situations, problem-solving is a necessary component, and simply assisting the client in exploring and discussing their perspectives on a problem can spark potential solutions. Satir (1967) outlined how crucial the client's involvement is to generating practical and significant solutions to problems, noting that frequently just assisting the client in discussing and exploring his or her perceptions of a problem stimulates potential solutions. The client may fear growth and change if someone else gives them advice on how to solve their problems and prevents them from participating, learning how to solve problems, and creating change-making pathways. When a nurse offers guidance or instructions on how to solve an issue, they are preventing the client from participating in the process and are implying that the client is not very capable. The client's self-esteem is lowered by this process and they begin to feel powerless and out of control. To feel in control again, the client might even defy the instructions. Involving a client more in the process of problem-solving increases the likelihood that the solutions will be implemented. In addition to helping the client create new coping mechanisms and sustaining or boosting their self-esteem, the nurse who supports the client in problem-solving techniques also shows that they believe the client is capable of changing. Any client would find it comfortable to feel competent and effective, which is why these objectives help the client broaden their skill set. While problem-solving techniques are widely employed in crisis intervention, they are also useful in everyday situations. When a client is having trouble coming up with a solution or when working with a group of people whose differing points of view make it difficult to find a solution, the problem-solving process is employed. It involves several steps:

- Identify the problem.
- Brainstorm all possible solutions.
- Select the best alternative.
- Implement the selected alternative.
- Evaluate the situation.
- If dissatisfied with results, select another alternative and continue the process.

It's critical to keep in mind that the nurse is supporting the client's ability to solve problems. Even though the nurse does not think the client is selecting the best or most efficient course of action, it is still critical that the nurse accepts the client's decision and helps the client put the chosen course of action into action. If the client makes a mistake or the chosen course of action fails, the nurse can encourage the client to try again and offer support. To solve problems effectively, one must assist the client in becoming as independent as possible in solving their own problems.

3.11. Assertive Communication

The capacity for direct, honest, and open expression of both positive and negative thoughts and emotions is known as assertive communication. It is helpful in a variety of circumstances, including settling disputes, finding solutions to issues, and expressing emotions or ideas that some people find difficult to articulate. It also acknowledges the rights of both parties. Dealing with conflicts with family, friends, or coworkers can be made easier with assertive communication. It is especially beneficial for those who find it difficult to say no to requests from others, express their anger or frustration, or interact with authority figures. In addition to teaching and practicing assertive communication techniques, nurses can help patients use them to interact with other nurses and healthcare professionals. It is applicable in both private and business contexts. The best ways for an assertive speaker to communicate are when they are composed, focus on "I" statements, and make precise, factual statements. One of the nurses on your unit, for instance, consistently arrives at work a few minutes late, arriving hurriedly and interfering with the change-of-shift report. There are four types of responses that coworkers can have to this situation:

- **Aggressive:** After saying nothing for several days, one nurse jumps up and yells, "You're always late! That is so rude! Why can't you be on time like everyone else?" Then the nurse stomps out of the room, leaving everyone uncomfortable.
- **Passive–aggressive:** A coworker says to another nurse, "So nice of her to join us! Aren't we lucky?" Everyone sits in uncomfortable silence.
- **Passive:** One nurse doesn't say anything at the time, but later tells coworkers, "She's always late. I had to tell her what she missed. I have so much work of my own to do." But this nurse doesn't say anything to the nurse who was late.
- **Assertive:** After the report, one nurse says, "When you are late, the report is disrupted, and I don't like having to repeat information that was already discussed." This nurse has communicated feelings about the specific situation calmly with no accusations or inflammatory comments.

While using assertive communication does not ensure that things will get better, it does give the speaker the opportunity to communicate honestly in a direct, honest, and courteous manner. This makes the speaker feel good about expressing their emotions and could start a conversation about possible solutions. People occasionally find it difficult to say no or turn down requests from other people. The person may later feel guilty about accepting and become resentful or overworked. Even when the person making the request is persistent, the use of assertive communication can assist the person in saying no in a courteous but firm manner.

We refer to this as the "broken record technique". Rather than reacting to further details, like concert tickets, not having any plans or emotional appeals, the speaker just reiterates the response without providing an explanation or justification. With time, the person may grow accustomed to turning down requests without feeling bad about it or obliged to give an explanation. By doing this, they may be able to prevent tension from being overly dedicated or resentful from fulfilling a request for which they later become resentful. It takes practice to communicate assertively. "Rehearsing" remarks or answers beforehand is frequently beneficial, particularly if expressing emotions or addressing conflict is challenging. In addition, others might not appreciate your assertive communication style if it differs from their previous way of communicating. Using assertive communication doesn't always yield positive results. However, the speaker can be sure that they respected the rights of both parties and expressed their thoughts and feelings honestly and openly.

3.12. Community-Based Care

The role of the nurse is growing along with the level of community care provided to individuals with both physical and mental health issues. The nurse may take on a more prominent role as the primary caregiver and resource for families and increasingly high-risk patients receiving in-home treatment. They may also be held more accountable for primary prevention in wellness and health maintenance. The ability to effectively manage clients in the community requires the use of therapeutic communication techniques and skills. Providing care for elderly individuals within families and communities is a significant nursing concern and duty in the modern world. Evaluating family relationships is crucial, and figuring out where they agree and disagree can have a big impact on how well clients are treated. The nurse must interact with clients, build a therapeutic relationship, and be receptive to their needs for care and support as well as those of their families.

A nurse must be self-aware and knowledgeable about cultural differences to practice in the community. Since the nurse is an outsider in each family's home when they visit, they must learn to negotiate their cultural context by learning about their values, traditions, and ways of life rather than passing judgment on them based solely on their own. The nurse shows her sincerity and unwavering positive regard for the family by asking for assistance in learning about their culture. In addition to showing a great deal of patience and forgiveness for the cultural blunders that nurses may make when adjusting to new customs and behaviors, families from diverse cultural backgrounds frequently respect nurses and healthcare professionals. To ensure that cultural health practices do not impede or change recommended treatment plans, nurses also need to be aware of and knowledgeable about these practices. Certain cultural healing methods, cures, and even food habits can change a patient's immune system and interfere with prescription drugs.

As a member of the healthcare team, the community care nurse must develop communication skills with the client, family, and other healthcare professionals who are involved in the client's care, including doctors, physical therapists, psychologists, and home health aides. In community care, working with multiple people concurrently is the norm rather than just with the client. For clients to receive effective care in a community setting, self-awareness and sensitivity to the opinions, actions, and feelings of others are essential. (Luft, 1970' Knapp, 1980)

A Closer Look

Therapeutic Touch

Therapeutic touch is a complementary therapy that involves the practitioner using their hands to promote healing and relaxation in the recipient. Rooted in the belief that the body has an inherent ability to heal itself, therapeutic touch aims to restore balance and harmony to the body's energy fields. This practice is based on the concept that disruptions or imbalances in the body's energy can lead to physical or emotional distress, and by manipulating these energy fields, practitioners can facilitate the healing process.

During a therapeutic touch session, the practitioner typically begins by centering themselves and entering a focused state of awareness. They then gently move their hands over the recipient's body, often without direct contact, sensing for areas of imbalance or blockage in the energy fields. Through a series of gentle movements and techniques, such as smoothing, lifting, or compressing, the practitioner seeks to clear these blockages and restore the flow of energy throughout the body.

Therapeutic touch is commonly used to promote relaxation, reduce stress, alleviate pain, and support the body's natural healing processes. Research suggests that it may help improve symptoms associated with various conditions, including anxiety, depression, chronic pain, and side effects of cancer treatment. While the mechanisms underlying therapeutic touch are not fully understood, proponents suggest that it works by balancing the body's energy fields and enhancing the body's innate healing mechanisms.

Critics of therapeutic touch argue that its efficacy is based on placebo effects rather than any measurable physiological changes. Skeptics point to the lack of scientific evidence supporting its mechanisms and outcomes, as well as concerns about the potential for practitioners to unintentionally influence the recipient's experience through subtle cues or biases.

Despite these criticisms, therapeutic touch continues to be practiced and studied in both clinical and research settings. Many healthcare institutions offer therapeutic touch as part of integrative care programs, alongside conventional medical treatments. Research into therapeutic touch is ongoing, with studies exploring its effects on various health conditions and its potential mechanisms of action.

In conclusion, therapeutic touch is a complementary therapy that involves the manipulation of the body's energy fields to promote healing and relaxation. While its mechanisms and efficacy remain the subject of debate, many people find it to be a valuable tool for managing stress, pain, and other health conditions. Further research is needed to better understand how therapeutic touch works and its role in integrative healthcare approaches.

Summary

- Empathy is the ability of the nurse to perceive the meanings and feelings of the client and to communicate that understanding to the client. It is considered one of the essential skills a nurse must develop to provide high-quality, compassionate care.
- A social relationship is primarily initiated for friendship, socialization, companionship, or accomplishment of a task. Communication, which may be superficial, usually focuses on sharing ideas, feelings, and experiences and meets the basic need for people to interact.
- A healthy intimate relationship involves two people who are emotionally committed to each other. Both parties are concerned about having their individual needs met and helping each other meet the needs as well.
- The therapeutic relationship differs from the social or intimate relationship in many ways because it focuses on the needs, experiences, feelings, and ideas of the client only. The nurse and client agree about the areas to work on and evaluate the outcomes.
- Confidentiality means respecting the client's right to keep private any information about his or her mental and physical health and related care. It means allowing only those dealing with the client's care to have access to the information that the client divulges.
- The nurse–client relationship can be jeopardized if the nurse finds the client's behavior unacceptable or distasteful and allows those feelings to show by avoiding the client or making verbal responses or facial expressions of annoyance or turning away from the client.
- In the advocate role, the nurse informs the client and then supports him or her in whatever decision he or she makes. In psychiatric–mental health nursing, advocacy is a bit different from medical–surgical settings because of the nature of the client's illness.
- Therapeutic communication is an interpersonal interaction between the nurse and the client during which the nurse focuses on the client's specific needs to promote an effective exchange of information.
- Nonverbal communication is the behavior a person exhibits while delivering verbal content. It includes facial expression, eye contact, space, time, boundaries, and body movements.
- The human face produces the most visible, complex, and sometimes confusing nonverbal messages. Facial movements connect with words to illustrate meaning' this connection demonstrates the speaker's internal dialogue.

References

1. Andrews, M., & Boyle, J. (2015). *Transcultural Concepts in Nursing Care* (7th ed.). Lippincott Williams & Wilkins.
2. Carper, B. (1978). Fundamental patterns of knowing in nursing. *Advances in Nursing Science, 1*(1), 13–23.
3. Cetrano, G., Tedeschi, F., Rabbi, L., Gosetti, G., Lora, A., Lamonaca, D., & Amaddeo, F. (2017). How are compassion fatigue, burnout, and compassion satisfaction affected by quality of

working life? Findings from a survey of mental health staff in Italy. *BMC Health Services Research, 17*(1), 755.

4. Choi, J. (2018). The value of psychosocial group activity in nursing education: A qualitative analysis. *Nurse Education Today, 64*, 65–70.
5. Hall, E. (1963). Proxemics: The study of man's spatial relationships. In J. Gladstone (Ed.), *Man's Image in Medicine and Anthropology* (pp. 109–120). Mosby.
6. Knapp, M. L. (1980). *Essentials of Nonverbal Communication*. Holt, Rinehart & Winston.
7. Luft, J. (1970). *Group Processes: An Introduction in Group Dynamics*. National Press Books.
8. McCall, C. (2017). Mapping social interactions: The science of proxemics. *Current Topics in Behavioral Neuroscience, 30*, 295–308.
9. Munhall, P. (1993). Unknowing: Toward another pattern of knowing in nursing. *Nursing Outlook, 41*(3), 125–128.
10. Papageorgiou, A., Loke, Y. K., & Fromage, M. (2017). Communication skills training for mental health professionals working with people with severe mental illness. *The Cochrane Database of Systematic Reviews, (6)*, CD010006. https://doi.org/10.1002/14651858.CD010006.pub2.
11. Peplau, H. (1952). *Interpersonal Relations in Nursing*. G. P. Putnam.
12. Peplau, H. E. (1952). *Interpersonal Relations in Nursing*. G. P. Putnam's Sons.
13. Satir, V. (1967). *Conjoint Family Therapy: A Guide to Theory and Technique* (Rev. ed.). Science and Behavior Books.
14. Wasajja, J. K. (2018). *Communication Tools for Nurses: Therapeutic Communication*. CreateSpace Independent Publishing Platform.
15. Wood, A. E., Prins, A., Bush, N. E., Hsia, J. F., Bourn, L. E., Earley, M. D., & Ruzek, J. (2017). Reduction in burnout in mental health care providers using the provider resilience mobile application. *Community Mental Health Journal, 53*(4), 452–459.

Chapter

ANGER, HOSTILITY, AGGRESSION, AND VIOLENCE

4

Contents

Introduction

A natural human emotion, anger is a strong, uneasy reaction to an actual or perceived provocation. Feelings such as frustration, hurt, or fear give rise to anger. Anger can be a useful tool when it is controlled, managed assertively, and used to help solve problems, settle disputes, and make decisions. Anger triggers the sympathetic nervous system's "fight-or-flight" response, energizing the body physically for self-defense when necessary. However, anger can disrupt relationships or result in physical or emotional issues when it is improperly expressed or repressed.

Verbal aggression, another name for hostility, is an emotion that manifests as verbal abuse, disobedience, breaking rules or conventions, or acting in a threatening manner (Schultz and Videbeck, 2013). When someone feels helpless or threatened, they may become hostile. Hostile behavior can escalate into physical aggression and is meant to intimidate or hurt someone emotionally. Physical aggression refers to actions where an individual assaults, hurts, or destroys property. Aggression, whether verbal or physical, is intended to injure, punish, or coerce another individual into doing something. Certain patients suffering from mental illnesses exhibit antagonistic or physically violent conduct, which poses a risk to nurses and other healthcare personnel.

Orientation and Directional Terms

Term	Definition	Illustration
Mental illnesses	Mental illnesses are health conditions involving changes in emotion, thinking or behavior (or a combination of these). Mental illnesses can be associated with distress and/or problems functioning in social, work or family activities.	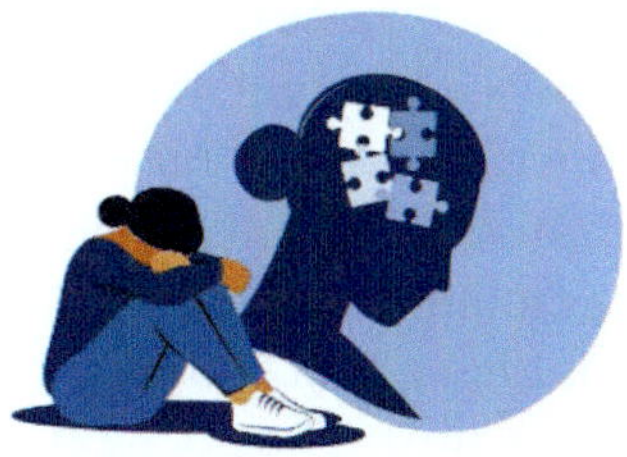
Intermittent explosive disorder (IED)	Intermittent explosive disorder (IED) is a mental health condition marked by frequent impulsive anger outbursts or aggression. The episodes are out of proportion to the situation that triggered them and cause significant distress.	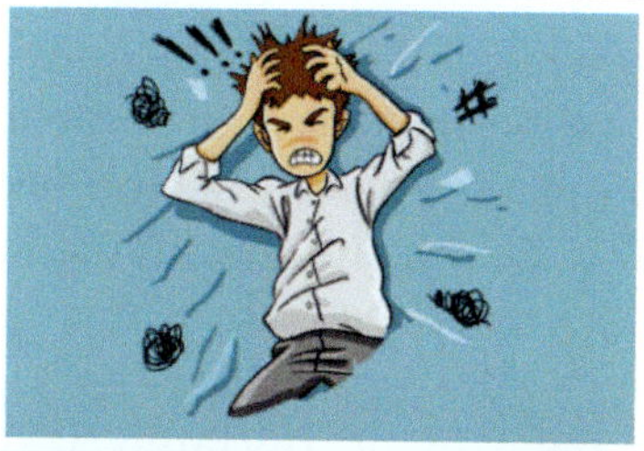
Family violence	Family violence is considered to be any form of abuse, mistreatment or neglect that a child or adult experiences from a family member, or from someone with whom they have an intimate relationship.	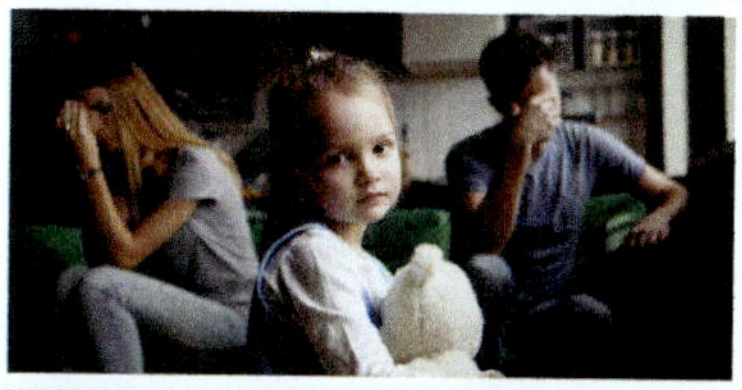
Self-neglect	Self-neglect is a behavioral condition in which an individual neglects to attend to their basic needs, such as personal hygiene, appropriate clothing, feeding, or tending appropriately to any medical conditions they have. More generally, any lack of self-care in terms of personal health, hygiene and living conditions can be referred to as self-neglect.	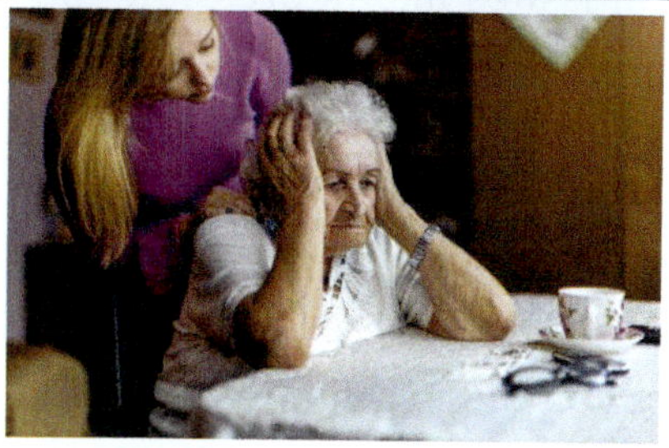
Dementia	Dementia is a syndrome that can be caused by a number of diseases which over time destroy nerve cells and damage the brain, typically leading to deterioration in cognitive function (i.e. the ability to process thought) beyond what might be expected from the usual consequences of biological ageing.	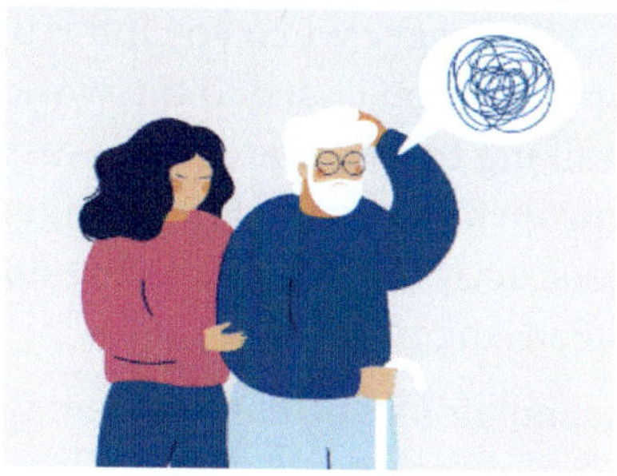

4.1. Onset and Clinical Course

4.1.1. Anger

Even though it's a natural emotion, anger is frequently viewed negatively. Many find it uncomfortable to express their anger in this way. However, when conditions or events are unfair or unjust, when individual rights are violated, or when reasonable expectations are not fulfilled, anger can be a normal and healthy response. Effective communication of anger can facilitate problem-solving and conflict resolution. Feelings of anger are neither wrong nor bad. Denying or attempting to completely stop feeling angry is unhealthy. Positively identifying, expressing, and handling anger is crucial for overall well-being. When someone suppresses, denies, or expresses anger inappropriately, it turns into a negative emotion. One may choose to suppress or deny (i.e., suppress) furious emotions if the person finds it difficult to communicate their anger. Physical issues like migraine headaches, ulcers, or coronary artery disease, as well as emotional issues like depression and low self-esteem, could result.

Anger that is expressed inappropriately can lead to hostility and aggression. The nurse can help clients express anger appropriately by serving as a model and by role-playing assertive communication techniques. Assertive communication uses "I" statements that express feelings and are specific to the situation, for example, "I feel angry when you interrupt me," or "I am angry that you changed the work schedule without talking to me." Statements such as these allow appropriate expression of anger and can lead to productive problem-solving discussions and reduced anger.

Some individuals attempt to vent their anger by hitting a punching bag or yelling—violent but safe behaviors. These so-called cathartic activities are meant to help people let go of their anger. Catharsis, however, can exacerbate anger rather than lessen it. For this reason, cathartic activities might not be appropriate for irate clients. Walking or conversing with someone else are examples of non-aggressive activities that are more likely to be successful in reducing anger. Distraction, problem-solving, perspective-changing, and reframing are some of the cognitive behavioral therapy strategies that can be useful in handling circumstances or issues that make one feel angry (Horiuchi, Tsuda, Aoki, Yoneda, and Sawaguchi, 2018).

Anger and hostility are linked to a higher risk of hypertension and coronary artery disease. Anger outbursts that are ineffective for expressing anger can result from hostility. Affirmative communication and mindfulness practices are two effective ways to communicate anger that should take the place of violent, angry outbursts of temper like hurling objects or screaming. Controlling one's temper or effectively managing anger should not be confused with suppressing angry feelings, which can result in the issues previously mentioned. Suppressing angry feelings can have a negative impact on the management of hypertension. Social inhibition and anger-related personality traits are linked to the existence and severity of coronary artery disease. Women are particularly prone to suppressing their anger since they have been taught to value and preserve interpersonal relationships while avoiding expressing what are perceived to be negative or unfeminine emotions like rage. When people treat women unfairly, withhold resources or power from them, or act carelessly around them, it frequently enrages women. Girls in school report being treated disrespectfully, written off, and denied the ability to express their rage. The perpetrators are typically their closest intimates rather than strangers. Women are more likely than men to exhibit physical complaints and psychological issues as signs of suppressed anger. Women need to understand that to grow and develop, they must be able to express and recognize their anger.

4.1.2. Hostility and Aggression

Aggressive and hostile conduct can appear out of the blue. However, there are frequently stages or phases that can be distinguished in aggressive incidents: an escalation phase, a crisis phase, a recovery phase, and a postcrisis phase. Triggered incidents are defined as those that initiate an aggressive response. Behavior escalation can result in physical aggression as a client loses the ability to accurately perceive events, solve problems, express feelings appropriately, and control their behavior as they approach the crisis phase. Therefore, the best way to stop physically aggressive behavior is to intervene during the triggering and escalation phases.

4.2. Related Disorders

Aggressive people with mental illnesses receive a lot of attention from the media. This misleads the public into believing that the majority of those suffering from mental illness are violent and ought to be feared. In actuality, patients with mental illnesses have a significantly higher risk of harming themselves than others. Although the majority of patients with mental illnesses do not behave aggressively, patients with a range of mental illnesses can act hostilely, angrily, and violently. Individuals suffering from paranoid delusions might think that someone is trying to harm them, so they might react aggressively or hostilely in self-defense. Some clients experience auditory hallucinations in which they are told to harm other people. Clients suffering from dementia, delirium, head injuries, alcohol or drug intoxication, antisocial and borderline personality disorders, and other conditions can also exhibit aggressive behavior. When compared to nonviolent patients, violent patients typically exhibit a greater degree of symptomatology, worse functioning, and a pronounced lack of insight (Zhu, Li, and Wang, 2016).

Anger outbursts are experienced by some depressed clients. These brief, intense outbursts of rage usually happen when the depressed person feels emotionally imprisoned. Anger attacks don't involve any physical violence' instead, they involve verbal displays of rage or anger. Clients characterize these out-of-character outbursts of rage as inappropriate behavior that is followed by regret. Anger outbursts that some depressed clients experience could be linked to irritability, exaggerating small irritations, and a diminished capacity for coping.

A rare psychiatric diagnosis known as intermittent explosive disorder (IED) is marked by isolated episodes of violent impulses that end in violent crimes or property destruction. The individual exhibits aggressive behavior that is wildly out of proportion to any provocation or aggravating circumstance. As previously mentioned, this diagnosis is only made if the client does not have any other comorbid psychiatric disorders. The individual talks about how an aggressive outburst seemed to relieve a period of tension or arousal. But afterward, the individual feels guilty and ashamed, and there are no indications of hostility in between the incidents (Ramesh, Hassamal, and Moeller, 2017). Between late adolescence and the third decade of life, IED develops. Men with dependent personality traits who have violent outbursts in response to feelings of helplessness or ineffectiveness are frequently the clients of IED.

Acting out is a defensive mechanism used by immature people to deal with emotional conflicts or stressors by acting out rather than thinking things through or feeling them. Acting out, such as using physical or verbal aggression, is the person's way of making themselves feel temporarily less weak or powerless. When kids and teenagers are unable to verbally resolve emotional conflict or manage strong emotions, they frequently "act out". It's critical to take into account both the circumstances and the individual's capacity for managing emotions to comprehend acting-out behaviors. In the US, there are a lot of reports of violence against both people and groups. It is common to characterize the identified suspects or perpetrators as suffering from mental illness or unresolved anger. It's crucial to keep in mind that these reports could come from neighbors or family members who are reporting from their own subjective points of view. Other people occasionally make assumptions about the reasons behind these violent acts. It's not always the case that someone has a mental illness just because they do something that seems hard to understand.

4.3. Etiology

4.3.1. Neurobiologic Theories

A single cause of aggression in humans and animals has not been found despite research on the role of neurotransmitters in the behavior. Reduced serotonin levels may cause aggressive behavior to increase because research indicates that serotonin plays a significant inhibitory role in hostility. The rage episodes that some depressed clients experience may be connected to this finding. Likewise, there is a correlation between an increase in impulsively violent behavior and elevated brain dopamine and norepinephrine activity. According to Victoroff (2017), an individual's capacity to control their aggression may be compromised by anatomical harm to the limbic system, frontal lobes, or temporal lobes of the brain. This can result in an increase in violent conduct.

4.3.2. Psychosocial Theories

It is typical for infants and toddlers to express themselves loudly and intensely during these developmental stages. Toddlers who have their wishes denied frequently react with temper tantrums. A child is supposed to grow up with impulse control—the capacity to postpone gratification—and socially acceptable behavior. The development of these attributes is facilitated by having successful academic careers, positive relationships with parents, teachers, and peers, as well as the capacity for self-reliance. Youngsters who grow up in dysfunctional homes with inadequate parenting, kids who experience mixed results from their actions, and kids from lower socioeconomic backgrounds are more likely to struggle to learn socially acceptable behavior. A person who lacks development may be impetuous, quickly irritated, and more likely to act aggressively.

The connection between interpersonal rejection and aggression can contribute to difficulties in regulating and managing emotions over the long term, including anger and other emotions. Rejection may result in feelings of anger and aggression when it causes emotional distress or challenges self-esteem. Aggressive behavior is often used as a way to regain control, enhance mood, or seek revenge, yet these methods usually do not achieve the desired outcomes (Victoroff, 2017).

To provide care that is culturally competent, the nurse must be aware of cultural norms. Women in the US have historically been prohibited from openly and directly expressing their anger because doing so would be seen as "feminine" and would go against the authority of men. Over the past few decades, there has been a gradual shift in that cultural norm. Some cultures, like Asian and Native American cultures, view expressing anger as impolite or disrespectful, and they will do everything to avoid it. It would be improper in these cultures to try to assist a client in verbally expressing their anger to a higher authority.

When it comes to the diagnosis and treatment of mental illness, ethnic or minority status can be significant. Regardless of race, patients with dark skin may be seen as more dangerous than those with lighter skin, which makes them more likely to require mandatory hospital stays, more frequent use of restraints, higher dosages of medication, and other similar outcomes. Interpersonal violence episodes are disproportionately associated with people of color. But when socioeconomic variables were taken into account, poverty and other socioeconomic factors—rather than race—explained the variation, and race was no longer a significant factor (Victoroff, 2017). To provide immigrants and patients from minority groups with high-quality care, education toward cultural competency is necessary.

The culturally specific syndrome known as Hwa-Byung, or hwabyeong, literally translates as "fire illness" or "angry syndrome," and it's linked to suppressing anger (Lee et al., 2018). It is common in Korea, mostly affecting women, and is characterized by sighing, tenseness, anxiety, depression, and abdominal pain as well as insomnia. Psychiatrists in the West would probably diagnose it as somatization disorder or depression. Two other culture-bound syndromes involve aggression. Bouffée délirante is a condition that has been reported in Haiti and West Africa. It is typified by psychomotor excitement, marked confusion, and abrupt outbursts of agitated and aggressive behavior. These episodes can include brief psychotic episodes-like paranoid ideation and auditory and visual hallucinations. According to Lewis-Fernandez, Kirmayer, Guarrnaccia, and Ruiz (2017), amok is a dissociative episode that is typified by a period of brooding followed by an outburst of violent, aggressive, or homicidal behavior directed towards other people and objects. This behavior is unique to men and is triggered by something perceived as a slight or insult. Similar behavior patterns, first documented in Malaysia, have also been observed in Papua New Guinea, Laos, the Philippines, Polynesia (cafard), Puerto Rico (mal de pelea), and among the Navajo (iich'aa).

4.4. Treatment

When treating aggressive clients, underlying or co-occurring mental diagnoses like bipolar disorder or schizophrenia are frequently treated first. Aggressive behavior can be successfully treated when comorbid disorders are successfully treated. Children with conduct disorders, intellectual disabilities, and aggressive bipolar disorder patients have all found success with lithium treatment. Aggression related to dementia, psychosis, and personality disorders is treated with carbamazepine (Tegretol) and valproate (Depakote). Aggressive clients with dementia, brain injury, intellectual disability, and personality disorders have found success with atypical antipsychotic agents like clozapine (Clozaril), risperidone (Risperdal), and olanzapine (Zyprexa). While benzodiazepines can help older adults with dementia feel less agitated and irritable, they can also cause other aggressive clients to lose their social inhibition, which makes their aggression worse rather than better.

To lessen agitation or aggression as well as psychotic symptoms, haloperidol (Haldol) and lorazepam (Ativan) are frequently combined. Lorazepam, available in 2-mg doses every 45–60 minutes, is most effective in treating patients who are agitated and aggressive but not psychotic. Vicktoroff (2017) found that for aggressive and psychotic clients, atypical antipsychotics are more effective than conventional antipsychotics. Since benztropine (Cogentin) can be used promptly to treat extrapyramidal side effects, using antipsychotic medications requires careful monitoring of their development. In the crisis stage of the aggression cycle, the client and others may need to be temporarily segregated or restrained' this is not a treatment per se, but it is necessary to keep them safe. Utilizing seclusion and restraint is subject to numerous ethical and legal protections.

4.4.1. Application of the Nursing Process

Aggressive episodes can frequently be avoided by properly assessing and intervening with clients who are hostile or angry. Early detection, careful medication administration, and talking to an angry client can frequently stop anger from turning into physical aggression.

4.4.1.1. Assessment

A nurse working in a psychiatric setting or unit should be aware of the variables that affect aggression. Strong mental leadership, defined staff responsibilities, and well-planned and sufficient events, like activities and staff-client interaction, are all associated with a lower incidence of aggressive behavior on psychiatric units. On the other hand, clients frequently experience frustration and boredom and become more aggressive when meetings, groups, and staff-client interactions are unpredictable. More likely to incite aggression than a lack of physical space is a lack of psychological space, such as not being able to enjoy privacy or get enough sleep.

The nurse must carefully evaluate each client in addition to the unit environment. One of the best indicators of future aggression is a violent or aggressive past. Helping a client with a history of aggression control or non-aggressively manage their anger requires understanding how the client deals with anger and what they feel is beneficial. Anger, frustration, and the feeling that no one is paying attention to them can make clients act more hostilely or aggressively. A client is more likely to act aggressively if they have a history of violence in the past as well as a history of personal victimization and/or substance abuse. The nurse may be able to identify impending aggressive behavior with the aid of specific cues. Aggressive behavior is more common in clients who think their hallucinations are all-powerful, evil, and irresistible. These indicators consist of the following: the client's words' variations in voice quality (volume, pitch, and speed)' shifts in the client's expression' and shifts in the client's actions.

In order to implement appropriate interventions, the nurse should evaluate the client's behavior to ascertain which phase of the aggression cycle the client is currently in. Table 4.1 lists the indications, symptoms, and behaviors associated with each of the five phases of aggression. Client assessments must be conducted safely away from the client. To ensure that the client doesn't feel confined or in danger, the nurse can approach them while keeping a safe distance. Two staff members approaching the client might be a good idea in order to protect worker safety and demonstrate teamwork.

Table 4.1. *Five-Phase Aggression Cycle*

Phase	Definition	Signs, Symptoms, and Behaviors
Triggering	An event or circumstances in the environment initiates the client's response, which is often anger or hostility.	Restlessness, anxiety, irritability, pacing, muscle tension, rapid breathing, perspiration, loud voice, anger
Escalation	The client's responses represent escalating behaviors that indicate movement toward a loss of control.	Pale or flushed face, yelling, swearing, agitation, threatening, demanding, clenched fists, threatening gestures, hostility, loss of ability to solve the problem or think clearly
Crisis	During an emotional and physical crisis, the client loses control.	Loss of emotional and physical control, throwing objects, kicking, hitting, spitting, biting, scratching, shrieking, screaming, inability to communicate clearly
Recovery	The client regains physical and emotional control.	Lowering of voice; decreased muscle tension; clearer, more rational communication; physical relaxation
Postcrisis	The client attempts reconciliation with others and returns to the level of functioning before the aggressive incident and its antecedents.	Remorse; apologies; crying; quiet, withdrawn behavior

Source: Adapted from Keltner, N. L., Bostrom, C. E., & McGinness, T. (2010). Psychiatric nursing (6th ed.). St. Louis, MO: Mosby.

4.4.1.2. Data Analysis

Nursing diagnoses commonly used when working with aggressive clients include:

- Risk for other-directed violence;
- Ineffective coping.

If the client is intoxicated, depressed, or psychotic, additional nursing diagnoses may be indicated.

Outcome Identification

Expected outcomes for aggressive clients may include the following:

- The client will not harm or threaten others.
- The client will refrain from behaviors that are intimidating or frightening to others.
- The client will describe his or her feelings and concerns without aggression.
- The client will comply with treatment.

4.4.2. Intervention

Even seasoned nurses may find verbally abusive or hostile behavior frightening or intimidating. Additionally dangerous to other clients, staff members, and outside guests are clients who display these behaviors. The most common reaction to hostile individuals in social settings is to avoid them as much as possible. However, the best way to stop the hostile behavior from turning into physical aggression in a psychiatric setting is to have a conversation with the person. Early in the cycle of aggression is when interventions are most effective and least restrictive. This section includes targeted interventions for each stage of the aggression cycle as well as milieu management strategies that are beneficial to all clients in any setting.

4.4.2.1. Managing the Environment

When attempting to lessen or completely eradicate aggressive behavior, it is critical to take into account the surroundings of each client. When clients are at ease, they can discuss events or problems informally or in groups through planned activities like card games, movies, and viewing and discussion sessions. Activities reduce boredom and involve clients in the therapeutic process. Setting up one-on-one meetings with patients shows that the nurse genuinely cares about them and is prepared to hear their worries, ideas, and emotions. The client feels more secure when they know what to expect. The nurse can provide a problem-solving or conflict-resolution opportunity if clients conflict with one another. Important skills that clients can practice include negotiating a solution, using assertive communication statements, and appropriately expressing anger. When the client returns to the community, these skills will be helpful. The safety and security of other clients, who might require protection from the invasive or threatening demeanor of a psychotic, hyperactive, or inebriated client, must be taken into consideration by the nurse when dealing with such clients. It's beneficial to discuss feelings with other clients, and it's crucial to keep a close eye on the client who may become aggressive.

4.4.2.2. Managing Aggressive Behavior

To deescalate the client's emotions and behavior during the triggering phase, the nurse should approach the client in a calm, nonthreatening manner. It's critical to show empathy for the client's annoyance or frustration. The nurse can support the patient in verbally expressing their anger, implying that the patient still has control and can continue to do so. Using succinct, straightforward sentences is beneficial. The client should be given space to express themselves, according to the nurse. To reduce stimulation, the nurse may advise the client to move to a quiet area or ask for help moving other clients. If prescribed, medications (PRN or as needed) ought to be made available. The nurse can assist the patient in using relaxation techniques and exploring conflict resolution options as the patient's anger fades. Walking is one type of physical activity that can aid in the client's relaxation and calmness.

If these methods prove ineffective and the client enters the escalation phase—a phase in which the client gradually loses control—the nurse has to step in and take charge of the circumstance. The client should receive instructions from the nurse in a firm, calm voice. It is advisable to instruct the client to take a moment to relax in a quiet place or in their own room. The nurse should explain to the client that she is there to help them regain control and that aggressive behavior is not acceptable. The nurse should reoffer the medications if the client turns them down during the triggering phase. The nurse should ask other staff members for help if the client's behavior doesn't improve and they won't follow instructions to go to a quiet place. Four to six staff members should initially stay available and near the client, but not as close as the primary nurse who is conversing with them. This tactic, sometimes referred to as a "show of force," tells the client that if they are unable to take control of the situation, the staff will. Occasionally, the client is persuaded to accept medication and take the required break to regain control by the presence of additional staff members. For the protection of the client, staff, and other clients, the staff must take command of the situation when the client exhibits physical aggression (crisis phase). Only personnel who have received such training should be involved in the physical restraint of a client who is aggressive. Psychiatric facilities provide training and practice in safe techniques for managing behavioral emergencies. The facility's protocols and standards for restraint and seclusion should be the basis for the nurse's decision to employ either. When the nurse decides to use seclusion or restraint, they should get a doctor's order as soon as possible.

A client who is aggressive needs to be safely restrained by four to six trained staff members. Young clients, teenagers, and female clients can exhibit aggression on par with that of adult male clients. The client is told that the staff is taking charge to ensure safety and prevent harm because their behavior is out of control. One staff member shields the client's head, four staff members take turns taking a limb, and one staff member assists in controlling the client's torso when necessary. After being carried to a seclusion room or transported in a gurney, the client is restrained on all limbs and secured to the bed frame. In this kind of emergency, the nurse may get an order for intramuscular (IM) medication if PRN medication hasn't been taken earlier. As was previously mentioned, the nurse closely examines the patient while they are being restrained or in seclusion and records their activities. The client is encouraged to discuss the circumstances or triggers that preceded the aggressive behavior as soon as they regain control (the recovery phase). The nurse should assist the patient in unwinding, falling asleep, and regaining composure. Asking the client or staff what they can do the next time to prevent an aggressive episode will help them explore alternatives to aggressive behavior. Along with checking for staff injuries, the nurse should complete all necessary paperwork, including flow sheets and incident reports. Every staff member participates in a debriefing to talk about the aggressive incident, how it was handled, what went well or could have been improved, and how the situation could have been defused more skillfully. Encouraging other clients to discuss their feelings about the incident is also crucial. It is not advisable to discuss the aggressive client in detail with other clients, though. When the client satisfies the behavioral criteria, they are taken out of seclusion or restraint during the post-crisis phase. Instead of lecturing or berating the client for the aggressive behavior, the nurse ought to have a cool, collected conversation about it. In the hopes that the client will be able to deal with emotions or situations in the future without becoming aggressive, feedback for regaining control can be given. As soon as the client can participate, he or she should be reintegrated into the environment and its activities.

4.4.3. Evaluation

When a client's anger can be subsided early on, care is most effective' however, in certain cases, physical aggression requires seclusion or restraint. The intention is to teach clients who are irate, hostile, and possibly aggressive how to verbally and safely express their feelings without endangering others or causing property damage.

4.5. Workplace Hostility

A sentinel event alert was released by The Joint Commission on Accreditation of Healthcare Organizations (JCAHO) in July 2008, addressing "intimidating and disruptive behaviors" that compromise a safety culture and result in errors, lower patient satisfaction, avoidable negative outcomes, higher Healthcare costs, and the departure of qualified staff. These undesirable behaviors include both overt ones, like verbal or physical abuse and threats, and passive ones, like refusing to do chores that are assigned to you or acting in an uncooperative manner. Disruptive and intimidating behaviors, which can include impatience, condescending or intimidating language or voice tone/volume, and reluctance to answer questions, return calls, or answer pages, are frequently displayed by Healthcare providers in positions of power.

In 2016, the JCAHO expanded this initiative to include workplace bullying, which is also referred to as lateral or horizontal violence. Bullying is characterized as violent behavior that interferes with the performance of tasks by using threats, intimidation, or humiliation, as well as verbal abuse. Because of this issue, the JCAHO implemented new leadership standards in January 2009. A code of conduct outlining acceptable, disruptive, and inappropriate behaviors is now required for any accredited healthcare organization. Furthermore, JCAHO (2016) states that leaders in these organizations need to develop and put into place a procedure for handling disruptive and improper behavior.

Several action steps have been suggested to accomplish this new standard of behavior, including:

- A code of conduct outlines acceptable and inappropriate/ unacceptable behavior;
- A process for managers to handle disruptive or unacceptable behavior;
- Education of all team members on expected professional behavior;
- Zero tolerance for unacceptable behaviors, meaning all persons are held accountable.

4.6. Community-Based Care

The key to controlling aggression for many clients who exhibit aggressive behavior is to effectively manage the co-occurring psychiatric disorder. Stability is aided by the client's participation in community support programs, adherence to medication regimen, and regular follow-up appointments. There are anger management groups available to assist clients in learning problem-solving and conflict-resolution strategies as well as in expressing their emotions. Research on assaults by patients on community staff is becoming more and more significant as more patients are being discharged from inpatient or acute care settings quickly. The community saw an increase in client assaults due in part to stressful living conditions, easier access to drugs and alcohol, the availability of deadly weapons, and medication noncompliance. Acute psychosis, overstimulating, and denial of services were frequently the causes of assault episodes.

Flannery (2012) investigated verbal threats, nonverbal intimidation, and physical or sexual assaults committed by residents of community homes. Male clients with schizophrenia who were older and younger clients with personality disorders were more likely to be aggressive. To assist staff victims in overcoming the psychological fallout from assaults by clients in community-based residential programs, the Assaulted Staff Action Program (ASAP) was founded in Massachusetts. Additionally, ASAP collaborates with staff to identify more effective ways to manage aggressive client situations and ways to enhance community safety. This program can now be purchased by any interested staff member and implemented across the United States.

4.7. Abuse and Violence

Since violent behavior affects more than 2 million people annually in the US, it has been designated as a national health priority and a target for intervention. The most concerning figures concern domestic violence and abuse, which include misusing and mistreating someone else. Based on statistical data, the majority of abuse cases involve a victim's acquaintance. Abuse victims can include children, elderly parents, spouses or partners, and people of all ages.

4.7.1. Clinical Picture of Abuse and Violence

In addition to psychological injuries that can cause a wide range of reactions, victims of abuse or violence can also suffer physical injuries that require medical attention. A few clients appear restless and obviously disturbed, while others are distant and reclusive, seemingly unaware of their environment. Because victims are afraid of their abusers, domestic violence frequently goes unreported for months or even years. Often, victims bottle up their rage and bitterness and keep it to themselves. This is especially true when there has been sexual abuse of children.

Abuse survivors frequently suffer in silence and harbor resentment and guilt. In particular, children start to feel that they are to blame for the abuse, that they somehow deserved it or provoked it. They have a higher probability of missing school, a lower likelihood of going to college, and problems that persist from adolescence into adulthood. As adults, they typically experience shame or guilt for failing to intervene to stop the abuse. Survivors experience dehumanization, humiliation, and degradation. They think they are unlovable and have very low self-esteem. They think they are polluted, ruined, or unaccepted by others. Suicidal thoughts and actions, depression, and marital and sexual problems are prevalent.

Abuse survivors and victims may struggle in their relationships with other people. They have a hard time trusting people, especially those in positions of authority. Their emotional responses are likely to be erratic, intense, and viewed as unpredictable in relationships. Intimate partnerships have the potential to elicit strong emotional reactions like terror, panic, anxiety, and fear. Even when abuse survivors want a close relationship, they could view a real relationship as obtrusive and dangerous. The need of the abused client to feel safe, secure, and in control of his or her body should be especially acknowledged by nurses. When approaching a client for any reason, they should be cautious to respect their personal space, gauge their degree of anxiety, and get their consent before touching them. Nursing professionals should exercise caution when working with clients in mental health settings, as they may not always be aware of a history of abuse.

4.7.2. Characteristics of Violent Families

Family violence includes elder abuse, marital rape, physical, emotional, and sexual abuse of children, as well as battering spouses. Frequently, family members put up with violent and abusive behavior from relatives that they would never put up with from outsiders. The home, which is typically a place of love and safety for victims of abuse, may actually be the most dangerous place for them.

4.7.2.1. Social Isolation

Social isolation is one trait of violent families. These families tend to be private, not to let people into their homes or share information with others. Abusers frequently threaten victims with even more harm if they divulge the information. Children may be told that if anyone outside the family finds out about the abuse, a parent, sibling, or pet will perish. Then, out of fear, kids keep the secret, keeping others from "interfering with private family business."

4.7.2.2. Abuse of Power and Control

The victim—a child, a spouse, or an elderly parent—is nearly always in a position of power and control over the abusive family member. In addition to using physical force, the abuser also controls society and the economy. Frequently, he or she is the only family member who engages in decision-making, financial transactions, or social interactions outside the home. The abuser frequently uses threats and emotional blackmail to denigrate and place the blame on the victim. Violence typically increases when the abuser detects any hint of independence or disobedience from the victim, whether it be imagined or real. Intimate partner violence (IPV) is a contributing factor to 14% of all fatalities. 30% were men and 70% were women among these deaths (Centers for Disease Control and Prevention [CDC], 2017). Just 16% of female homicide victims in the US were killed by a stranger' half of all female homicide victims were killed by a romantic partner, either current or past.

4.7.2.3. Alcohol and Other Drug Abuse

Family violence and substance abuse, particularly alcoholism, have been linked. This result does not suggest a cause-and-effect connection. It is more likely for an abusive person to use alcohol or other drugs than alcohol makes them abusive. Most victims of intimate partner violence state that alcohol played a role in the violent incident. Women who had abusive relationships with alcohol had a higher risk of being abused by their partners than other women. Many researchers think that alcohol may lower inhibitions and increase the intensity or frequency of violent behavior, even though it may not be the cause of the abuse (Stromberg, 2017). Drinking has also been linked to date or acquaintance rape. Both the attacker and the victim frequently admitted to consuming alcohol before the attack. Additionally, it's becoming more common to subdue possible victims with the illegal drug flunitrazepam (Rohypnol) or other "date rape drugs."

4.7.2.4. Intergenerational Transmission Process

The process of intergenerational transmission demonstrates how social learning and role modeling help to sustain violent patterns from one generation to the next (Bartlett, Kotake, Fauth, and Easterbrooks, 2017). Family violence may be a taught pattern of behavior, according to intergenerational transmission. Children who see violence between their parents, for instance, come to understand that violence is a necessary component of close relationships and a means of resolving conflict. According to statistics, one-third of abusive men are probably from violent homes where they either experienced abuse firsthand or witnessed abuse. Women who experience domestic violence as children are 50% more likely to anticipate or put up with violence in their own relationships. Nonetheless, not every individual who witnesses domestic abuse grows up to be violent or abusive. For this reason, the persistence of violent behavior cannot be explained by a single factor. All racial and ethnic groups, age groups, national origins, sexual orientations, religious beliefs, and socioeconomic statuses are affected by domestic abuse' however, immigrant women are a particularly vulnerable group. Battered immigrant women face legal, social, and economic problems different from the U.S. citizens who are battered and from people of other cultural, racial, and ethnic origins who are not battered.

- The battered woman may come from a culture that accepts domestic violence.
- She may believe she has less access to legal and social services than do U.S. citizens.
- If she is not a citizen, she may be forced to leave the United States if she seeks legal sanctions against her abuser or attempts to leave him or her.
- She is isolated by cultural dynamics that do not permit her to leave her abuser' economically, she may be unable to gather the resources to leave, work, or go to school.
- Language barriers may interfere with her ability to call 911' learn about her rights or legal options' and obtain shelter, financial assistance, or food.

To address these additional concerns, the nurse may need to get the help of a trusted interpreter, refer the woman to legal services, and help her get in touch with the Department of Immigration.

4.8. Intimate Partner Violence

The abuse or mistreatment of one person by another in the setting of a close, emotionally connected relationship is known as intimate partner violence. Relationships can be spousal, partner-to-partner, boyfriend-girlfriend, or even strained. The abuse may be physical, sexual, emotional, psychological, or—as is frequently the case—a combination of these. Name-calling, belittling, screaming, yelling, destroying property, threatening, and more subtle forms, like ignoring or refusing to speak to the victim, are examples of psychological abuse, also known as emotional abuse. Physical abuse can result in broken limbs and ribs, internal bleeding, brain damage, and even homicide. It can also involve pushing, shoving, and severe battering and choking. Attacks that occur during sexual relations, such as rape, slapping and hitting, hair pulling, and biting of the nipples, are considered sexual abuse.

In the US, one in seven men and one in four women say they have at some point in their lives suffered severe physical abuse at the hands of an intimate partner. According to the CDC (2017), one in six women and one in fourteen men have been sexually abused by an intimate partner. Violence against pregnant women rises during their pregnancies. Negative outcomes, including miscarriage and stillbirth, as well as additional physical and psychological issues for the woman, are associated with battering during pregnancy. The partner's jealousy, possessiveness, insecurity, and decreased physical and emotional availability of the expectant mother are frequently the causes of the rise in violence (Stromberg, 2017).

The statistical frequency of domestic violence in same-sex relationships is equal to that of heterosexual relationships. Even though same-sex battering is just as common as heterosexual battering, its victims are not as protected. Victims who are same-sex are not included in the definition of domestic violence in seven states. Although the Supreme Court struck down sodomy (anal intercourse) laws in 2003, twelve states still have sodomy laws in place that criminalize the practice. The fear of disclosing the partner's homosexuality to friends, family, employers, or the public is an extra tool in the same-sex batterer's arsenal.

4.8.1. Clinical Picture

This section uses the example of a husband abusing his wife because that is a common occurrence. Nonetheless, same-sex relationships, unmarried couples, and wives who mistreat their husbands all exhibit similar tendencies. An abusive spouse frequently feels that his wife is his property and will only get more violent and abusive if she exhibits any signs of independence, like getting a job or making threats to leave. The abuser usually has poor social and problem-solving abilities, low self-esteem, and intense feelings of inadequacy. He is needy, irrationally jealous, possessive, and emotionally immature. He might even beat both his children and his wife out of jealousy over her attention to their own children. The abuser frequently feels a sense of power and control by physically abusing the family—a feeling he rarely gets outside the house. As a result, engaging in violent behavior frequently pays off and raises his self-esteem.

The most prevalent characteristic among abused wives who continue to live with their husbands is dependency. Women frequently give financial and emotional dependence as explanations for why it is so difficult for them to leave abusive relationships. No matter how gifted or talented the victim is, she believes she cannot survive without her spouse. She also frequently experiences low self-esteem and measures her personal success by her capacity to stick with her spouse and "make it work". Some women internalize criticism and think they are the ones who are at fault. Women also worry that if they attempt to flee, their abusers will murder them. This fear is understandable considering that national statistics indicate that women who leave abusive relationships face a significantly higher risk of murder than those who remain.

4.8.2. Cycle of Abuse and Violence

Women frequently cite the cycle of violence or abuse as another reason why they find it difficult to leave abusive relationships. There is a typical pattern here: after the initial violent or abusive episode, there is typically a period during which the abuser apologizes, expresses regret, and vows that it won't happen again. He declares his love for his spouse and occasionally indulges in amorous actions, such as purchasing flowers and gifts. The honeymoon period refers to this phase of regret or repentance. Naturally, the woman hopes the violence was an isolated incident and wants to believe her husband. The honeymoon phase ends, and the tension-building phase starts' there might be fights, stony silence, or husband complaints. The abuser feels regret and remorse once more and promises to change after the tension is released with another violent episode. This vicious cycle keeps happening again. The victim maintains the hope that the violence will end each time.

The woman may think that her husband has changed and their relationship has improved during the first few weeks or even months of their marriage. But as time passes, the frequency of violent episodes increases, the feeling of regret completely vanishes, and the degree of violence and damage increases. Violence eventually becomes the norm, occurring multiple times a week or even every day. Although it is the most prevalent pattern of IPV, the cycle of violence is not applicable in all circumstances. Many survivors only mention one or two aspects of the pattern. For instance, there might only be sporadic violent outbursts and no noticeable honeymoon phase or rising tension afterwards.

4.8.3. Assessment

Nurses must assist in identifying abused women in a variety of settings because the majority of these women do not seek out direct assistance for the issue. Nurses working in pediatricians' offices, emergency rooms, or clinics may come across women who have been abused. It's possible that some victims are pregnant or seeking care for other health issues unrelated to the abuse. The Department of Health and Human Services has made it a high priority to identify abused women who require assistance. It is not expected of the generalist nurse to handle this challenging issue by themselves. Nonetheless, he or she can provide recommendations and put in touch with suitable medical specialists who have experience treating abused women. Above all, the nurse can provide the victim with support and care during the visit. The strategies for assisting victims of partner violence are compiled in Table 4.2.

Table 4.2. *Dos and Don'ts of Working with Victims of Partner Abuse*

Don'ts	Dos
Don't tell the victim what to do.	Do believe the victim.
Don't express disgust, disbelief, or anger.	Do ensure and maintain the client's confidentiality.
Don't disclose client communications without the client's consent.	Do listen, affirm, and say, "I am sorry you have been hurt."
Don't preach, moralize, or imply that you doubt the client.	Do express, "I'm concerned for your safety."
Don't minimize the impact of violence.	Do tell the victim, "You have a right to be safe and respected."
Don't express outrage with the perpetrator.	Do say, "The abuse is not your fault."
Don't imply that the client is responsible for the abuse.	Do recommend a support group or individual counseling.
Don't recommend couples' counseling.	Do identify community resources, and encourage the client to develop a safety plan.
Don't direct the client to leave the relationship.	Do offer to help the client contact a shelter, the police, or other resources.
Don't take charge and do everything for the client.	Do accept and respect the victim's decision.
	Do encourage development of a safety plan.

Source: Sheila L. Videbeck, Psychiatric-Mental Health Nursing, ISBN-10: 1-975116-37-2.

It is imperative to find out if people feel safe in their relationships or at home. The nurse will be stereotyping and might overlook someone who truly needs assistance if they only ask those who are thought to be "likely victims". As part of any health history or intake interview, women are frequently questioned about safety concerns by hospitals, clinics, and physician offices. Nursing professionals need to be adept at posing pertinent questions regarding abuse because this is a delicate and sensitive subject, and many women who have been abused are embarrassed or afraid to acknowledge the issue.

4.8.4. Treatment and Intervention

The United States has laws requiring police to make arrests for at least some domestic violence crimes in more than half of the states. All states permit police to make arrests in cases of domestic violence. The abuser may occasionally be permitted to stay at home after police are called, provided they have spoken with them and have calmed down. When an arrest is made, the abuser may only be detained for a few hours or even overnight. Women have a right to be afraid of reporting abuse to the police because the abuser frequently retaliates after being freed. Arresting the batterer may decrease immediate violence but may increase long-term violence, according to studies.

A restraining order, also known as a protection order, can be obtained by a woman from her county of residence, which forbids the abuser from making contact or approaching her. However, a restraining order offers very little defense. Before the authorities can step in, the abuser may choose to disobey the order and murder or seriously hurt the victim. A few states have passed legislation requiring the removal of firearms from individuals listed on protection orders. However, some states have unclear procedures for notifying someone of the firearm ban or retrieving the firearm (Fleury-Steiner, Miller, and Carcirieri, 2017).

When combined with other interventions like advocacy counseling, shelter, or consultations with medical professionals, civil orders of protection have a greater impact on averting future acts of violence. Successful women who leave abusive relationships are more likely to do so if both their legal and psychological needs are met at the same time.

Issues might persist even after a beaten person has "ended" the relationship. It's problematic when someone tries to force unwelcome communication or contact on someone else—stalking. Apart from abusive partners who stalk their partners when the breakup is not acceptable, there are also "would-be lovers" who pursue relationships that never happened, doctors who are stalked by patients, and famous people who are stalked by "fans". One in six women and one in 19 men will experience stalking at some point in their lives. 12% to 13% of college students said they had experienced stalking (Violence Prevention and Action Center/John Carroll University, 2018). Cyberstalking includes following, monitoring, or breaking into someone else's social media accounts' adopting a false identity to re-enter the person's life' and using a cell phone to track the victim's whereabouts. All of these have increased in frequency in recent years, and identifying the stalker has grown more challenging (Lund and Ross, 2017).

When battered women and their children decide to leave the abusive relationship, battered women's shelters can offer them food and temporary housing. But in many cities, shelters are overcrowded, and the temporary relief they offer is accompanied by waiting lists in some cases. The woman quitting an abusive relationship can be unsupported financially and have little experience or training in her line of work. She frequently has dependent kids. Overcoming these obstacles is challenging, and there is little support from the public or private sectors. Women who are abused may sustain numerous physical wounds, but there are also psychological and emotional fallout. Women who have experienced abuse can begin to heal from their trauma and form new, healthier relationships with the support of support and self-help groups, group therapy, or individual psychotherapy or counseling.

4.9. Child Abuse

The intentional harming of a child is the general definition of child abuse or maltreatment. It can involve sexual assault or intrusion, overt torture or maiming, physical abuse or injuries, neglect or a failure to stop harm, a lack of proper physical or emotional care or supervision, and abandonment. Every state in the union defines child abuse, specifies how reports must be made and sets up mechanisms for providing services. State laws differ greatly from one another even though they share many similarities. Because of this, it is challenging to find precise information about the kind, prevalence, and intensity of child abuse across the nation. In the US, 702,000 victims were found in 2014 out of over 6.6 million reports. Seventy-five% of these cases involved neglect, followed by physical abuse (17%), sexual abuse (8), and emotional/psychological maltreatment (6%). An estimated 1,580 children under the age of three died as a result of maltreatment (Bernet and Freeman, 2017). Girls are frequently abused by fathers, stepfathers, uncles, elder siblings, and the child's mother's live-in partner. Mother-son incest is far less common than father-daughter incest, which accounts for about 75% of reported cases. An estimated 15 million American women experienced sexual abuse during their childhood, with one-third of victims having been molested before the age of nine. Since many cases of sexual abuse go unreported out of embarrassment and shame, accurate statistics are hard to come by. In other instances, women wait until they are adults to confess to being sexually abused. Adults who experienced sexual abuse as children are more likely to experience depression, attempt suicide, have marital issues, marry an alcoholic, smoke, abuse alcohol, experience chronic pain, and have medically unexplained symptoms (Steine et al., 2017).

4.9.1. Types of Child Abuse

Abuse of children physically usually stems from excessively harsh physical discipline or unwarranted punishment, like hitting a baby for cries or soiled diapers. Children can be intentionally and purposefully harmed by being burned, bit, cut, poked, having limbs twisted, or being scalded with hot water. The victim frequently possesses evidence of past injuries (such as scars, untreated fractures, or numerous bruises of varying ages) that is insufficiently explained by the victim's parents or caregivers' medical histories.

- When an adult performs sexual acts on a child under the age of eighteen, it is considered sexual abuse. Examples include acts of molestation such as rubbing, fondling, or exposing an adult's genitalia, as well as incest, rape, and sodomy that are carried out either directly by the perpetrator or with the aid of an object. Sexual abuse can take the form of one event or several over an extended period of time. A second form of sexual abuse entails coercing minors to perform obscene acts and using them as props in pornography that is made, promoted, or sold.
- The deliberate or careless withholding of a child's physical, emotional, or educational needs is known as neglect. The most common form of maltreatment is child abuse by neglect, which includes the following: abandonment' insufficient supervision' reckless disregard for the child's safety' punitive, exploitative, or abusive emotional treatment' spousal abuse in the child's presence' permission to be truant' or failure to enroll the child in school.
- Emotional abuse, also known as psychological abuse, encompasses various forms of maltreatment such as name-calling, blaming, screaming, and using sarcasm' ongoing family strife marked by shouting, fighting, and chaos' and emotional deprivation or withholding of normal experiences that foster acceptance, love, security, and self-worth. Other forms of abuse (such as physical abuse) frequently coexist with emotional abuse

(either physical or sexual). This also includes being exposed to parental drug or alcohol abuse, prostitution, or alcoholism, as well as the neglect that follows.

4.9.2. Clinical Picture

Abusing parents frequently lack basic parenting abilities and knowledge. They might not know what their kids need, or they might not know what to do with their emotions or money, and that makes them angry or frustrated. While poverty and illiteracy are factors in child abuse and neglect, they do not fully account for the phenomenon. Families that appear to have it all—well-educated parents who have successful careers, a stable income—are frequently the victims of abuse and violence.

Abusing parents are frequently emotionally immature, needy, and unable to provide for their own needs, let alone a child's. Similar to domestic abuse, child abuse often occurs because the abuser sees the victim's children as their own. The abuser doesn't think of the kids as sentient beings with feelings and rights. Sometimes a parent feels that having children is necessary to make up for the flawed and unsatisfactory upbringing they experienced as a child' they want to experience the love that exists between a child and parent, which they were unable to experience as a child. However, these irrational expectations are typically dashed by the reality of the enormous emotional, physical, and financial demands that come with raising children. When the parent's irrational expectations are not satisfied, he or she frequently turns back to the strategies employed by their own parents. The cycle of family violence is sustained by adults' propensity to raise their offspring in the same manner in which they were raised. Adults who experienced abuse as kids often mistreat their own kids.

4.9.3. Assessment

The first steps in dealing with any kind of family violence are detection and precise identification. Burns and scalds can be easily recognized by their distinctive shapes, like cigarette marks, or by the distribution of a "stocking and glove," which denotes scalding. When a baby has a severe skull fracture, the parent may say that the child "rolled off the couch," even though the injury is too severe or the child is too young to be able to do so. Bruises can resemble well-known and identifiable shapes, like belt buckles or teeth marks.

Warning Signs of Abused/Neglected Children:

- Serious injuries such as fractures, burns, or lacerations with no reported history of trauma;
- Delay in seeking treatment for a significant injury;
- Child or parent giving a history inconsistent with the severity of the injury, such as a baby with contrecoup injuries to the brain (shaken baby syndrome) that the parents claim happened when the infant rolled off the sofa;
- Inconsistencies or changes in the child's history during the evaluation by either the child or the adult;
- Unusual injuries for the child's age and level of development, such as a fractured femur in a 2-month-old or a dislocated shoulder in a 2- 2-year-old;
- High incidence of urinary tract infections' bruised, red, or swollen genitalia' tears or bruising of rectum or vagina;
- Evidence of old injuries not reported, such as scars, fractures

not treated, and multiple bruises that parent/caregiver cannot explain adequately.

Urinary tract infections, tears in the rectum or vagina, swollen, red, or bruised genitalia, and bruising are all possible symptoms of sexual abuse of children. These kids react emotionally in very different ways. These kids frequently act or speak in ways that suggest they have a deeper understanding of sexual issues than is reasonable given their age. Sometimes they are scared and nervous, and they might completely reject adult attention or cling to an adult. Recognizing when a child behaves differently than what is typical for their age and developmental stage is crucial. Abuse may be indicated by seemingly inexplicable behavior, such as refusing to eat or acting aggressively toward peers.

The nurse is not required to determine for sure whether abuse has taken place. Nurses must report any suspicions of child abuse while accurately and completely documenting the results of their assessments. There are laws in all 50 states that compel nurses to report suspected abuse' these laws are also known as mandatory reporting laws. The nurse working alone or in conjunction with other members of the health team (e.g., doctors, or social workers) may notify the relevant local government authorities about suspicions of abuse. In certain states, the Department of Health, Children and Family Services, or Child Protective Services have this authority. You can look up the number to call in the local phone book. If desired, the reporting party may maintain their anonymity. Employees in these organizations have specialized training in abuse investigation. It is important to ask questions in a way that doesn't exacerbate the child's trauma or obstruct any potential legal action. There may be more harm than good if the generalist nurse investigates the child.

4.9.4. Treatment and Intervention

Making sure the child is safe and healthy comes first in the treatment of abuse or neglect of children. Removing the child from the home may be necessary for this, which can also be traumatizing. A comprehensive psychiatric evaluation is also recommended due to the elevated likelihood of psychological issues. The therapist-child relationship must be one of trust in order to support the child in healing from the trauma of abuse. Therapy may be necessary for a considerable amount of time, depending on the child's reaction and the extent and duration of the abuse.

In most cases, the child will require long-term care from specialists in multiple fields, including psychology, social work, and psychiatry. For a very young child, play therapy may be the most effective means of communication. Instead of talking about what has happened or how they are feeling, the child uses puppets or dolls to draw or act out scenarios. Depending on whether the parents can demonstrate that they will benefit from treatment, social service agencies are involved in deciding whether it is feasible to return the child to the parental home. If the family can be reunited, family therapy might be recommended. Treatment for mental illness or drug addiction may be necessary for parents. Foster care services, whether short- or long-term, may be necessary if it seems unlikely that the child will return home.

4.10. Elder Abuse

The mistreatment of elderly people by family members or other caregivers is known as elder abuse. It can involve neglect, self-neglect, financial exploitation, physical and sexual abuse, psychological abuse, and denial of appropriate medical care. One in ten adults over 65 are thought to be mistreated, neglected, abused, or exploited by their careers, although few of these incidents are ever reported. The abusers most likely have psychological or legal issues in addition to living with the victim and/or being related to the victim. The majority of elder abuse victims are 75 years of age or older, with 60%–65% of them being female. Elder abuse is more common in cases where the victim has several ongoing physical and mental health issues as well as when they are dependent on others for basic daily needs like food and medical attention (Greenwood, Haroun, and Naimark, 2017).

When someone abuses an elderly person, it's usually because they are a caregiver or the elderly are dependent on them. Elder abuse typically happens when one elderly spouse looks after another. Spousal abuse of this kind typically occurs over a long period of time after a handicap prevents the victimized spouse from taking care of themselves. It is twice as likely to be a son as a daughter when the abuser is an adult child. Elder abuse may worsen in cases of mental illness or substance misuse. Bullying has also been reported amongst residents in senior living facilities. Social and verbal bullying is most prevalent. According to Andresen and Buchanan (2017), there were physical and cognitive impairments reported in both the offenders and the victims. Programs for education on safe responses to resident bullying are recommended.

Even when they can report abuse, elders are frequently reluctant to do so because the abuse typically involves family members that the elder wants to keep safe. Victims frequently worry about being committed to an institution and losing their support system. There are no national estimates available regarding elder abuse in institutions. Nonetheless, ombudsmen are permitted to visit nursing homes to verify the care of the elderly following a 1978 federal mandate. Although not all allegations of elder abuse in institutions are verified, these ombudsmen report that such complaints are frequent.

4.10.1. Clinical Picture

The victim might be deprived of food, drink, or medication' they might have fractures or bruises' they might not have the necessary eyeglasses or hearing aids' they might be restrained in a chair or bed. While the elderly victim cannot afford food or medication, the abuser may use the victim's financial resources for personal gain. Elder abusers may refuse to treat an elderly person who is ill, either acutely or chronically. The inability of the elderly person to take care of oneself is known as self-neglect.

4.10.2. Assessment

Elder abuse must be identified by carefully evaluating elderly people and the relationships that surround their care. It can be challenging to distinguish between elder abuse and the deterioration brought on by a chronic illness. Many possible abuse indicators need to be carefully considered and further assessed. However, these symptoms don't always indicate abuse or neglect on their own. Possible Indicators of Elder Abuse includes:

4.10.2.1. Physical Abuse Indicators

- Frequent, unexplained injuries accompanied by a habit of seeking medical assistance from various locations;
- Reluctance to seek medical treatment for injuries or denial of their existence;
- Disorientation or grogginess indicating misuse of medications;
- Fear or edginess in the presence of a family member or caregiver.

4.10.2.2. Psychosocial Abuse Indicators

- Change in the elder's general mood or usual behavior;
- Isolated from previous friends or family;
- Sudden lack of contact with other people outside the elder's home;
- Helplessness;
- Hesitance to talk openly;
- Anger or agitation;
- Withdrawal or depression.

4.10.2.3. Material Abuse Indicators

- Unpaid bills;
- The standard of living below the elder's means;
- Sudden sale or disposal of the elder's property/possessions;
- Unusual or inappropriate activity in bank accounts;
- Signatures on checks that differ from the elder's;
- Recent changes in will or power of attorney when the elder is not capable of making those decisions;
- Missing valuable belongings that are not just misplaced;
- Lack of television, clothes, or personal items that are easily affordable;
- Unusual concern by the caregiver over the expense of the elder's treatment when it is not the caregiver's money being spent.

4.10.2.4. Neglect Indicators

- Poor personal hygiene;
- Lack of needed medications or therapies;
- Dirt, fecal or urine smell, or other health hazards in the elder's living environment;
- Rashes, sores, or lice on the elder;
- The elder has an untreated medical condition or is malnourished or dehydrated not related to a known illness;
- Inadequate material items, such as clothing, blankets, furniture, and television.

4.10.2.5. Indicators of Self-Neglect

- Inability to manage personal finances, such as hoarding, squandering, or giving away money while not paying bills;
- Inability to manage activities of daily living, such as personal care, shopping, or housework;
- Wandering, refusing needed medical attention, isolation, and substance use;
- Failure to keep needed medical appointments;
- Confusion, memory loss, and unresponsiveness;
- Lack of toilet facilities, or living quarters infested with animals or vermin.

4.10.2.6. Warning Indicators From Caregiver

- The elder is not given an opportunity to speak for self, have visitors, or see anyone without the presence of the caregiver;

- Attitudes of indifference or anger toward the elder;
- Blaming the elder for his or her illness or limitations;
- Defensiveness;
- Conflicting accounts of elder's abilities, problems, and so forth;
- Previous history of abuse or problems with alcohol or drugs.

If injuries are concealed, untreated, or inconsistent with the given explanation, the nurse should suspect abuse. Cuts, lacerations, puncture wounds, bruises, welts, and burns are examples of these types of injuries. Burns can include those from cigarettes, scalds, burns from acid or caustic substances, or friction burns on the ankles or wrists from being bound by clothes, ropes, or chains. A persistent stench of feces or urine, dirt, rashes, sores, lice, or insufficient clothing are all indicators of physical neglect. Malnourishment or dehydration that is not associated with a particular disease also strongly suggests abuse.

An elderly person who is fearful, withdrawn, depressed, and helpless, or who is reluctant to speak candidly with the nurse, may be exhibiting signs of emotional or psychological abuse. The elderly person may also seem agitated or angry for no apparent reason. Even if the facts clearly show otherwise, he or she may still deny any issues. The inability to manage finances (hoarding or squandering while neglecting to pay bills), the incapacity to carry out daily tasks (personal care, shopping, food preparation, and cleaning), and cognitive abnormalities (confusion, disorientation, inappropriate responses, memory loss, and isolation) are all potential signs of self-neglect. Additional clues of self-neglect include bodily rashes or sores, an unpleasant stench from urine or feces, signs of malnourishment or dehydration, and missing important doctor's appointments. The elderly person must be assessed as being unable to manage daily affairs and take care of themselves for self-neglect to be diagnosed. It is insufficient to prove self-neglect based only on family members' perceptions that the senior cannot handle money. For instance, just because an older adult donates sizable sums of money to a charity or organization, or engages in an endeavor that family members disapprove of, does not equate to self-neglect.

Signs of financial abuse or exploitation could include a lot of unpaid bills (even though the client has enough money to pay them), strange activity in bank accounts, checks that are not signed by the elder, or recent modifications to a power of attorney or will when the elder is unable to make such decisions. The elderly person might be without luxuries like a television, personal hygiene products, or clothes that they can afford. The elderly person may mention that they have lost important items and that they don't communicate with friends or family.

The caregiver's potential signs of abuse may also be picked up by the nurse. The caregiver might gripe about the elder's incontinence, feeding issues, high prescription costs, or how hard it is to care for them. He or she may act hostile or uncaring toward the elderly person and attempt to prevent the nurse from having a private conversation with them. If the caregiver has a history of alcohol or drug abuse or family violence, elder abuse is more likely to occur.

Adult protective services are governed by laws in each of the 50 states, the District of Columbia, Guam, Puerto Rico, and the Virgin Islands. These include senior citizens as well as adults who are deemed dependent, impaired, or disabled and who need assistance from others to meet their basic needs. This is the case in the majority of states. These laws offer a framework for identifying, disclosing, looking into, and helping victims of abuse. However, not all states and territories require reporting abuse to be reported in relation to elders or dependent adults. The regulations or statutes pertaining to reporting abuse in their individual states should be known to nurses. Numerous cases are still unreported. In compliance with state laws, the local agency on aging can offer procedures for reporting abuse. Go online and type in adult protective services to find local addresses and phone numbers in the area where you wish to report abuse. This will help you locate a local agency.

4.10.3. Treatment and Intervention

Elder abuse can occur when the responsibilities of caregiving become too much for the caregiver to handle physically or emotionally. By reducing the caregiver's stress and offering more support, the abusive behavior may be corrected and the caregiving relationship preserved. However, in some cases, the neglect or abuse is deliberate and aimed at benefiting the caregiver, like gaining access to the elder's money. In these instances, it may be necessary to remove either the elder or the caregiver from the situation.

4.11. Rape and Sexual Assault

Rape is the act of having sex with someone against their will and without their consent, regardless of whether that person's will is overridden by coercion, fear of coercion, drugs, or alcohol. Rape is a sexual offense that involves the use of force and humiliation against the victim. In addition, it qualifies as rape if the victim lacks the legal age of consent (which ranges from 14 to 18 years old in different states) or is mentally ill and unable to make rational decisions. A complete erection and ejaculation are not required for the crime of rape' only a slight penetration of the outer vulva or rectum is required. Even though forced oral sex and anal penetration often follow rape, they are legally classified as sodomy, which is still sexual assault. In addition to physical assault, the victim of a rape may sustain injuries.

Rape can happen between acquaintances, married people, strangers, and people of the same sex, though victims of same-sex relationships are not included in the definition of domestic violence in seven states. The percentage of rapes perpetrated by strangers is only 28%, with 7% of victims being children (Rape Abuse and Incest National Network [RAINN], 2018). Date rape, also known as acquaintance rape, is a phenomenon that can happen on a first date, during a ride home from a party, or after a while of getting to know someone. It's more common in or near college campuses. Both the victim's and the offender's increased alcohol consumption is linked to a higher rate of serious injuries from dating violence.

Less than 50% of rapes are thought to be reported, making it a severely underreported crime. The reasons behind the underreporting are the victim's sense of helplessness and guilt, their fear of getting hurt again, and their conviction that they have no legal options. Rape victims can be of any age' cases that have been reported have included victims as young as 15 months old as old as 82. Girls and women between the ages of 16 and 24 have the highest incidence. In 80% of recorded rapes, the victims were girls under the age of 20 (Stromberg, 2017). The victim's neighborhood is most frequently the scene of rape, frequently inside or close to the home. Most rapes are planned crimes. Up to 50% of female victims minimize their experiences as minor incidents or misunderstandings, refusing to report their sexual assault (Stromberg, 2017). This is especially true if the offender is someone the woman knows or who holds a position of authority, like a family member, respected member of the community, or a manager at work. Another crime that is notably underreported and underacknowledged is male rape. It happens most frequently in institutions like prisons, but it can also happen between gay partners or strangers. An estimated 80,000 male prisoners are sexually assaulted annually, though this number could be considerably higher given that 60% of these crimes are committed by staff members of prisons or jails. The dynamics of power and control in this kind of rape are similar to those in heterosexual rape, and it is especially violent (RAINN, 2018).

4.11.1. Dynamics of Rape

Men who commit rape comprise 50% of those who are 30 years of age or older and 25% of those who are 21 to 29. Of all races, white people make up 57%. In 34% of cases, alcohol is a factor. Crimes of violence frequently coexist with rape. Nearly 75% of rapists who are apprehended have a history of previous criminal activity, which includes homicides, robberies, assaults, and rapes (RAINN, 2018). Rape and those who commit it have historically been explained in terms of dynamics or motivations (e.g., power, anger, opportunity). These categories weren't very helpful because they were based on the idea of "rape by a stranger," which isn't usually the case. It is widely acknowledged that rape is not a sexual crime, but rather the exercise of power and control, the infliction of pain, or retribution for perceived transgressions.

According to feminist theory, women have historically been the targets of violence since they were considered the legal property of men, along with children. When a married man was found guilty of raping his wife in 1982, it was the first instance of the idea that sexual relations could not be refused in a married relationship ending. Women who are sexually assaulted often find themselves in dangerous situations, and their main goal is to survive. Sometimes the attacker is resisted or fought back, but other times fighting and screaming lead to more serious injuries or even death. The degree of submission increases if the assailant is brandishing a knife or gun. The more aggressive rapist may also forcefully penetrate her, urinate or defecate on her, or insert foreign objects into her rectum and vagina. Rape victims experience severe physical and psychological trauma. Acute injuries, STDs, pregnancy, and persistent medical issues are examples of related medical issues. Women who had been raped rated their own health significantly lower, saw doctors twice as frequently and had medical expenses more than twice as high as those of women who had not been victimized by crime, according to a cross-sectional study of patients. It was discovered that the degree of violence encountered during the assault was a strong indicator of the need for medical care in the future. Fear, helplessness, shock, disbelief, guilt, humiliation, and embarrassment are common emotions experienced by rape victims. In addition, they might stay away from the scene or circumstances of the rape' give up previously enjoyable hobbies' suffer from melancholy, anxiety, PTSD, sexual dysfunction, insomnia, and memory loss' or think about taking their own life (Ba and Bhopal, 2017). The rights of victims of rape were frequently disregarded until recently. For instance, rape victims frequently encountered skepticism and awkward inquiries from police when they reported a rape to the authorities. The courts did not uphold the rights of victims' for instance, a woman's previous sexual history could be introduced in court even though her alleged attacker's prior criminal history could not. Since the middle of the 1980s, state-by-state legislation has been passed to address these issues, and it is still being passed. While there has been progress in the last twenty years in both the prosecution and the treatment of rape victims, many people still hold the belief that a woman's actions can incite rape and that she bears some responsibility for the crime.

4.11.2. Assessment

The physical examination should take place before the victim has taken a shower, brushed their teeth, changed into new clothes, or had anything to drink to preserve any potential evidence. Given that the victim might have done some of these things before seeking care, this might not be achievable. Rinsing the mouth or consuming liquids can be allowed right away if there has been no report of oral sex. The nurse asks the victim to explain what happened so that she can evaluate the patient's physical condition. If the patient is unable to do so, the nurse may carefully and gently ask the necessary questions. The majority of emergency department settings offer rape kits and protocols, which include the tools and guidelines required to gather tangible evidence. This portion of the examination is mainly the responsibility of the doctor or a sexual assault nurse examiner with specialized training.

4.11.3. Treatment and Intervention

Rape victims do best when they receive prompt assistance and can communicate their fear and rage to family members, caregivers, medical professionals, and law enforcement officers who will believe them. Law enforcement, the general public, and medical professionals must continue to receive education about rape and the needs of victims.

There are relationship abuse warning indicators. The characteristics of those who are likely to commit dating violence can be identified by these indicators, which can also serve as a warning to others and students about date rape. Instances comprise disparaging remarks directed towards women, being stern, drinking excessively, showing jealousy, expressing fury, and employing intimidation.

Warning Signs of Relationship Violence:

- Emotionally abuses you (insults, makes belittling comments, or acts sulky or angry when you initiate an idea or activity);
- Tells you with whom you may be friends or how you should dress or tries to control other elements of your life;
- Talks negatively about women in general;
- Gets jealous for no reason;
- Drinks heavily, uses drugs, or tries to get you drunk;
- Acts in an intimidating way by invading your personal space such as standing too close or touching you when you don't want that;
- Cannot handle sexual or emotional frustration without becoming angry;
- Does not view you as an equal: sees self as smarter or socially superior;
- Guards masculinity by acting tough;
- Is angry or threatening to the point that you have changed your life or yourself so you won't anger him;
- Goes through extreme highs and lows: is kind one minute, cruel the next;
- Berates you for not getting drunk or high, or not wanting to have sex;
- Is physically aggressive, grabbing and holding you, or pushing and shoving.

The victims benefit most from rape treatment centers, which are emergency services that work with law enforcement agencies to coordinate psychiatric, gynecologic, and physical trauma services in one location. When it comes to offering the victim emotional support in an emergency situation, the nurse is a vital member of the team. The victim should not be rushed through any interview or examination processes' instead, the nurse should let them go at their own pace. Restoring the victim's control as much as possible is crucial. One way to achieve this is to give them the freedom to decide for themselves when it comes to who to call, what to do next, what they would like done, and other matters. Whether or not to press charges and provide testimony against the offender is up to the victim. Before taking pictures or taking samples of the victim's hair and nails for potential use as evidence, the victim must sign consent forms.

Treatment for sexually transmitted infections is provided prophylactically. It is economical to do this because many rape victims won't come back for conclusive test results for these illnesses. Since seroconversion to positive status takes time, HIV testing is highly advised at predetermined intervals. Until the results of HIV testing are known, victims are also urged to practice safe sexual behavior. To avoid pregnancy, prophylaxis with norgestrel (Ovral) and ethinyl estradiol may be recommended. Some women may decide to postpone seeking help until after they miss a menstrual cycle or receive a positive pregnancy test result.

From the emergency room to longer-term follow-up, a counselor or volunteer is frequently available to accompany victims through rape crisis centers, advocacy groups, and other local resources. This person can be completely available to the victim, offers emotional support, and acts as an advocate for them throughout the process. This kind of all-encompassing, unwavering support is frequently essential to healing. The goal of therapy is usually to help the victim regain control over their life' to deal with feelings of guilt, shame, and anger' to improve everyday functioning' to relieve feelings of helplessness, dependency, and obsession with the assault that often follow rape' and to rebuild trust. Group therapy with other raped victims is a particularly successful form of treatment. Some patients go to group and individual therapy sessions.

4.12. Community Violence

The most current information regarding school safety and crime comes from the 2017 report, which is released annually by the National Center for Education Statistics. Less than 3% of deaths at schools are caused by homicide. However, a single shooter's multiple killings have become more frequent in recent years than a single school shooting. News of multiple shootings is reported globally. To address safety concerns, schools have increased security in many ways and train students on what to do in the event of an active shooter. The CDC has been collaborating with schools to create curricula that prioritize the development of social skills, anger management, and problem-solving abilities in an effort to prevent school violence. Furthermore, mentoring programs for youth and parenting initiatives that foster a strong bond between parents and children as well as conflict resolution in the home have the potential to address school-related violence. A small number of those who commit acts of such violence have been identified as having a mental illness, most frequently conduct disorder. But this violence seems to happen most often when there is a predominance of alienation, indifference to others, and low regard for oneself. Bullying at school encompasses various forms of aggression, such as verbal abuse, physical acts such as shoving or breaking bones, targeting a student to cause them to be shunned or ignored by others, and cyberbullying, which involves sending unwanted emails, texts, or posting pictures online. Bullying is associated with adolescent suicide, substance abuse, thoughts and acts of self-harm, and moderate-to-severe depressive symptoms.

Ostracism, which involves excluding and ignoring the target person, has become one of the more prevalent and harmful types of bullying in recent times. The victim feels as though their sense of control, self-worth, sense of belonging, and meaningful existence are in danger. More than bullying, racism may be a bigger threat to children's ability to adjust (Heithaus, Twyman, and Braddock, 2017). Almost one-third of Americans. S. Students claim to have been bullied, either as the victim or the aggressor. Bullying occurred most frequently in grades six through eight. Children who were bullied also had higher rates of poor grades, alcohol and tobacco use, and loneliness. Bullied children also reported having a harder time making friends. Bullying is more common among children who require special physical health care, and it is also more likely to affect children who have ongoing emotional, behavioral, or developmental issues.

Initiation rites, also known as hazing, are common in both high school and college. Victims could be the target of degrading or even unlawful behavior. Negative effects of hazing include fighting, getting hurt, hurting other people, performing poorly in school, having trouble eating, sleeping, or focusing, and feeling confused, angry, embarrassed, or guilty. Hazing incidents are typically linked to sports teams, fraternities, or other organizations that provide a sense of exclusivity, status, admiration, and/or recognition. Along with the potential drawbacks of refusing, the promise of these advantages serves to entice students to participate. Hazing behaviors include drinking, being teased, being alone, not getting enough sleep, and having sex acts. These behaviors are not exclusive to athletics or fraternities among student organizations. Children and young adults are profoundly impacted by exposure to communal violence.

Children who witness violence exhibit symptoms of stress that worsen in proportion to the violence they witness. Furthermore, experiencing violence can set the stage for issues with aggression, depression, relationships, success, and drug and alcohol abuse in the future. Resolving the issue of exposure to violence could potentially mitigate the vicious cycle of dysfunction and subsequent violence. Large-scale acts of violence, like the terrorist attacks that occurred in Pennsylvania, Washington, and New York in 2001, also have a profound impact on the populace. Children were terrified to go to school or to have their parents leave them for any reason in the immediate aftermath. Adults found it challenging to travel by public transit, fly, leave their homes, and go to work. A year later, 532,240 cases of PTSD had been reported in the New York City metropolitan area alone, and 10% of people in the New York area still experienced post-September 11 stress and depression. Furthermore, a greater number of people reported relapses from anxiety and depression.

Despite initial concerns, there was no nationwide rise in PTSD cases as a result of people watching the attacks and related television coverage. Even after 15 years, there is still a high prevalence of depression and PTSD (Adams et al., 2019). To address victims of violence, early intervention and treatment are crucial. Referrals, counseling, and continuous treatment were implemented right away to assist individuals affected in coping with the horrific events that followed multiple shootings at schools or workplaces. Working with survivors, families, and other affected parties since the terrorist attacks of 2001 have been groups of doctors, therapists, and other health professionals (many of whom are connected to colleges and hospitals).

A Closer Look

Relational Aggression

Relational aggression, often termed "social aggression," is a form of behavior aimed at harming others through manipulation and damage to their social relationships or social standing. Unlike physical aggression, which involves direct harm to someone's body, relational aggression is more subtle and can be just as harmful. It typically involves behaviors such as spreading rumors, exclusion from social groups, silent treatment, and backstabbing. These tactics are designed to undermine an individual's social connections and self-esteem, leading to significant emotional and psychological distress.

Relational aggression is most commonly observed in social settings such as schools, workplaces, and online platforms. It is particularly prevalent among adolescents, especially girls, although boys can also engage in and be victims of such behavior. In schools, for example, relational aggression can manifest as cliques that exclude certain individuals or as the spreading of harmful gossip intended to isolate a peer. In the workplace, it can involve undermining colleagues through rumors or deliberately excluding them from important meetings and social activities.

The motivations behind relational aggression can vary. Often, individuals engage in this behavior to gain or maintain social status, power, or control within a group. It can also stem from jealousy, insecurity, or a desire for revenge. Those who engage in relational aggression may have learned these behaviors from their social environment, observing and mimicking others who use such tactics effectively.

The impact of relational aggression on victims can be profound and long-lasting. Victims often experience feelings of loneliness, depression, anxiety, and low self-esteem. The emotional toll can lead to difficulties in forming and maintaining healthy relationships, both during adolescence and into adulthood. In severe cases, the stress and isolation caused by relational aggression can contribute to academic or professional decline, and even suicidal thoughts or behaviors.

Addressing relational aggression requires a multi-faceted approach. In educational settings, programs that promote social-emotional learning (SEL) can be effective. These programs teach empathy, communication skills, and conflict resolution, helping students understand the impact of their actions and fostering a more inclusive environment. Anti-bullying policies and interventions that involve the whole school community, including staff training and peer support systems, are also crucial.

In the workplace, addressing relational aggression involves creating a culture of respect and inclusivity. Employers can implement clear policies against workplace bullying and harassment, provide training on recognizing and responding to relational aggression, and establish confidential reporting mechanisms. Encouraging open communication and team-building activities can also help reduce the incidence of relational aggression by promoting a more supportive and collaborative work environment.

Parental and community involvement is also essential in addressing relational aggression. Parents can model healthy relational behaviors and guide managing conflicts constructively. Community programs that offer support and education on relational aggression can raise awareness and equip individuals with the tools to recognize and counteract such behaviors.

In conclusion, relational aggression is a pervasive and damaging form of social manipulation that can significantly impact the emotional and psychological well-being of individuals. Understanding its manifestations, motivations, and consequences is crucial for developing effective prevention and intervention strategies. By fostering environments that emphasize empathy, respect, and open communication, schools, workplaces, and communities can mitigate the harmful effects of relational aggression and promote healthier, more inclusive social interactions.

Summary

- Anger is an emotion that nearly everyone feels from time to time in their lives. It is not wrong or bad to feel anger, but it is a negative emotion meaning that it tends to bring a person's mood down.
- Hostility or aggression is a behavior, often the direct result of anger that goes unchecked. Most people believe that they have little to no control over their hostility or aggression and even less control over anger.
- Anger is a normal emotion experienced by everyone at different times. It is, in fact, a natural response to a threat, helping prime ourselves for protection or stand up for ourselves. It can also be useful to motivate people to meet challenges or make changes.
- Victims of abuse or violence can certainly have physical injuries needing medical attention, but they also experience psychological injuries with a broad range of responses. Some clients are agitated and visibly upset' others are withdrawn and aloof, appearing numb or oblivious to their surroundings.
- Family violence encompasses spouse battering' neglect and physical, emotional, or sexual abuse of children' elder abuse' and marital rape. In many cases, family members tolerate abusive and violent behavior from relatives they would never accept from strangers.
- Intimate partner violence is the mistreatment or misuse of one person by another in the context of an emotionally intimate relationship. The relationship may be spousal, between partners, boyfriend, girlfriend, or an estranged relationship.
- Child abuse or maltreatment generally is defined as the intentional injury of a child. It can include physical abuse or injuries, neglect or failure to prevent harm, failure to provide adequate physical or emotional care or supervision, abandonment, sexual assault or intrusion, and overt torture or maiming.
- Elder abuse is the maltreatment of older adults by family members or others in a caregiver role. It may include physical and sexual abuse, psychological abuse, neglect, self-neglect, financial exploitation, and denial of adequate medical treatment.
- Rape is the perpetration of an act of sexual intercourse with a person against his or her will and without her consent, whether that will is overcome by force, fear of force, drugs, or intoxicants. Rape is a crime of violence and humiliation of the victim expressed through sexual means.
- Victims of rape fare best when they receive immediate support and can express fear and rage to family members, nurses, physicians, and law enforcement officials who believe them.

References

1. Adams, S. W., Bowler, R. M., Russell, K., Brackbill, R. M., Li, J., & Cone, J. E. (2019). PTSD and comorbid depression: Social support and self-efficacy in World Trade Center survivors 14–15 years after 9/11. *Psychological Trauma, 11*(2), 156–164.
2. Andresen, F. J., & Buchanan, J. A. (2017). Bullying in senior living facilities: Perspectives of long-term care staff. *Journal of Gerontological Nursing, 43*(7), 34–41.
3. Ba, I., & Bhopal, R. S. (2017). Physical, mental and social consequences in civilians who have experienced war-related sexual violence: A systematic review (1981–2014). *Public Health, 142*, 121–135.
4. Bartlett, J. D., Kotake, C., Fauth, R., & Easterbrooks, M. A. (2017). Intergenerational transmission of child abuse and neglect: Do maltreatment type, perpetrator, and substantiation status matter? *Child Abuse & Neglect, 63*, 84–94.
5. Bernet, W., & Freeman, B. W. (2017). Child maltreatment. In B. J. Sadock, V. A. Sadock, & P. Ruiz (Eds.), *Comprehensive Textbook of Psychiatry* (Vol. 2, 10th ed., pp. 3828–3842). Wolters Kluwer/Lippincott, Williams, & Wilkins.
6. Byrne, E., Vessey, J. A., & Pfeifer, L. (2018). Cyberbullying and social media: Information and interventions for school nurses working with victims, students, and families. *Journal of School Nursing, 34*(1), 38–50.
7. Centers for Disease Control and Prevention. (2017). Preventing intimate partner violence. Retrieved from: http://www.cdc.gov/violenceprevention/intimatepartnerviolence/index.html (accessed on 7 September 2024).
8. Coccaro, E. F., Beman, M. E., & McCloskey, M. S. (2017). Development of a screening questionnaire for DSM-5 intermittent explosive disorder (IED-SQ). *Comprehensive Psychiatry, 74*, 21–26.
9. Crosswell, A. D., Moreno, P. I., Raposa, E. B., Motivala, S. J., Stanton, A. L., Ganz, P. A., & Bower, J. E. (2017). Effects of mindfulness training on emotional and physiologic recovery from induced negative effect. *Psychoneuroendocrinology, 86*, 78–86.
10. Fisher, K. (2016). Inpatient violence. *Psychiatric Clinics of North America, 39*(4), 567–577.
11. Flannery, R. B. Jr. (2012). *The Assaulted Staff Action Program (ASAP): Psychological Counseling for Victims of Violence*. American Health Foundation. Retrieved from: http://Americanmentalhealthfoundation.org/2012/04/the-assaulted-staff-action-program-asap-psychological-counseling-for-victims-of-violence (accessed on 7 September 2024).
12. Fleury-Steiner, R. E., Miller, S. L., & Carireri, A. (2017). Calling the shots: How family courts address the firearms ban in protection orders. *Violence Against Women, 23*(9), 1140–1151.
13. Greenwood, P. R., Haroun, A. M., & Naimark, D. (2017). The legal and ethical analysis of elder abuse. In B. J. Sadock, V. A. Sadock, & P. Ruiz (Eds.), *Comprehensive Textbook of Psychiatry* (Vol. 2, 10th ed., pp. 4250–4255). Wolters Kluwer/Lippincott, Williams, & Wilkins.
14. Harden, B. J., Buhler, A., & Parra, L. J. (2016). Maltreatment in infancy: A developmental perspective on prevention and intervention. *Trauma, Violence & Abuse, 17*(4), 366–386.
15. Heithaus, J. L., Twyman, K. A., & Braddock, B. A. (2017). Ostracism and peer victimization in adolescents with and without mental health diagnoses in a public middle school setting. *Clinical Pediatrics, 56*(14), 1301–1311.

16. Horiuchi, S., Tsuda, A., Aoki, S., Yoneda, K., & Sawaguchi, Y. (2018). Coping as a mediator of the relationship between stress mindset and psychological stress response: A pilot study. *Psychology Research and Behavior Management, 11*, 47–54.

17. Jeckell, A. S., Copenhaver, E. A., & Diamond, A. B. (2018). The spectrum of hazing and peer sexual abuse in sports: A current perspective. *Sports Health, 10*(6), 558–564.

18. Joint Commission on Accreditation of Healthcare Organizations. (2016). Bullying has no place in healthcare. Retrieved from: https://www.jointcommission.org/assets/1/23/Quick_Safety_Issue_24_June_2016.pdf (accessed on 7 September 2024).

19. Lee, H. Y., Kim, J. E., Kim, M., Kim, A. R., Park, H. J., Kwon, O. J., & Kim, J. H. (2018). Effect and safety of acupuncture for Hwa-byung, an anger syndrome: A study protocol of a randomized controlled pilot study. *Trials, 19*(1), 98.

20. Lewis-Fernandez, R. L., Kirmayer, L. J., Guarnaccia, P. J., & Ruiz, P. (2017). Cultural concepts of distress and assessment. In B. J. Sadock, V. A. Sadock, & P. Ruiz (Eds.), *Comprehensive Textbook of Psychiatry* (Vol. 2, 10th ed., pp. 2443–2470). Wolters Kluwer/Lippincott, Williams, & Wilkins.

21. Lin, I. M., Wang, S. Y., Chu, I. H., Lu, Y. H., Lee, C. S., Lin, T. H., & Fan, S. Y. (2017). The association of Type D personality with heart rate variability and lipid profiles among patients with coronary artery disease. *International Journal of Behavioral Medicine, 24*(1), 101–109.

22. Lund, E. M., & Ross, S. W. (2017). Bullying perpetration, victimization, and demographic differences in college students: A review of the literature. *Trauma, Violence & Abuse, 18*(3), 348–360.

23. Pinquart, M. (2017). Systematic review: Bullying involvement of children with and without chronic physical illness and/or physical/sensory disability—A meta-analytic comparison with healthy nondisabled peers. *Journal of Pediatric Psychology, 42*(3), 245–259.

24. Ramesh, D., Hassamal, S., & Moeller, F. G. (2017). Intermittent explosive disorder. In B. J. Sadock, V. A. Sadock, & P. Ruiz (Eds.), *Comprehensive Textbook of Psychiatry* (Vol. 1, 10th ed., pp. 2110–2113). Wolters Kluwer/Lippincott, Williams, & Wilkins.

25. Rape Abuse & Incest National Network (RAINN). (2018). Perpetrators of sexual violence: Statistics. Retrieved from: https://www.rainn.org/statistics/perpetrators-sexual-violence (accessed on 7 September 2024).

26. Schultz, J. M., & Videbeck, S. L. (2013). *Lippincott's Manual of Psychiatric Nursing Care Plans* (9th ed.). Lippincott Williams & Wilkins.

27. Steine, I. M., Winje, D., Krystal, J. H., Bjorvatn, B., Milde, A. M., Grønli, J., & Pallesen, S. (2017). Cumulative childhood maltreatment and its dose-response relation with adult symptomatology: Findings in a sample of adult survivors of sexual abuse. *Child Abuse & Neglect, 65*, 99–111.

28. Stromberg, S. F. (2017). Physical and sexual abuse of adults. In B. J. Sadock, V. A. Sadock, & P. Ruiz (Eds.), *Comprehensive Textbook of Psychiatry* (Vol. 2, 10th ed., pp. 2538–2542). Wolters Kluwer/Lippincott, Williams, & Wilkins.

29. U.S. Department of Education, National Center for Education Statistics. (2017). Indicators of school crime and safety, 2017. Retrieved from: http://nces.ed.gov/programs/crimeindicators/ind_01.asp (accessed on 7 September 2024).

30. Victoroff, J. (2017). The neuropsychiatry of human aggression. In B. J. Sadock, V. A. Sadock, & P. Ruiz (Eds.), *Comprehensive Textbook of Psychiatry* (Vol. 2, 10th ed., pp. 2471–2504). Wolters Kluwer/Lippincott, Williams, & Wilkins.

31. Violence Prevention and Action Center/John Carroll University. (2018). Stalking statistics. Retrieved from: http://sites.jcu.edu/vpac/pages/educate-yourself/stalking/stalking-statistics (accessed on 7 September 2024).

32. Woodlock, D. (2017). The abuse of technology in domestic violence and stalking. *Violence Against Women, 23*(5), 584–602.

33. Zhu, X., Li, W., & Wang, X. (2016). Characteristics of aggressive behavior among male inpatients with schizophrenia. *Shanghai Archives of Psychiatry, 28*(5), 280–288.

Chapter

5

TRAUMA, ANXIETY, AND STRESSOR-RELATED PSYCHIATRIC DISORDERS

Contents

Introduction

A person's life may contain incidents that are exceptionally severe or intense, far beyond the strain of day-to-day living. Not just those who are predisposed to mental health problems or issues, but everyone who experiences these traumatic events or stressors should be expected to have their lives disrupted. A person with a history of childhood abuse, a child recently diagnosed with type 1 diabetes, or an adult suffering from an acute coronary syndrome, such as a myocardial infarction or unstable angina, maybe the only one affected by the trauma or incident. A traumatic event, like a war, terrorist attack, or natural disaster like a flood, hurricane, or tsunami, can affect a large number of people or groups of people. Worldwide, PTSD, or posttraumatic stress disorder, is a common condition.

While everyone who experiences something like this exhibits anxiety, insomnia, trouble coping, grief, or any other number of reactions, the majority of people get through the experience and return to their typical levels of equilibrium and coping—possibly even improved coping as a result of handling the event. Nonetheless, some people still struggle to cope, control their emotions and stress, or go back to their regular activities. They might experience PTSD, dissociative disorder, adjustment disorder, or acute stress disorder. Anxiety is a generalized sensation of dread or apprehension that can manifest as behavioral, emotional, cognitive, or physical symptoms in response to internal or external stimuli. Fear is a different emotion from anxiety' fear is the feeling of being afraid or threatened by an obvious external stimulus that one believes poses a threat to oneself. In life, anxiety is inevitable and can have a lot of beneficial effects, like inspiring someone to act to address a crisis or solve a problem. When it fits the context, it's regarded as normal, and once the issue has been settled, it goes away. A set of conditions known as anxiety disorders are characterized by excessive anxiety and the corresponding behavioral, emotional, cognitive, and physiological reactions. Individuals with anxiety disorders may exhibit peculiar behaviors like uncontrollable shaking, unfounded fear of things or situations, or excessive or inexplicable worry. Over time, the disorder causes them great distress, and it seriously affects their ability to go about their daily lives, interact with others, and perform their jobs.

Orientation and Directional Terms

Term	Definition	Illustration
Acute stress disorder	Acute stress disorder is a psychological response to a terrifying, traumatic or surprising experience. Combat stress reaction is a similar response to the trauma of war.	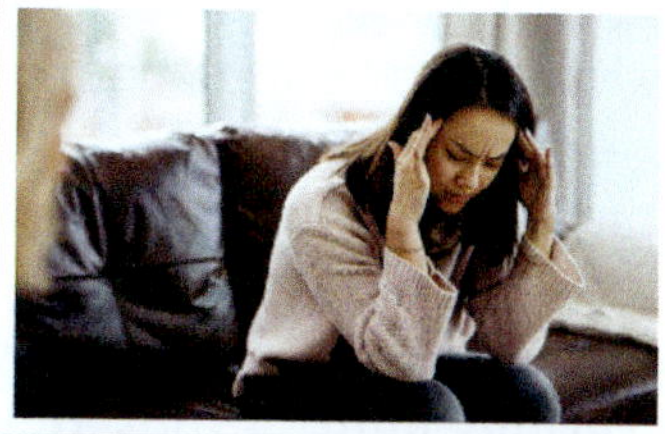
Anxiety	Anxiety is a feeling of fear, dread, and uneasiness. It might cause you to sweat, feel restless and tense, and have a rapid heartbeat. It can be a normal reaction to stress.	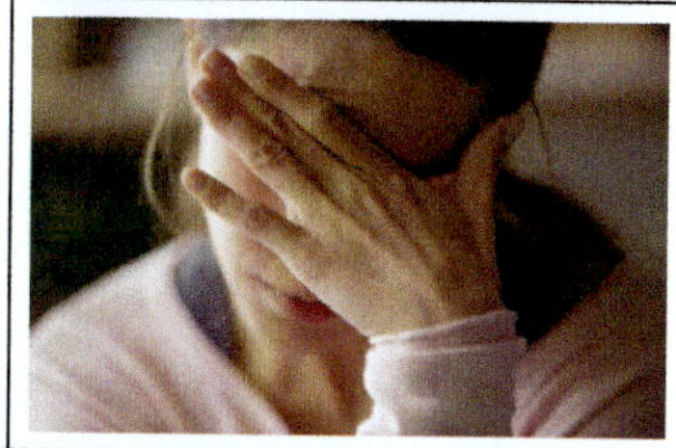
Posttraumatic stress disorder (PTSD)	Posttraumatic stress disorder (PTSD) is a psychiatric disorder that may occur in people who have experienced or witnessed a traumatic event, series of events or set of circumstances. An individual may experience this as emotionally or physically harmful or life-threatening and may affect mental, physical, social, and/or spiritual well-being.	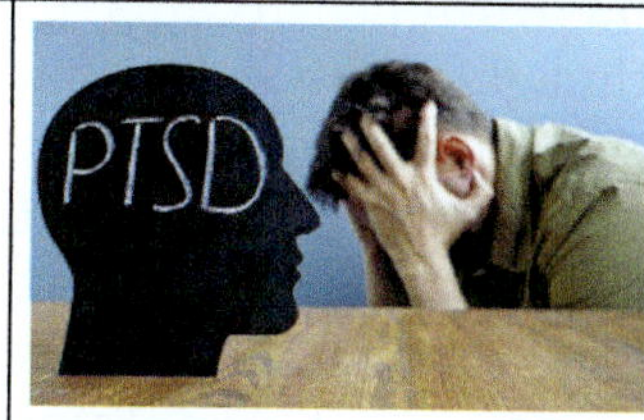
Trauma	Trauma is an emotional response to a terrible event like an accident, crime, natural disaster, physical or emotional abuse, neglect, experiencing or witnessing violence, death of a loved one, war, and more. Immediately after the event, shock and denial are typical.	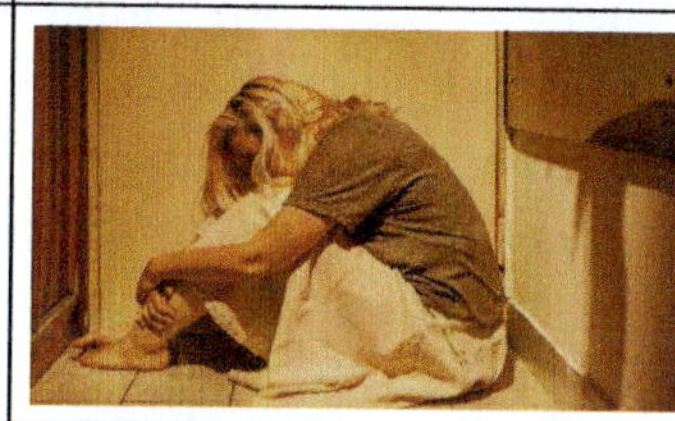
Reactive attachment disorder (RAD)	Reactive attachment disorder (RAD) is a rare condition where children don't form an emotional bond with their caretakers. Children who are adopted may experience RAD. Treatment focuses on repairing and/or creating emotionally healthy family bonds.	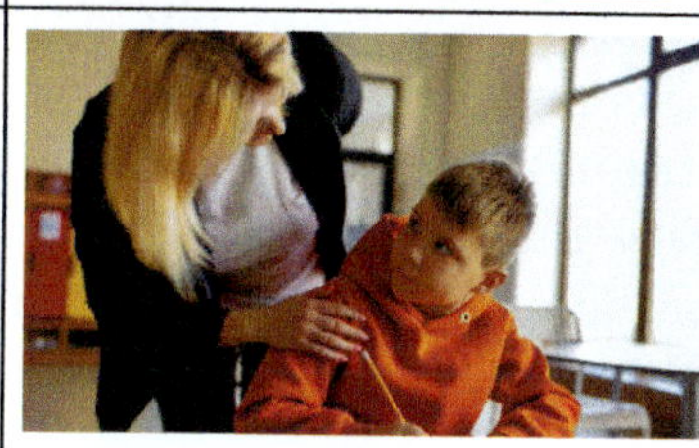
Dissociative amnesia	Dissociative amnesia is when your mind blocks out important information about yourself, causing "gaps" in your memory. One of the most common reasons your mind blocks out things is to protect you from unpleasant, distressing or traumatic experiences.	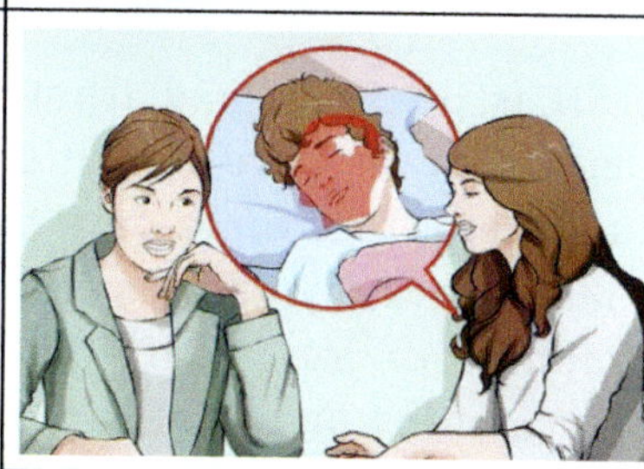

5.1. Posttraumatic Stress Disorder

A person with posttraumatic stress disorder (PTSD) exhibits a troubling pattern of behavior after experiencing, witnessing, or coming into contact with a traumatic event, such as an assault, a natural disaster, or combat. An event that actually or potentially threatened death or serious injury exposed a person with PTSD, and they reacted with extreme fear, helplessness, or terror. According to Shalev and Marmar (2017), there are four subcategories of symptoms associated with post-traumatic stress disorder (PTSD): avoidance, negative cognition or thoughts, hyperarousal, and reliving the trauma through dreams or persistent, intrusive thoughts. The individual consistently relives the trauma through flashbacks, dreams, memories, or responses to outside cues about what happened, and as a result, they avoid situations that are linked to the trauma. In addition to persistent symptoms of elevated arousal, such as insomnia, hypervigilance or hyperarousal, irritability, or violent outbursts, the victim experiences a numbing of general responsiveness. He or she claims to have lost control over and a sense of connection to life. This may result in avoidance behavior, or a desire to stay away from any locations, people, or circumstances that could bring up memories of the trauma. While seeking solace, security, and safety, the person may, in fact, grow more and more alone over time, which may intensify the unpleasant emotions they were attempting to suppress.

PTSD is distinguished from acute stress disorder, which can have similar symptoms but lasts anywhere from three days to one month, by the fact that the symptoms of PTSD manifest three months or longer after the trauma. It may take months or even years for the onset to occur. Although symptoms of PTSD can vary in intensity and severity and worsen during stressful times, they are usually chronic in nature. PTSD symptoms are frequently made worse by other life events. Furthermore, many PTSD patients go on to experience other mental health issues like depression, anxiety disorders, or drug and alcohol abuse (Shalev and Marmar, 2017). Any age can experience PTSD, even in early childhood. Up to 60% of those who are vulnerable, such as veterans of armed conflicts, victims of violent crimes, and victims of natural disasters, are thought to experience PTSD. For roughly 50% of individuals, full recovery happens in three months. The most significant variables influencing the risk of developing PTSD are the trauma's intensity and duration as well as the individual's proximity to the incident. PTSD affects one-fourth of all assault victims who sustain physical harm. Rape victims experience PTSD at one of the highest rates—roughly 70%—of any other group.

5.1.1. Related Disorders

5.1.1.1. Adjustment Disorder

An individual with adjustment disorder may react negatively to a stressful event that leaves them with difficulties. The person typically struggles more than one might anticipate to deal with the incident or integrate it into their life. The most frequent occurrences are stressors pertaining to money, relationships, and employment. Within a month, the symptoms start to appear and last for no more than six months. Either the adjustment was successful at that point, or the patient moves on to a different diagnosis (Katzman and Geppert, 2017). Treatment that is most popular and effective is outpatient counseling or therapy. Reliving the trauma, avoidance, and hyperarousal that transpire three days to four weeks after the trauma are symptoms of acute stress disorder. It may appear before PTSD. The development of PTSD can be stopped with cognitive-behavioral therapy (CBT), which combines anxiety management and exposure (Carpenter et al., 2018).

5.1.1.2. Reactive Attachment Disorder (RAD) and Disinhibited Social Engagement Disorder (DSED)

In reaction to the trauma of child abuse or neglect, also known as grossly pathogenic care, children under the age of five develop reactive attachment disorder (RAD) and disinhibited social engagement disorder (DSED). In the majority of circumstances, the child exhibits disturbed inappropriate social relatedness. The child with RAD shows minimal social and emotional responses to others, lacks a positive effect, and maybe sad, irritable, or afraid for no apparent reason, instead of turning to a small group of emotionally attached caregivers for solace. Unselective socialization is exhibited by the DSED child, who accepts or tolerates social interaction with both strangers and caregivers. Unlike most children their age, they don't hesitate to approach or strike up a conversation with strangers. Institutionalization and egregiously inadequate parenting are the two most frequent circumstances leading to this disorder.

5.1.2. Etiology

Although they are distinct from other diagnoses in that category, PTSD and acute stress disorder were previously included in the category of anxiety disorders. However, they are currently placed in their own category. Unlike anxiety disorders, which do not require a prior occurrence of a causative trauma or event, PTSD requires one. PTSD is a condition more commonly found in adults and linked to exposure to events than to personal traits. To put it another way, for most people, the effects of the trauma at the time—such as being directly involved, getting hurt, or losing loved ones—are stronger indicators of PTSD than the actual trauma itself. This is especially true for trauma that is the result of a single event, or triggering event, like natural disasters. However, when they are present pretrauma, peri-trauma dissociation, prior psychiatric history, and personality factors can increase the risk of PTSD even more. Furthermore, posttrauma counseling immediately following the event reduces the likelihood of developing PTSD in participants. (Lies, Lau, Jones, Jensen, and Tan, 2017)

Adolescents are more likely than children or adults to experience PTSD, according to studies on PTSD sufferers. Increased rates of PTSD are associated with age, gender, type of trauma, and repeated trauma. Teens suffering from PTSD are more vulnerable to substance misuse, academic difficulties, poor physical health, low social support, and suicide. Both community-based and educational settings can benefit from trauma-focused cognitive behavioral therapy (CBT). Additionally, it provides long-term benefits for PTSD and other co-occurring disorders (Gutemann, Schwartzkopff, and Stell, 2017). Adolescents with PTSD may experience long-term emotional and behavioral problems that necessitate episodic or continuous therapy to address pertinent issues. PTSD may also disrupt biologic maturation processes. In cases of parental major depression and childhood abuse, children are at a higher risk of developing post-traumatic stress disorder (PTSD). Parental psychopathology creates a stressful environment for the child and increases the likelihood that the child will be diagnosed with PTSD. Postevent counseling reduces these risks when it is received soon after the trauma. For traumatized children, parental involvement in treatment greatly increases the benefits of CBT. It also lessened the common depressive symptoms that parents experience.

5.1.3. Treatment

People with acute stress disorder who receive individual or group counseling or therapy may be able to avoid developing PTSD. The recommended course of treatment for PTSD is outpatient therapy. Certain drugs may also help with a successful outcome, particularly if they are used to treat a particular condition like insomnia. The best outcomes are obtained when both therapies are used in combination (Greenbaum, Neylan, and Rosen, 2017). While brief inpatient stays may be required during severe crises, inpatient treatment is not recommended for clients with PTSD. This usually happens when a client is suffering from suicidal thoughts or is experiencing overwhelming flashbacks or other reliving events. The most popular and effective forms of formal treatment are cognitive behavioral therapy (CBT) and specialty therapy programs that incorporate CBT components. The type of trauma and whether to seek formal individual or group counseling can influence the therapy selection. Self-help groups provide a safe space for emotional sharing and support.

The goals of exposure therapy are to help the client confront uncomfortable thoughts and feelings, regain some degree of control over their thoughts and feelings, and stop the avoidance behavior associated with PTSD. Instead of trying to escape the feared feelings, circumstances, and thoughts connected to the trauma, the client faces them head-on. To help the client tolerate and control the anxiety response, a variety of relaxation techniques are used. Exposure therapy can involve confronting the event in real life, such as going back to the location of the assault, or it can involve imagined confrontation, which involves mentally putting oneself in the traumatic circumstance. Both veterans and active military personnel have found great success with prolonged exposure therapy. The military created adaptive disclosure, a specialized CBT technique, to provide active-duty military personnel with PTSD with focused, brief therapy. It combines the empty chair technique, in which the person says whatever they need to say to anyone, living or dead, with exposure therapy. This is comparable to Gestalt therapy methods. This method appears to be well-tolerated and successful in lowering PTSD symptoms and encouraging posttrauma growth, despite the brief six-session schedule.

Cognitive processing therapy has proven effective in treating both combat veterans and rape survivors with post-traumatic stress disorder. A written account of the most traumatic experience is read aloud during the therapy course. Participants will also learn how to recognize generalized thinking, such as the idea that "No one can be trusted," and regain more realistic and balanced perspectives on the world and themselves. The course focuses on examining beliefs that are false or interfere with daily life, such as guilt and self-blame, such as "It was my fault, I should have fought harder" or "I should have died with my fellow Marines". Clients with PTSD may use medication to treat symptoms like anxiety, insomnia, or hyperarousal. Second-generation antipsychotics, like risperidone, are less effective than SSRIs and serotonin and norepinephrine reuptake inhibitors (SNRIs) as antidepressants, according to studies. Benzodiazepines are commonly used in clinical practice, but there is insufficient evidence to support their effectiveness (Friedman and Bernardy, 2017). It is thought that taking both drugs and CBT at the same time is more beneficial than doing so separately.

5.1.4. Community-Based Care

Most care provided to people in the aftermath of traumatic experiences is done on an outpatient basis. Individual therapy, group therapy, and self-help groups are among the most common treatment modalities. In addition, both clients and families can implement many self-care interventions to promote physical and emotional well-being.

5.1.5. Mental Health Promotion

Many of the traumatic life events that have the potential to cause mental health issues are unavoidable. Natural catastrophes like hurricanes and earthquakes are uncontrollable by humans. Additionally, not all man-made traumatic events can be avoided' trauma has been experienced by people while out shopping, watching a movie, or engaging in any other routine daily activity. Dealing with trauma effectively as soon as it occurs is one of the best ways to prevent pathologic reactions to trauma. Counselors are frequently on hand in addition to first responders in the event of a disaster to assist individuals in processing their emotional and behavioral reactions.

Some people find it easier to talk about difficult, distressing, or overwhelming experiences and to express their feelings. They might do this in the company of friends, family, or experts. Some people find it harder to be vulnerable and share their innermost thoughts. They are more prone to downplay emotions, downplay the significance of the incident, or declare, "I'm fine' I'm over it". They raise the possibility of developing issues like PTSD in the future by doing that. Having a precise diagnosis of PTSD is crucial. Whereas PTSD develops gradually, stress that arises right after an incident is known as an acute stress disorder. Some people claim to be "having PTSD," but they actually self-diagnose. They could be experiencing grief, autism spectrum disorder, or any number of other issues. A precise, expert diagnosis is the only thing that allows for effective treatment.

5.2. Dissociative Disorders

Dissociation is a subconscious defense mechanism that helps a person prevent their emotional self from fully realizing the impact of a terrifying or traumatic event by enabling their mind to block out or forget the upsetting circumstance or memory. Dissociation may happen during or following the incident. Dissociating gets easier with practice, just like any other protective coping strategy. A disruption in the typically integrated functions of identity, consciousness, memory, or environmental perception is a fundamental feature of dissociative disorders. This frequently makes it difficult for the individual to maintain relationships, go about their everyday lives, and deal with the consequences of the traumatic or abusive experience. People experience this disturbance at varying degrees of intensity, and it can start suddenly or gradually, temporarily or permanently. According to Lowenstein, Frewen, and Lewis-Fernandez (2017), clients with PTSD experience dissociative symptoms.

- **Dissociative Amnesia:** The client cannot remember important personal information (usually of a traumatic or stressful nature). This category includes a fugue experience where the client suddenly moves to a new geographic location with no memory of past events and often the assumption of a new identity.
- **Dissociative Identity Disorder (Formerly Multiple Personality Disorder):** The client displays two or more distinct identities or personality states that recurrently take control of his or her behavior. This is accompanied by the inability to recall important personal information.
- **Depersonalization/Derealization Disorder:** The client has a persistent or recurrent feeling of being detached from his or her mental processes or body

(depersonalization) or the sensation of being in a dream-like state in which the environment seems foggy or unreal (derealization). The client is not psychotic nor out of touch with reality.

Dissociative disorders are comparatively uncommon in the general population, but they are far more common in people who experienced physical and/or sexual abuse as children. Some people think that because mental health professionals are becoming more aware of dissociative disorders, there has been a recent rise in the diagnosis of these disorders in the US. Psychiatrists who specialize in the diagnosis of dissociative identity disorder disagree about whether it is a valid diagnosis.

The idea that abuse victims have repressed memories has received a lot of attention from the media. Many experts think that victims of childhood abuse can be assisted in recovering from or remembering such traumatic experiences, even though the memories may be repressed or buried deep in the subconscious mind because they are too painful for the victims to acknowledge. A mental health professional may assist a person in recalling or recovering memories of abuse if they are experiencing severe relationship difficulties, PTSD symptoms, or abuse-related flashbacks. There is a risk in psychotherapy, according to some mental health professionals, of creating false memories of childhood sexual abuse through imagination. Families have experienced issues as a result of this so-called false memory syndrome when clients have leveled unfounded allegations of abuse. However, there is a concern that those who experienced childhood abuse may be less inclined to disclose their past because they believe no one will listen to them. Other therapists contend that individuals diagnosed with dissociative identity disorder are experiencing intrusive thoughts and feelings, anxiety, and terror and should be helped' therefore, the therapist should maintain an open mind regarding the diagnosis.

5.2.1. Treatment and Interventions

Dissociative disorder survivors who have experienced abuse are frequently enrolled in community-based group or individual therapy programs to address the lasting effects of their trauma. Reassociation, or reassembling consciousness, is the main goal of therapy for dissociative clients. Dissociative symptoms rooted in trauma are addressed by this specialized treatment. Reduction of symptoms, enhanced functional abilities, and improved quality of life are the objectives of therapy. Patients with dissociative disorders may receive symptomatic treatment, meaning they may be prescribed drugs for depression or anxiety, or both, depending on which symptoms are more severe.

5.2.1.1. Short Hospital Treatment for Survivors of Trauma and Abuse

Dissociative disorders and PTSD patients can be found in every setting of healthcare, including clinics and primary care offices. In acute care settings, the nurse is most likely to see these patients only when there are worries about their own safety or the safety of others, or when acute symptoms have become severe enough to require stabilization. Acute care patients typically receive short-term care before transitioning back to community-based therapy as soon as is practical.

5.2.2. Nursing Care Plan: For A Client with PTSD

5.2.2.1. Nursing Diagnosis

A persistent, maladaptive pattern of behavior following a traumatic event that threatened the person's wellbeing is known as post-trauma syndrome.

- 5.2.2.2. Assessment Data
- Flashbacks or reexperiencing the traumatic event(s);
- Nightmares or recurrent dreams of the event or other trauma;
- Sleep disturbances (e.g., insomnia, early awakening, or crying out in sleep);
- Depression;
- Denial of feelings or emotional numbness;
- Projection of feelings;
- Difficulty in expressing feelings;
- Anger (may not be overt);
- Guilt or remorse;
- Low self-esteem;
- Frustration and irritability;
- Anxiety, panic, or separation anxiety;
- Fears—may be displaced or generalized (as in fear of men by survivors who have been raped by men);
- Decreased concentration;
- Difficulty expressing love or empathy;
- Difficulty experiencing pleasure;
- Difficulty with interpersonal relationships, marital problems, and divorce;
- Abuse in relationships;
- Sexual problems;
- Substance use;
- Employment problems;
- Physical symptoms.

5.2.2.3. Expected Outcomes

- Immediate

The client will:

- Identify the traumatic event within 24 to 48 hours.
- Demonstrate decreased physical symptoms within 2 to 3 days.
- Verbalize the need to grieve loss(es) within 3 to 4 days.
- Establish an adequate balance of rest, sleep, and activity' for example, sleep at least 4 hours per night within 3 to 4 days.
- Demonstrate decreased anxiety, fear, guilt, and so forth within 4 to 5 days.
- Participate in a treatment program' for example, join in a group activity or talk with staff for at least 30 minutes twice a day within 4 to 5 days.

Stabilization

The client will

- Begin the grieving process' for example, talk with staff about grief-related feelings and acknowledge the loss or event.
- Express feelings directly and openly in nondestructive ways.
- Identify strengths and weaknesses realistically' for example, make a list of abilities and review with staff.
- Demonstrate an increased ability to cope with stress.
- Eliminate substance use.
- Verbalize knowledge of illness, treatment plan, or safe use of medications, if any.

Community

The client will:

- Demonstrate initial integration of the traumatic experience into his or her life outside the hospital.
- Identify a support system outside the treatment setting' for example, identify specific support groups, friends, or family, and establish contact.
- Implement plans for follow-up or ongoing therapy, if indicated' for example, identify a therapist and schedule an appointment before discharge.

5.2.2.4. Implementation

Nursing Interventions	Rationale
When you approach the client, be nonthreatening and professional.	The client's fears may be triggered by authority figures with different characteristics (e.g., gender and ethnicity).
Initially, assign the same staff members to the client if possible' try to respect the client's fears and feelings. Gradually increase the number and variety of staff members interacting with the client.	Limiting the number of staff members who interact with the client at first will facilitate familiarity and trust. The client may have strong feelings of fear or mistrust about working with staff members with certain characteristics. These feelings may have been reinforced in previous encounters with professionals and may interfere with the therapeutic relationship.
Educate yourself and other staff members about the client's experience and about posttraumatic behavior.	Learning about the client's experience will help prepare you for the client's feelings and the details of his or her experience.
Examine and remain aware of your own feelings regarding both the client's traumatic experience and his or her feelings and behavior. Talk with other staff members to work through your feelings.	Traumatic events engender strong feelings in others and may be quite threatening. You may be reminded of a related experience or of your own vulnerability, or issues related to sexuality, morality, safety, or well-being. It is essential that you remain aware of your feelings so that you do not unconsciously project feelings, avoid issues, or be otherwise nontherapeutic with the client.
Remain nonjudgmental in your interactions with the client.	It is important not to reinforce blame that the client may have internalized related to the experience.
Be consistent with the client' convey acceptance of him or her as a person while setting and maintaining limits regarding behaviors.	The client may test limits of the therapeutic relationship. Problems with acceptance, trust, or authority often occur with posttraumatic behavior.

Assess the client's history of substance use (information from significant others might be helpful)	Some clients may use substances to help repress (or release) emotions.
Be aware of the client's use or abuse of substances. Set limits and consequences for this behavior' it may be helpful to allow the client or group to have input into these decisions.	Substance use undermines therapy and may endanger the client's health. Allowing input from the client or group may minimize power struggles.
If substance use is a major problem, refer the client to a substance-dependent treatment program.	Substance use must be dealt with because it may affect all other areas of the client's life.
Encourage the client to talk about his or her experience(s)' be accepting and nonjudgmental of the client's accounts and perceptions.	Retelling the experience can help the client identify the reality of what has happened and help identify and work through related feelings.
Encourage the client to express his or her feelings through talking, writing, crying, or other ways in which the client is comfortable.	Identification and expression of feelings are central to the grieving process.
Especially encourage the expression of anger, guilt, and rage.	These feelings often occur in clients who have experienced trauma. The client may feel survivor's guilt that he or she survived when others did not or guilt about the behavior he or she undertook to survive (killing others in combat, enduring a rape, or not saving others).
Give the client positive feedback for expressing feelings and sharing experiences' remain nonjudgmental toward the client.	The client may feel that he or she is burdening others with his or her problems. It is important not to reinforce the client's internalized blame.
Teach the client and the family or significant others about posttraumatic behavior and treatment.	Knowledge about posttraumatic behavior may help alleviate anxiety or guilt and may increase hope for recovery.
Help the client learn and practice stress management and relaxation techniques, assertiveness, self-defense training, or other skills as appropriate.	The client's traumatic experience may have resulted in a loss of or decrease in self-confidence, sense of safety, or ability to deal with stress.

As tolerated, encourage the client to share his or her feelings and experiences in group therapy, in a support group related to posttrauma, or with other clients informally.	The client needs to know that his or her feelings are acceptable to others and can be shared. Peer or support groups can offer understanding, support, and the opportunity for sharing experiences.
If the client has a religious or spiritual orientation, referral to a member of the clergy or a chaplain may be appropriate.	Guilt and forgiveness are often religious or spiritual issues for the client.
Encourage the client to make realistic plans for the future, integrating his or her traumatic experience.	Integrating traumatic experiences and making future plans are important resolution steps in the grief process.
Talk with the client about employment, job-related stress, and so forth. Refer the client to vocational services as needed.	Problems with employment frequently occur in clients with posttraumatic issues.
Help the client arrange for follow-up therapy as needed.	Recovering from trauma may be a long-term process. Follow-up therapy can offer continuing support in the client's recovery.
Encourage the client to identify relationships, or social or recreational situations that have been positive in the past.	The client may have withdrawn from social relationships and interest in recreational activities are common following trauma.
Encourage the client to pursue past relationships, personal interests, hobbies, or recreational activities that were positive in the past or that may appeal to the client.	The client may be reluctant to reach out to someone with whom he or she has had limited contact recently, and may benefit from encouragement to do so. Recreational activities can serve as a structure for the client to build social interactions as well as provide enjoyment.
Encourage the client to identify and contact supportive resources in the community or on the internet.	Many community or internet resources can be helpful to clients with PTSD and to their families or significant others.

Source: Adapted from Schultz, J. M., & Videbeck, S. L. (2013). Lippincott's manual of psychiatric nursing care plans (9th ed.). Philadelphia, PA: Lippincott Williams & Wilkins.

5.3. The Nursing Process

5.3.1. Assessment

The client's medical history indicates that there has been past trauma or abuse. It could be abuse experienced as a child or in a recent or ongoing relationship. In individual psychotherapy sessions, a thorough discussion of the actual abuse is typically conducted instead of the client reliving specific events of the abuse or trauma. This is generally not necessary or desirable.

5.3.1.1. General Appearance and Motor Behavior

The client's overall appearance and motor behavior are evaluated by the nurse. The client frequently exhibits hyperalert behavior, exhibiting a startled reaction to even tiny environmental noises. If the nurse approaches him or her too closely, he or she might feel uneasy and might need more space or privacy than the average person. The client may exhibit signs of anxiety or agitation, find it difficult to remain still, and frequently need to pace or move around the room. The client may occasionally sit motionless, appearing to curl up with their arms around their knees.

5.3.1.2. Mood and Affect

The nurse must keep in mind that a wide range of emotions, from passivity to anger, can be experienced when assessing mood and affect. Depending on what happened to them, the client may appear scared, agitated, or hostile. The client looks scared and may cry, scream, try to hide, or flee when they have a flashback. The client may speak in a different tone of voice or have a vacant stare when they are dissociating. The client might express extreme rage, anger, or a sense of being dead inside while being unable to name any other emotions.

5.3.1.3. Thought Process and Content

The nurse probes for content and thought processes. Clients who have experienced abuse or trauma report experiencing flashbacks or nightmares that bring back the trauma. The client experiences difficulty thinking about other things or focusing on day-to-day activities due to intrusive, persistent thoughts about the trauma. A few clients report hearing voices in their heads or experiencing hallucinations. Suicidal thoughts and urges are also frequent, as are self-destructive thoughts and behaviors. A number of clients report having fantasies about getting even with their abusers.

5.3.1.4. Sensorium and Intellectual Processes

The nurse typically observes that the client is aware of reality during the sensorium and intellectual processes assessment, unless the client is going through a dissociative episode or flashback. The client might not reply to the nurse during those encounters or might not be able to speak at all. Additionally, the nurse might discover that patients who have experienced abuse or trauma have memory gaps—a period of time for which they are unable to recall specific details. These intervals, which can be brief or long, are typically connected to the time of the trauma or abuse. Distracting thoughts or thoughts of self-harm frequently make it difficult for the client to focus or pay attention.

5.3.1.5. Judgment and Insight

The length of the client's dissociation or PTSD issues is frequently correlated with their level of insight. In the early stages of treatment, the client might not know much about how his or her current symptoms and issues relate to prior trauma. If they have advanced in their treatment, other clients might be highly informed. The client may have trouble deciding what to do or coming up with solutions.

5.3.1.6. Self-Concept

These clients probably have low self-esteem, the nurse will discover. They might think that they are horrible people who inadvertently cause or deserve the abuse. Many clients feel that because of their abusive experiences, they are damaged or undeserving and will never be valuable or worthwhile. Customers might think they're going insane, that they're out of control, and that there's no way back. It's possible for clients to feel worthless, hopeless, and powerless.

5.3.1.7. Roles and Relationships

The majority of clients say they struggle greatly in all kinds of relationships. Issues with authority figures frequently result in issues at work, such as the inability to follow instructions or have someone else keep an eye on performance. Because of the client's severely compromised ability to trust others, close relationships are either impossible or very difficult. The client is frequently divorced from family members and has either quit or been fired. The client may find it difficult to socialize with friends or family due to intrusive thoughts, flashbacks, or dissociative episodes, and avoidant behavior may prevent the client from attending family or social gatherings.

5.3.1.8. Physiologic Considerations

The majority of clients say that nightmares or anxiety related to having nightmares keep them from sleeping. It's also typical to overeat or not feel like eating. These clients often try to block out disturbing memories or thoughts by using alcohol or other drugs to help them fall asleep.

5.3.2. Data Analysis

Nursing diagnoses commonly used in the acute care setting when working with clients who dissociate or have PTSD related to trauma or abuse include:

- Risk of self-Mutilation;
- Risk of Suicide;
- Ineffective Coping;
- Posttrauma Response;
- Chronic Low Self-Esteem;
- Powerlessness.

In addition, the following nursing diagnoses may be pertinent to clients over longer periods, although not all diagnoses apply to each client:

- Disturbed Sleep Pattern;
- Sexual Dysfunction;
- Rape-Trauma Syndrome;
- Spiritual Distress;
- Social Isolation.

5.3.3. Outcome Identification

Treatment outcomes for clients who have survived trauma or abuse may include:

- The client will be physically safe.
- The client will distinguish between ideas of self-harm and taking action on those ideas.
- The client will demonstrate healthy, effective ways of dealing with stress.
- The client will express emotions nondestructively.
- The client will establish a social support system in the community.

5.3.4. Intervention

5.3.4.1. Promoting the Client's Safety

The security of the client comes first. The nurse must continuously evaluate the client's risk of suicide or self-harm and adjust their care accordingly. When the client is unable to provide safety measures, the nurse and treatment team must step in. The client needs to start managing safety needs as soon as possible in order to increase their sense of personal control. The nurse can discuss with the patient the distinction between thinking about harming oneself and acting on those thoughts' the patient does not have to act on these thoughts just because they are present. The nurse can gradually assist the patient in learning to cope with the thoughts until their intensity lessens.

5.3.5. Nursing Interventions

5.3.5.1. Promote Client's Safety

- Discuss self-harm thoughts.
- Help the client develop a plan for going to a safe place when having destructive thoughts or impulses.

5.3.5.2. Help Client Cope with Stress and Emotions

- Use grounding techniques to help client who is dissociating or experiencing flashbacks.
- Validate client's feelings of fear, but try to increase contact with reality.
- During dissociative experience or flashback, help the client change body position, but do not grab or force the client to stand up or move.
- Use supportive touch if the client responds well to it.
- Teach deep breathing and relaxation techniques.
- Use distraction techniques such as participating in physical exercise, listening to music, talking with others, or engaging in a hobby or other enjoyable activity.
- Help to make a list of activities and keep materials on hand to engage the client when the client's feelings are intense.

5.3.5.3. Help Promote Client's Self-Esteem

- Refer to the client as "survivor" rather than "victim."
- Establish a social support system in the community.
- Make a list of people and activities in the community for the client to contact when he or she needs help.

To calm down and wait for destructive thoughts and impulses to pass, the nurse can assist the client in learning how to find a safe place to retreat to when they arise. This could initially just entail sitting next to the nurse or in a group. Afterwards, the client can locate a small room or closet in their house that they feel comfortable being in. For comfort, the client might want to keep pillows and blankets there, and pictures or a tape recording could be useful as a reminder of the present.

5.3.5.4. Helping the Client Cope with Stress and Emotions

When a client is dissociating or going through a flashback, grounding techniques can be useful. By using grounding techniques, the client is reminded that they are safe, mature, and in the present moment. "I know this is frightening, but you are safe now," is a crucial way to validate the client's feelings during these experiences. "

In addition, the nurse can increase contact with reality and diminish the dissociative experience by helping the client focus on what he or she is currently experiencing through the senses:

- "What are you feeling?"
- "Are you hearing something?"
- "What are you touching?"
- "Can you see me and the room we're in?"

- "Do you feel your feet on the floor?"
- "Do you feel your arm on the chair?"
- "Do you feel the watch on your wrist?"

For the client experiencing dissociative symptoms, the nurse can use grounding techniques to focus the client on the present. For example, the nurse approaches the client and speaks in a calm reassuring tone. First, the nurse calls the client by name and then introduces him or herself by name and role. If the area is dark, the nurse turns on the lights. He or she can reorient the client by saying the following:

"Hello, Janet, I'm here with you. My name is Sheila. I'm the nurse working with you today. Today is Wednesday, September 18, 2019. You're here in the hospital. This is your room at the hospital. Can you open your eyes and look at me? Janet, my name is Sheila."

The nurse repeats this reorienting information as needed. Asking the client to look around the room encourages the client to move his or her eyes and avoid being locked in a daze or flashback.

The nurse urges the patient to switch positions as soon as possible. The client often curls up in a defensive position during a flashback. To help the client overcome the dissociative or flashback experience, get them to stand and move around. The client can now concentrate on moving his or her feet across the floor or swinging their arms. It is forbidden for the nurse to grab the patient or make any attempt to make them stand up or move. When a client has a flashback, they could react to the attempts by acting defensively or aggressively, possibly even attacking the nurse. To determine whether using touch is helpful for a client, the nurse should ideally ask how the client reacts to touch when dissociating or having a flashback before one happens. In addition, the nurse might ask the patient to touch her arm. Supportive touch is advantageous for the client if they comply.

A lot of clients struggle to recognize or measure the strength of their emotions. They might also say that sudden, strong emotions strike without warning. With the use of a journal or log, the nurse can assist patients in connecting with their emotions. Initially, clients might choose to select the emotion that most closely aligns with their experience by using a "feelings list". The client is encouraged by the nurse to record their feelings on paper at predetermined times during the day, such as every 30 minutes. Following the identification of their emotions, clients can rate each feeling on a scale from 1 to 10, for example, to determine how strong those emotions are. Through the use of this process, clients become more conscious of their emotions and their varying intensities' this is a crucial step in the management and expression of those emotions.

Clients can start looking for triggers, or feelings that come before flashbacks or dissociative episodes, after they have identified feelings and their intensities. Next, in order to lessen or prevent these episodes, clients can start using grounding techniques. To help them deal with the emotions, they can practice deep breathing and relaxation, pay attention to environmental stimuli or sensory data, or find constructive diversion. Exercise, listening to music, conversing with people, and partaking in hobbies or other pastimes are a few examples of such distractions. Once clients have determined which distractions are most effective for them, they should write them down and keep the list and the supplies needed for the activities handy. When severe emotions start to surface, clients can refer to the list and take one of several actions, like reading a book, listening to a tape, or drawing.

5.3.5.5. Helping Promote the Client's Self-Esteem

Instead of seeing the client as a victim, it is frequently helpful to see them as a survivor of trauma or abuse. It helps these clients shift their perspective from being victims to survivors because they may feel helpless and powerless over the circumstances. By identifying as survivors, they enable themselves to believe that they are resilient enough to endure their experiences. Seeing oneself as a victim is not as empowering as this perception.

5.3.5.6. Establishing Social Support

The client must locate community resources or activities. The client can compile a list of supporters with the assistance of the nurse. Stress makes it harder for these clients to solve problems, so having a prepared list reduces uncertainty or anxiety. Included on this list should be a local crisis hotline that the client can contact if they have thoughts or urges to harm themselves, as well as friends or family to contact in times of loneliness or depression. Additionally, the client can pinpoint neighborhood clubs or activities that offer a change of pace and an opportunity to leave the house. Establishing community supports is necessary for the client to lessen their reliance on medical professionals. Contacting the Department of Health and Human Services or the county or city mental health services will help you find local support groups. The internet offers a wide range of support groups that are both in-person and virtual.

5.3.6. Evaluation

For patients who have endured trauma or abuse, long-term treatment results could take several years to attain. These clients typically make slow but steady progress in learning self-defense techniques, stress and emotion management skills, and day-to-day living skills. Even though individuals learn to control their emotions and reactions, trauma and abuse can have long-lasting, profound effects.

5.4. Anxiety as a Response To Stress

Stress is the physical deterioration brought on by life (Selye, 1956). It happens when someone finds it difficult to manage goals, challenges, and life circumstances. Everybody responds to stress differently' while some people thrive in certain circumstances, others find them to be extremely distressing. For instance, public speaking is often associated with fear, but for educators and performers, it's a common and joyful experience. Among the things that can cause stress are getting married, having kids, flying, snakes, starting a new job or school, and moving away from home.

The physiological components of stress were recognized by endocrinologist Hans Selye (1956, 1974), who named this condition "general adaptation syndrome". The stages of the body's physical reactions to pain, heat, toxins, and restraint, as well as the mind's emotional reactions to actual or imagined stressors, were all measured by him using laboratory animals. He identified three stages of stress reactions:

- In the alarm reaction stage, stress stimulates the body to send messages from the hypothalamus to the glands (such as the adrenal gland, to send out adrenaline and norepinephrine for fuel) and organs (such as the liver, to reconvert glycogen stores to glucose for food) to prepare for potential defense needs.
- In the resistance stage, the digestive system reduces function to shunt blood to areas needed for defense. The lungs take in more air, and

the heart beats faster and harder so that it can circulate this highly oxygenated and highly nourished blood to the muscles to defend the body by fight, flight, or freeze behaviors. If the person adapts to the stress, the body's responses relax, and the gland, organ, and systemic responses abate.

- The exhaustion stage occurs when the person has responded negatively to anxiety and stress' body stores are depleted or the emotional components are not resolved, resulting in continual arousal of the physiological responses and little reserve capacity.

Responses of the autonomic nervous system to anxiety and fear cause the body to engage in involuntary self-preservation behaviors. At the first sign of danger, sympathetic nerve fibers "charge up" the vital signs to get the body ready for defense. In addition to constricting peripheral vessels, diverting blood from the gastrointestinal (GI) and reproductive systems, and increasing glycogenolysis to release glucose for energy for the heart, muscles, and central nervous system, the adrenal glands release adrenaline, also known as adrenaline (epinephrine), which causes the body to absorb more oxygen, dilate the pupils, and increase arterial pressure and heart rate. Parasympathetic nerve fibers stop this process once the threat has passed, allowing the body to function normally until the next threat triggers sympathetic reactions again.

Symptoms of anxiety include elevated vital signs, difficulty thinking logically, and agitated motor activity. Anxiety also causes uncomfortable cognitive, psychomotor, and physiological reactions. The person attempts to adopt new adaptive behaviors or defense mechanisms in an attempt to lessen the degree of discomfort in order to lessen these unpleasant feelings. Positive adaptive behaviors can aid in learning. Some examples include practicing sequential body relaxation from head to toe, breathing slowly and steadily to lower stress levels in the muscles, and using visualization techniques to draw attention back to a pleasant scene. Pain syndromes, tension headaches, and stress-related reactions are examples of maladaptive behaviors that can arise from negative reactions to anxiety and lower immune system effectiveness.

Anxiety can be expressed to others both orally and nonverbally. When someone yells "fire," those in the vicinity may start to get nervous as they imagine a fire and the potential threat it poses. Seeing a distressed parent in a mall searching for their missing child can make others anxious because they can only imagine the fear and panic the parent is going through. By empathy—the ability to temporarily put oneself in another person's shoes—they can communicate their feelings of anxiety without using words (Sullivan, 1952). Examples of nonverbal empathetic communication include when a nurse reads a client's cry for assistance, when a patient feels the tension in a room where two people have been fighting and are now not speaking to each other, or when the family of a patient undergoing surgery can deduce the death of their loved one from the doctor's body language.

5.4.1. Levels of Anxiety

Depending on the level and duration of the anxiety as well as the individual's ability to manage it, anxiety can have both beneficial and detrimental effects. There are four stages of anxiety: panic, moderate, severe, and mild. Every level modifies the person's physiology as well as their emotions (Table 5.1).

Table 5.1. Levels of Anxiety

<table>
<tr><th>Anxiety Level</th><th>Psychological Responses</th><th>Physiological Responses</th></tr>
<tr><td>Mild</td><td>Wide perceptual field
Sharpened senses
Increased motivation
Effective problem-solving
Increased learning ability
Irritability</td><td>Restlessness
Fidgeting
GI "butterflies"
Difficulty sleeping
Hypersensitivity to noise</td></tr>
<tr><td>Moderate</td><td>Perceptual field narrowed to immediate task
Selectively attentive
Cannot connect thoughts or events independently
Increased use of automatisms</td><td>Muscle tension
Diaphoresis
Pounding pulse
Headache
Dry mouth
High voice pitch
Faster rate of speech
GI upset
Frequent urination</td></tr>
<tr><td>Severe</td><td>Perceptual field reduced to one detail or scattered details
Cannot complete tasks
Cannot solve problems or learn effectively
Behavior geared toward anxiety relief and is usually ineffective
Doesn't respond to redirection
Feels awe, dread, or horror
Cries
Ritualistic behavior</td><td>Severe headache
Nausea, vomiting, and diarrhea
Trembling
Rigid stance
Vertigo
Pale
Tachycardia
Chest pain</td></tr>
<tr><td>Panic</td><td>Perceptual field reduced to focus on self
Cannot process any environmental stimuli
Distorted perceptions
Loss of rational thought
Doesn't recognize potential danger
Can't communicate verbally
Possible delusions and hallucination
May be suicidal</td><td>May bolt and run or totally immobile and mute
Dilated pupils
Increased blood pressure and pulse
Flight, fight, or freeze</td></tr>
</table>

Source: https://tms.iau.ir/file/download/download/1660127163-psychiatric-mental-health-nursing-8th-edition-2020-.pdf.

5.4.2. Levels of anxiety

5.4.2.1. Mild Anxiety

The feeling that something is unusual and needs extra care is known as mild anxiety. Increased sensory stimulation aids in concentration, which is necessary for learning, problem-solving, thinking, acting, feeling, and self-defense. People with mild anxiety are frequently inspired to make changes or take part in goal-directed activities. For instance, it aids pupils in maintaining concentration when preparing for a test.

5.4.2.2. Moderate Anxiety

A person experiencing moderate anxiety feels uneasy and agitated as if there is a clear problem. With the help of others, an individual experiencing moderate anxiety can still process information, work through issues, and pick up new skills. Although he or she can be directed to the topic, they struggle to focus on their own. For instance, the nurse may be providing preoperative instructions to a patient who is nervous about the impending surgery. The client's focus may stray while the nurse is instructing, but the nurse can pull the client back on track by guiding him or her. Severe anxiety and panic lead to a decline in cognitive abilities, the emergence of defensive reactions, and the use of more rudimentary survival skills. Severe anxiety impairs one's ability to reason and think clearly. Vital indicators rise as muscles tense. The person pacing, restless, agitated, and angry, or employing other comparable emotional–psychomotor ways to let go of pent-up tension. Panic is primarily an emotional-psychomotor state with corresponding freeze, flight, or fight responses. An adrenaline rush significantly raises vital signs. The only cognitive process concentrates on the individual's defense, and pupils enlarge to allow in more light.

5.4.3. Working with Anxious Clients

In a range of settings, including emergency rooms, intensive care units (ICUs), offices, and clinics, nurses deal with nervous patients and their families. The nurse's primary responsibility is to determine the patient's level of anxiety as it dictates the most likely interventions. Moderate anxiety benefits the client and doesn't need direct assistance. Even those with mild anxiety are eager to learn new things and are capable of solving problems. When a client experiences mild anxiety, teaching can be beneficial. When a client exhibits moderate anxiety, the nurse needs to make sure the client is listening to her instructions. Over time, the client may experience some difficulty focusing and their attention may wander. It works well for the nurse to speak in short, clear, and understandable sentences' however, she must pause occasionally to make sure the client is still processing the information correctly. If the patient veers off topic, the nurse might have to bring them back on track. Severe anxiety makes it impossible for the client to focus or process information. Before doing anything further, the nurse's objective must be to bring the patient's anxiety down to a moderate or mild level. Staying with the person is also crucial because leaving them alone is likely to make their anxiety worse. It can be beneficial to speak with the client in a soft, soothing voice. Walking alongside the person while conversing can be beneficial if they are unable to remain still. It doesn't really matter what the nurse says—what matters is how they say it. Taking even, deep breaths with the person can help reduce anxiety.

The person's safety is the main priority when experiencing panic anxiety. He or she might not be able to think rationally and is incapable of sensing possible harm. Even though the client is unable to comprehend what the nurse is saying, the nurse must continue to speak to them in a consoling way. Visiting a small, calm, and unstimulating place could aid in lowering anxiety. The nurse can comfort the patient, telling them that they are in a safe place and that this is just anxiety that will pass. The client should stay under the nurse's care until the panic subsides. The duration of panic-level anxiety varies, ranging from five to thirty minutes. The nurse needs to be conscious of their own level of anxiety when working with someone who is nervous. The nurse can easily start to feel more and more nervous. To effectively work with the client, the nurse must maintain composure and control. Anxiolytic drugs can be used to treat transient anxiety. Benzodiazepines, which are often prescribed for anxiety, make up the majority of these medications.

Table 5.2. *Anxiolytic Drugs*

Generic (Trade) Name	Speed of Onset	Half-Life (Hours)	Side Effects	Nursing Implications
Benzodiazepines				
Diazepam (Valium) Alprazolam (Xanax)	Fast	20–100	Dizziness, clumsiness, sedation, headache, fatigue, sexual dysfunction, blurred vision, dry throat and mouth, constipation, high potential for abuse and dependence	Avoid other CNS depressants, such as antihistamines and alcohol. Avoid caffeine. Take care with potentially hazardous activities, such as driving. Rise slowly from lying or sitting position. Use sugar-free beverages or hard candy. Drink adequate fluids. Take only as prescribed. Do not stop taking the drug abruptly.
Alprazolam (Xanax)	Intermediate	6–12		
Chlordiazepoxide (Librium)	Intermediate	5–30		
Lorazepam (Ativan)	Intermediate	10–20		
Clonazepam (Klonopin)	Slow	18–50		
Oxazepam (Serax)	Slow	4–15		
Nonbenzodiazepines				
Buspirone (BuSpar)	Very slow		Dizziness, restlessness, agitation, drowsiness, headache, weakness, nausea, vomiting, paradoxical excitement or euphoria	Rise slowly from sitting position. Take care with potentially hazardous activities, such as driving. Take with food. Report persistent restlessness, agitation, excitement, or euphoria to physician.
Meprobamate (Miltown,	Rapid			

Source: https://tms.iau.ir/file/download/download/1660127163-psychiatric-mental-health-nursing-8th-edition-2020-.pdf.

However, because of their high potential for abuse and dependence, benzodiazepines should only be used for brief periods of time—no more than four to six weeks. These medications are intended to reduce anxiety so that the patient can handle the stressful event or crisis more skillfully. Unfortunately, a lot of people continue to use these medications as a "cure" for anxiety rather than changing their behavior or acquiring better-coping mechanisms (Table 5.2).

5.4.4. Stress-Related Illness

A wide range of illnesses that are brought on by or make worse by persistent, unresolved stress are collectively referred to as stress-related illnesses. Eating disorders like bulimia and anorexia nervosa can be brought on by repressed chronic stress. If left untreated, traumatic stressors can result in PTSD at a later time or a brief, acute stress reaction. Somatic symptom disorders are physical symptoms caused by untreated or suppressed stress that do not correspond to an actual organic disease. In addition, a lot of medical conditions, including ulcerative colitis and hypertension, can have their symptoms made worse by stress. Anxiety disorder can also be attributed to persistent or recurrent anxiety brought on by stress.

5.5. Overview of Anxiety Disorders

When anxiety stops serving as a warning sign or a catalyst for necessary change and instead develops into a chronic condition that affects a significant portion of a person's life and leads to emotionally crippling behaviors and maladaptive behaviors, it is diagnosed as an anxiety disorder. Anxiety is the fundamental component of all anxiety disorders, despite their wide range of expressions. Types of anxiety disorders include the following:

- Agoraphobia;
- Panic Disorder;
- Specific Phobia;
- Social Anxiety Disorder (Social Phobia);
- Generalized Anxiety Disorder (GAD).

5.5.1. Nursing Care Plan: Anxious Behavior

5.5.1.1. Nursing Diagnosis

A vague feeling of dread or apprehension in response to external or internal stimuli resulting in emotional, physical, cognitive, and/or behavioral symptoms

5.5.1.2. Assessment Data

- Decreased Attention Span;
- Restlessness, Irritability;
- Poor Impulse Control;
- Feelings of Discomfort, Apprehension, or Helplessness;

- Hyperactivity, Pacing;
- Wringing Hands;
- Perceptual Field Deficits;
- Decreased Ability to Communicate Verbally.

5.5.1.3. Expected Outcomes

- Immediate

The client will:

- Be free from injury throughout hospitalization.
- Discuss feelings of dread, anxiety, and so forth within 24 to 48 hours.
- Respond to relaxation techniques with staff assistance and demonstrate a decreased anxiety level within 2 to 3 days.
- Stabilization

The client will

- Demonstrate the ability to perform relaxation techniques.
- Reduce own anxiety level without staff assistance.

Community

The client will

- Be free from anxiety attacks.
- Manage the anxiety response to stress effectively.

5.5.1.4. Implementation

Nursing Interventions	Rationale
Remain with the client at all times when levels of anxiety are high (severe or panic).	The client's safety is a priority. A highly anxious client should not be left alone' his or her anxiety will escalate.
Move the client to a quiet area with minimal or decreased stimuli such as a small room or seclusion area.	Anxious behavior can be escalated by external stimuli. In a large area, the client can feel lost and panicky, but a smaller room can enhance a sense of security.
PRN medications may be indicated for high levels of anxiety, delusions, disorganized thoughts, and so forth.	Medication may be necessary to decrease anxiety to a level at which the client can feel safe.
Remain calm in your approach to the client.	The client will feel more secure if you are calm and if the client feels you are in control of the situation.
Use short, simple, and clear statements.	The client's ability to deal with abstractions or complexity is impaired.

Avoid asking or forcing the client to make choices.	The client may not make sound decisions or may be unable to make decisions or solve problems.
Be aware of your own feelings and level of discomfort.	Anxiety is communicated interpersonally. Being with an anxious client can raise your own anxiety level.
Encourage the client's participation in relaxation exercises such as deep breathing, progressive muscle relaxation, meditation, and imagining being in a quiet, peaceful place.	Relaxation exercises are effective, nonchemical ways to reduce anxiety.
Teach the client to use relaxation techniques independently.	Using relaxation techniques can give the client confidence in having control over anxiety.
Help the client see that mild anxiety can be a positive catalyst for change and does not need to be avoided.	useful.
Encourage the client to identify and pursue relationships, personal interests, hobbies, or recreational activities that may appeal to the client.	The client's anxiety may have prevented him or her from engaging in relationships or activities recently, but these can be helpful in building confidence and having a focus on something other than anxiety.
Encourage the client to identify supportive resources in the community or on the internet.	Supportive resources can assist the client in the ongoing management of his or her anxiety and decrease social isolation.

Source: Adapted from Schultz, J. M., & Videbeck, S. L. (2013). Lippincott's Manual of Psychiatric Care Plans (9th ed.). Philadelphia, PA: Lippincott Williams & Wilkins.

The most prevalent of these, panic disorder, is the subject of this chapter. In many of the other anxiety disorders, severe or panic-like episodes can occur during times of extreme stress.

5.5.2. Incidence

Out of all mental disorders, anxiety disorders are most prevalent in adults and children in the United States. The prevalence of anxiety disorders in young people is comparable to that of nearly one in four adults in the United States. Women, those under 45, those who have recently separated or divorced, and those from lower socioeconomic backgrounds are more likely to suffer from anxiety disorders.

5.5.3. Related Disorders

When children who can speak are unable to communicate in social settings, it is known as selective mutism. They might not communicate with extended family or at school, but they might talk openly with their parents at home. Speech impairment affects both academic achievement and social communication. In these circumstances, social anxiety is highly prevalent.

When it is determined that the prominent symptoms of anxiety are caused directly by a physiological condition, anxiety disorder related to another medical condition is diagnosed. The individual may experience panic episodes, generalized anxiety, or compulsive behaviors. This disorder may be brought on by endocrine dysfunction, neurologic disorders, congestive heart failure, and chronic obstructive pulmonary disease.

Anxiety brought on directly by drug abuse, medication side effects, or exposure to toxins is known as substance- or medication-induced anxiety disorder. Prominent anxiety, panic attacks, phobias, obsessions, or compulsions are some of the symptoms. Medication-assisted treatment of anxiety disorders is only one aspect of the required strategy. It's critical to provide people with anxiety management skills and appropriate therapy referrals. Although it requires more effort and time to see the desired effects, this method is far more effective than medication alone. Excessive worry about being away from home or from loved ones—parents, caregivers, or other family members—is known as separation anxiety disorder. It happens before the age of eighteen and when it is no longer developmentally appropriate.

5.6. Etiology

5.6.1. Biologic Theories

5.6.1.1. Genetic Theories

First-degree relatives of clients with elevated anxiety have higher rates of developing anxiety, suggesting that anxiety may have an inherited component. Heritability refers to the proportion of a disorder that can be attributed to genetic factors:

- High heritabilities are greater than 0.6 and indicate that genetic influences dominate.
- Moderate heritabilities are 0.3 to 0.5 and suggest an even greater influence of genetic and non-genetic factors.
- Heritabilities less than 0.3 mean that genetics are negligible as a primary cause of the disorder.

There is a moderate heritability for panic disorder, social anxiety disorder, and particular phobias, such as agoraphobia. OCD and GAD are more likely to run in families, suggesting a significant genetic component, but more research is still needed. There is no straightforward Mendelian inheritance pattern for anxiety disorders. As of right now, research clearly points to a genetic predisposition or vulnerability for anxiety disorders' however, the actual development of these disorders requires the presence of other factors.

5.6.1.2. Neurochemical Theories

The amino acid neurotransmitter thought to be malfunctioning in anxiety disorders is gamma-aminobutyric acid (GABA). The body naturally combats anxiety through the inhibitory neurotransmitter GABA, which lowers cell excitability and, consequently, the rate of neuronal firing. One-third of nerve synapses have it, particularly those in the limbic system and the locus coeruleus, which is where norepinephrine, a neurotransmitter that stimulates cellular activity, is produced. Because norepinephrine increases anxiety and GABA decreases it, researchers think that anxiety disorders are caused by a disruption in the regulation of these neurotransmitters.

There are numerous subtypes of serotonin, an indolamine neurotransmitter that is frequently linked to mood disorders and psychosis. 5-Hydroxytryptamine type 1a influences aggression and mood in addition to contributing to anxiety. It is thought that serotonin has a specific function in GAD, OCD, and panic disorders. Excess norepinephrine is thought to be involved in PTSD, GAD, and panic disorders.

5.6.2. Psychodynamic Theories

5.6.2.1. Intrapsychic/Psychoanalytic Theories

According to Freud (1936), behavior is driven by an individual's innate anxiety. He defined defense mechanisms as an individual's effort to manage awareness of and lessen anxiety. Defense mechanisms are unconscious cognitive distortions that someone employs to reduce discomfort, deal with stress, and feel in control of a situation. Defense mechanisms are unconscious to the person because they come from the unconscious. Some individuals overuse their defense mechanisms, which prevents them from picking up useful skills for handling anxiety-inducing circumstances. Reliance on one or two defense mechanisms can also impede emotional development, result in subpar problem-solving abilities, and cause relationship problems.

5.6.2.2. Interpersonal Theory

According to Harry Stack Sullivan (1952), interpersonal relationship issues are what cause anxiety. Inadequate nurturing, agitation when holding or handling the child, and misinterpreted cues are some ways that caregivers can convey anxiety to babies or young children. Disruption, such as the inability to complete developmental tasks that are appropriate for one's age, can arise from this kind of expressed anxiety. Adults experience anxiety as a result of their desire to fit in with their cultural group's norms and values. The likelihood of developing anxiety disorders increases with anxiety level, as does one's capacity for problem-solving and communication. According to Hildegard Peplau (1952), a nurse can better assist a client in achieving health by attending to both the interpersonal and physiological domains in which humans exist. Based on Sullivan's interpersonal perspective of anxiety, she recognized the four stages of anxiety and created nursing interventions and interpersonal communication strategies. To establish and maintain the nurse-client relationship and to implement the nursing process, nurses now employ Peplau's interpersonal therapeutic communication techniques.

5.6.2.3. Behavioral Theory

According to behavioral theorists, anxiety is a skill that is acquired via experiences. On the other hand, novel experiences can cause people to "unlearn" or alter their behavior. Behaviorists think that without understanding the reasons behind maladaptive behaviors, people can change them. They argue that through repeated experiences under the supervision of a qualified therapist, troubling behaviors that arise and interfere with a person's life can be eliminated or unlearned.

5.6.3. Treatment

Medication and counseling are typically used in the treatment of anxiety disorders. According to Huppert and Foa (2017), this combination yields superior results than either one alone. Treating anxiety disorders with cognitive-behavioral therapy (CBT) has proven to be successful. Rephrasing negative messages into positive ones is known as positive reframing. The client learns from the therapist how to construct affirmations to utilize in times of panic. For instance, consider this instead of thinking, "My heart is racing. The client thinks, "I think I'm going to die, but I can handle this. This is nothing more than fear. It will disappear. The customer can jot down these notes and store them somewhere easy to find them, like in a wallet, calendar, or address book (Table 5.3).

When a therapist uses questions to assess a situation more realistically, it is known as decatastrophizing. "What is the worst thing that could happen? Is that likely? Could you survive that? Is that as bad as you imagine?" the therapist might ask. The client employs thought-stopping and distraction techniques to shake off unfavorable thoughts. Shouting, slapping a rubber band around the wrist, and sprinkling cold water on the face are a few ways to interrupt the negative thought pattern. A person can gain more control over life circumstances with the aid of assertiveness training. These methods support self-assurance and assist the person in navigating social situations. They entail expressing needs or concerns to others and identifying feelings through "I" statements. "I feel angry when you turn your back while I'm talking," "I would like to have an uninterrupted conversation about something important for five minutes," and "I would like to have about thirty minutes in the evening to relax without interruption" are a few examples."

Table 5.3. *Drugs Used to Treat Anxiety Disorders*

Generic (Trade) Drug Name	Classification	Used to Treat
Alprazolam (Xanax)	Benzodiazepine	Anxiety, panic disorder, social phobia, agoraphobia
Buspirone (BuSpar)	Nonbenzodiazepine anxiolytic	Anxiety, social phobia, GAD
Clorazepate (Tranxene)	Benzodiazepine	Anxiety
Chlordiazepoxide (Librium)	Benzodiazepine	Anxiety
Clonazepam (Klonopin)	Benzodiazepine	Anxiety, panic disorder
Clonidine (Catapres)	Beta-blocker	Anxiety, panic disorder
Diazepam (Valium)	Benzodiazepine	Anxiety, panic disorder
Fluoxetine (Prozac)	SSRI antidepressant	Panic disorder, GAD
Hydroxyzine (Vistaril, Atarax)	Antihistamine	Anxiety
Imipramine (Tofranil)	Tricyclic antidepressant	Anxiety, panic disorder, agoraphobia
Meprobamate (Miltown, Equanil)	Nonbenzodiazepine anxiolytic	Anxiety
Oxazepam (Serax)	Benzodiazepine	Anxiety
Paroxetine (Paxil)	SSRI antidepressant	Social phobia, GAD
Propranolol (Inderal)	Alpha-adrenergic agonist	Anxiety, panic disorder, GAD
Sertraline (Zoloft)	SSRI antidepressant	Panic disorder, social phobia, GAD

GAD, generalized anxiety disorder' SSRI, selective serotonin reuptake inhibitor.

Source: Sheila L. Videbeck, Psychiatric-Mental Health Nursing, ISBN-10: 1-975116-37-2.

5.6.4. Community-Based Care

Rather than inpatient settings, community settings are where nurses often come into contact with patients who have anxiety disorders. Formal treatment for these patients typically takes place in doctor's offices, community mental health clinics, psychiatric clinical specialists' offices, psychologists' offices, or other mental health counselors' offices. As the individual with anxiety disorder frequently assumes that the intermittent symptoms are caused by illness, the family doctor or advanced practice nurse may be the first medical professional to assess them. The nurse can better assist the client in receiving appropriate referrals for assessment, diagnosis, and treatment by knowing the community resources. For diagnosis, treatment, and medication, the nurse may recommend that the client see an advanced-practice psychiatric nurse or a psychiatrist. Additional community resources, like self-help or anxiety disorder support groups, can offer assistance and lessen the client's feelings of loneliness and isolation.

5.7. Mental Health Promotion

Anxiety is far too frequently seen negatively and avoided at all costs. In actuality, anxiety is often a sign that a person is not managing their stress well. A healthy way to handle the stress of everyday events is to learn to heed this warning and make the necessary changes. Life issues are not the only thing that cause stress and the anxiety that follows. Positive or desired events like moving away for college, landing your first job, getting married, and starting a family can be stressful and anxiety-inducing. Being healthy requires controlling the effects of stress and anxiety in one's life. Tips for managing stress include the following:

- Keep a positive attitude and believe in yourself.
- Accept there are events you cannot control.
- Communicate assertively with others: Talk about your feelings to others, and express your feelings through laughing, crying, and so forth.
- Learn to relax.
- Exercise regularly.
- Eat well-balanced meals.
- Limit intake of caffeine and alcohol.
- Get enough rest and sleep.
- Set realistic goals and expectations, and find a personally meaningful activity.
- Learn stress management techniques, such as relaxation, guided imagery, and meditation' practice them as part of your daily routine.

It is critical to stress that the goal for individuals with anxiety disorders is effective stress and anxiety management, not complete anxiety eradication. While medication plays a significant role in reducing excessive anxiety, the issue remains unresolved. Acquiring knowledge of anxiety management strategies and efficient coping mechanisms is crucial for enhancing life quality overall.

5.8. Panic Disorder

Discrete episodes of panic attacks, or 15 to 30 minutes of fast, intense, and intensifying anxiety during which the sufferer feels both extreme emotional fear and physical discomfort, are the components that make up panic disorder. An individual experiencing a panic attack typically experiences four or more of the following symptoms in addition to extremely high levels of anxiety: palpitations, sweating, trembling, shortness of breath, feeling as though they are being choked, nausea, abdominal discomfort, dizziness, paresthesias, chills, or hot flashes. A person is diagnosed with panic disorder if they experience frequent, unplanned panic attacks and then, for at least a month, they consistently worry about these attacks, their meaning, or any major behavioral changes they may cause. An environmental trigger-free initial attack occurs spontaneously in slightly over 75% of individuals with panic disorder. Agoraphobia coexists in half of cases of panic disorder. People who are single and have not completed their college education are more likely to suffer from panic disorder. Panic disorder sufferers are more likely to consider suicide. Research indicates that between 17% and 32% of people with panic disorder experience suicidal thoughts frequently, and one-third have attempted suicide before.

The late adolescent and mid-30s are the peak times for panic disorder onset. Panic disorder sufferers experience similar emotional and physiological reactions even in the absence of a life-threatening event, although panic anxiety may be normal in such cases. Avoidance behavior may result from the recall of the panic attack and the anxiety of experiencing another one. Sometimes the individual stays in a small area close to their home, like the block or the town limits, or they become housebound. This condition is called agoraphobia, which means "fear of the marketplace" or "fear of being outside". A panic attack could start as soon as they leave the house, which is why some agoraphobics are afraid to go outside the front door. Others who have a restricted area in which they feel safe from the anticipation of experiencing a panic attack can leave the house. Without panic episodes, agoraphobia can also manifest on its own.

The ideas of primary and secondary gain, which are connected to numerous anxiety disorders, are eloquently illustrated by the way agoraphobics behave. The primary benefit of engaging in a particular anxiety-driven behavior, like staying home to prevent the anxiety of leaving a safe place, is the relief of anxiety that is experienced. The attention one gets from others as a result of these behaviors is known as secondary gain. For instance, family members who also take on all of the duties of family life outside the home (such as work and shopping) may show the agoraphobic person attention and compassionate concern. In essence, the agoraphobic's self-imprisonment is made possible by these sympathetic significant others.

5.8.1. Treatment

Treatments for panic disorder include cognitive behavioral therapy (CBT), relaxation techniques, deep breathing, and prescription drugs like benzodiazepines, SSRIs, tricyclic antidepressants, and antihypertensives like propranolol (Inderal) and clonidine (Catapres).

5.8.2. The Nursing Process: Panic Disorder

After experiencing multiple panic attacks, the client typically seeks treatment for panic disorder. "I feel like I'm going crazy," the client might say. Although the doctor says it's anxiety, I thought I was having a heart attack. Usually, the client is unable to pinpoint a cause for these occurrences.

5.8.2.1. General Appearance and Motor Behavior

The client's overall appearance and motor behavior are evaluated by the nurse. If the client is worried about experiencing a panic attack in the near future, he or she may show no symptoms of anxiety or appear completely "normal". Anxious clients may speak more quickly, loudly, and with an increased pitch. They may also find it difficult to sit still in a chair. Automatisms are unconsciously performed, automatic behaviors that can be seen. Some examples are jingling keys, twisting hair, or tapping fingers. Automatisms are designed to reduce anxiety, and their frequency and intensity rise in proportion to the client's level of anxiety.

5.8.2.2. Mood and Affect

An evaluation of the client's mood and affect may indicate that they are tense, worried, depressed, serious, or melancholy. The client might become emotional when talking about the panic attacks. He or she might become upset with themselves for not being able to exercise self-control. The majority of clients are upset that anxiety attacks have entered their lives. The client may describe sensations of depersonalization (feeling cut off from oneself) or derealization (feeling as though something is not real) during a panic attack.

5.8.2.3. Thought Processes and Content

The client experiences overwhelming feelings during a panic attack, thinking they are losing control, dying, or "going insane". Even suicide may occur to the client. The client's capacity for rational thought is lost, and their thoughts become disorganized. At other times, the client might be preoccupied with anxiety over when or how to handle their next panic attack.

5.8.2.4. Sensorium and Intellectual Processes

A panic attack may cause the client to become disoriented and confused. He or she is unable to recognize cues from the surroundings and react correctly. The panic attack passes and these abilities return to normal.

5.8.2.5. Judgment and Insight

Panic attacks cause a person to lose their sense of judgment. In an attempt to flee, they may run out of a building and into the street in front of a speeding car before they can determine whether their safety has returned. It is only after the client has received education about panic disorder that they can gain insight into it. Even so, clients initially think they have no control over their anxiety attacks and are powerless.

5.8.2.6. Self-Concept

Nurses must evaluate their clients' self-concept when they suffer from panic disorder. These clients often express self-blame by saying things like, "I used to be a happy, well-adjusted person," or "I can't believe I'm so weak and out of control". They might have a poor opinion of themselves in every area of their lives. They might become paralyzed by fear of future attacks and find it impossible to perform many of the activities they used to be able to do before suffering from panic attacks.

5.8.2.7. Roles and Relationships

The patient may report changes in their social, professional, or familial lives due to the severe fear of experiencing another panic attack. People, places, and events linked to past panic attacks are usually avoided by the person. For example, if someone has experienced a panic attack on a bus, they might not be able to ride the bus anymore. The person may resort to even more drastic measures, like quitting work and staying at home, to avoid these objects, even though doing so does not stop the panic attacks. This is because they feel so powerless.

5.8.2.8. Physiological and Self-Care Concerns

The client frequently complains of difficulty eating and sleeping. Despite spending hours in bed, the fear and anxiety that follow a panic attack can prevent a person from getting enough good sleep. In an effort to reduce their anxiety, clients may lose their appetite or eat all the time.

5.8.2.9. Data Analysis

The following nursing diagnoses may apply to the client with panic disorder:

- Risk for injury;
- Anxiety;
- Situational low self-esteem (panic attacks);
- Ineffective coping;
- Powerlessness;
- Ineffective role performance;
- Disturbed sleep pattern.

5.8.2.10. Outcome Identification

Outcomes for clients with panic disorders include:

- The client will be free from injury.
- The client will verbalize feelings.
- The client will demonstrate the use of effective coping mechanisms.
- The client will demonstrate effective use of methods to manage anxiety response.
- The client will verbalize a sense of personal control.
- The client will reestablish adequate nutritional intake.
- The client will sleep at least 6 hours per night.

5.8.3. Intervention

5.8.3.1. Promoting Safety and Comfort

The nurse's top priorities when a client is having a panic attack are making sure they are in a safe space and protecting their privacy. The client should relocate to a less stimulating area if the current setting is too stimulating. A calm environment gives the client privacy and lessens anxiety. In addition to assessing the client's behaviors and concerns, the nurse stays with the client to assist in helping him or her relax. Once the client is focused, the nurse reassures him or her of their safety by speaking in a soothing, calm tone and providing brief instructions. Calm assurances and a composed attitude can ease nervousness. The nurse can reassure a client who feels out of control by stating that she is in charge until the client regains control.

5.8.3.2. Using Therapeutic Communication

A good rapport between the nurse and the client is crucial because patients with anxiety disorders can work with the nurse to plan and assess their care. Since a client with severe anxiety cannot focus on long messages and may pace to release energy, communication should be straightforward and calm. If the patient feels too sick to sit still and converse, the nurse can accompany them on walks. Because individuals with high levels of anxiety may perceive touch from an unfamiliar person as a threat and quickly withdraw, the nurse should carefully consider when and how to use touch.

5.8.3.3. Managing Anxiety

The client can learn relaxation techniques from the nurse to apply in times of stress or anxiety. Deep breathing is easy enough for everyone to do. To release tense muscles, try progressive relaxation and guided imagery. Using guided imagery, one can visualize a fun, safe space to unwind. In progressive relaxation, the practitioner uses rhythmic breathing to release tension from the body as they gradually tighten, hold, and then relax specific muscle groups. The client may benefit from using cognitive restructuring techniques, which were covered earlier in the text, to control their anxiety response. It is crucial that the client learns and uses any of these techniques when he or she is reasonably calm. The client is more likely to employ these strategies effectively during panic episodes or times of elevated anxiety if they are skilled at them. As they use these techniques to manage their anxiety, clients are likely to think that their ability to control themselves is returning. Clients' overall anxiety level decreases when they think they can control the panic attack and spend less time worrying and anticipating the next one.

5.8.4. Nursing Interventions

- Provide a safe environment and ensure the client's privacy during a panic attack.
- Remain with the client during a panic attack.

- Help the client focus on deep breathing.
- Talk to the client in a calm, reassuring voice.
- Teach the client to use relaxation techniques.
- Help the client use cognitive restructuring techniques.
- Engage the client to explore how to decrease stressors and anxiety-provoking situations.

5.8.4.1. Providing Client and Family Education

When working with clients who have anxiety disorders, education of the client and their family is crucial. The client gains knowledge on how to control their stress levels and deal with stressful events and reactions. The client can take charge of their own treatment for anxiety disorders if they are informed about the benefits of both medication and psychotherapy together as well as the side effects of the prescribed drug. The nurse must inform the patient and their family members about the physiological basis of anxiety as well as the advantages of combining medication management with psychotherapy. The client can learn to control these extreme reactions and develop self-control by using a combined treatment approach and stress reduction techniques. The nurse should assist the patient in realizing that these treatments and medications are tools to help them manage and control their disorder rather than a "cure". Education about medications for clients and their families should cover suggested dosage and schedule, anticipated effects, handling of side effects, and substances that interact or work in opposition to the drug. The client is urged to exercise on a regular basis by the nurse. Regular exercise lowers panic attacks, boosts endorphin production, and aids in the metabolism of adrenaline—all of which contribute to a better sense of well-being.

5.8.5. Phobias

A phobia is an unreasonable, severe, and enduring fear that interferes with daily functioning and produces great distress over a particular object or social circumstance. Typically, phobias are not brought on by unpleasant experiences in the past. It's possible that the phobic individual has never even laid eyes on the object of their fear. Individuals who suffer from phobias react in a way that is not appropriate for the circumstances or situation. People with phobias experience anticipatory anxiety even when they are merely considering the possibility of coming into contact with the dreaded object or situation. Some people may even realize that their fear is unusual and irrational, but they are still unable to overcome it. They have avoidance behaviors, which frequently drastically restrict their lives. Such avoidance behavior typically has a short-term negative effect on anticipatory anxiety.

There are three categories of phobias:

- **Agoraphobia** (discussed earlier in the text);
- **Specific Phobia:** which is an irrational fear of a particular object or a situation;
- **Social Anxiety or Phobia:** which is anxiety provoked by certain social or performance situations.

A lot of people talk about their "phobias" of snakes, spiders, rats, or similar things. These fears are focused, manageable, and worry- or anxiety-free. A phobic disorder is only diagnosed when a person's phobic behavior substantially disrupts their life, causing noticeable distress or making it difficult for them to function in social or professional situations.

Specific phobias are subdivided into the following categories:

- **Natural Environmental Phobias:** fear of storms, water, heights, or other natural phenomena;

- **Blood-injection Phobias:** fear of seeing one's own or others' blood, traumatic injury, or an invasive medical procedure such as an injection;
- **Situational Phobias:** fear of being in a specific situation such as on a bridge or in a tunnel, elevator, small room, hospital, or airplane;
- **Animal Phobia:** fear of animals or insects (usually a specific type' often, this fear develops in childhood and can continue through adulthood in both men and women' cats and dogs are the most common phobic objects);
- **Other Types of Specific Phobias:** for example, fear of getting lost while driving if not able to make all right (and no left) turns to get to one's destination.

When confronted with social situations, a person with social phobia, also called social anxiety disorder, experiences extreme anxiety that can render them incapacitated or panicked. Making a speech, going to a social event by yourself, interacting with people of the opposite sex or complete strangers, and voicing grievances are a few examples. The fear stems from low self-worth and worries about what other people will think of you. The person is afraid of coming off as nervous, unsocial, or of burping or spilling food, among other embarrassing things. Fears of eating in public, using restrooms in public, writing in public, and being the center of attention are examples of additional social phobias. An individual can suffer from one or more social phobias' the latter is referred to as generalized social phobia. Most cases of specific phobias happen in childhood or adolescence. Sometimes the fear comes from thinking about the object you fear or from handling a plastic model of it. 80% of the time, specific phobias that last into adulthood are lifelong. The peak age of onset for social phobia is middle adolescence' individuals who were shy as children may also develop social phobia. Social phobia frequently worsens over time, though it may lessen in severity as an adult. The degree of impairment varies according to demands and stress in life.

5.8.5.1. Treatment

Behavioral therapy is effective. Behavioral therapists first educate their clients on the definition of anxiety, how to recognize anxiety reactions in themselves, how to relax, how to set objectives, how to talk about achieving those goals, and how to picture situations that frighten them. Assertiveness training and positive reframing are two popular therapies that assist clients in gaining self-worth and self-control (explained earlier). Systematic (serial) desensitization is a behavioral therapy that is frequently used to treat phobias. In this method, the client is gradually exposed to the threatening object in a safe environment until their anxiety subsides. Each exposure progressively increases in complexity and intensity while lowering the client's level of anxiety. Until the anxiety is eventually gone, the decreased anxiety acts as a positive reinforcement. For instance, the therapist might encourage a client who is afraid of flying to hold a small model airplane and discuss their experiences' eventually, the client would hold a larger model airplane and discuss flying. Exposures could occur even later, such as when you stroll by an airport, sit in a parked aircraft, and finally take a quick flight. The challenge for each session is determined by how well the previous sessions went. A behavioral therapist will "flood" a client with the phobic object (a picture or the real thing) until the client is no longer afraid of it. This is a type of rapid desensitization. There isn't much reason to be afraid of the scenario now that the client's worst fear has been realized and they are not dead. In one or two sessions, the client is supposed to overcome the phobia. Because this approach greatly increases anxiety, it should only be used by a licensed psychotherapist in a controlled setting with the client's permission. (Sadock, Sadock & Ruiz).

A Closer Look

Trauma Therapy

Trauma therapy is an essential psychological intervention designed to help individuals process and recover from traumatic experiences. Trauma can result from various distressing events, such as physical or emotional abuse, accidents, natural disasters, or witnessing violence. The impact of trauma on mental health is profound, often leading to conditions like post-traumatic stress disorder (PTSD), anxiety, and depression. Effective trauma therapy involves a range of therapeutic approaches tailored to the individual's needs. One widely used method is Cognitive Behavioral Therapy (CBT), which helps individuals reframe negative thought patterns and develop healthier coping mechanisms. Another approach, Eye Movement Desensitization and Reprocessing (EMDR), involves guided eye movements to process and integrate traumatic memories, reducing their emotional impact. Additionally, somatic therapies focus on the connection between the mind and body, addressing how trauma is stored in the body and helping release physical tension associated with traumatic memories. Incorporating mindfulness and grounding techniques is also crucial in trauma therapy. These practices help individuals stay present and manage overwhelming emotions that arise from trauma. For example, mindfulness-based stress reduction (MBSR) teaches clients to observe their thoughts and feelings without judgment, promoting a sense of calm and control. Trauma therapy often involves a safe, supportive therapeutic environment where clients feel validated and heard. Establishing trust between the therapist and the client is fundamental, as it enables individuals to explore their traumatic experiences without fear of re-traumatization. Group therapy can also be beneficial, providing a sense of community and shared understanding among individuals who have experienced similar traumas. Sharing stories and coping strategies within a group setting can foster resilience and reduce feelings of isolation. Moreover, trauma therapy recognizes the importance of addressing not only the psychological but also the physiological effects of trauma. Techniques such as yoga, breathwork, and other body-based practices are integrated into treatment plans to help regulate the nervous system and promote overall well-being.

An emerging area in trauma therapy is the use of technology and virtual reality (VR). VR allows individuals to confront and work through traumatic memories in a controlled, immersive environment, offering new avenues for healing. Additionally, the integration of art and music therapy provides alternative means of expression and processing for those who may find verbal communication challenging. Trauma therapy is a dynamic and evolving field that underscores the importance of a holistic approach. It acknowledges that healing from trauma is not a linear process but a journey that requires patience, compassion, and a variety of therapeutic tools. The goal of trauma therapy is not only to alleviate symptoms but also to empower individuals, helping them reclaim their sense of safety, self-worth, and autonomy. By addressing the multifaceted nature of trauma, therapists can support clients in achieving meaningful and lasting recovery, fostering a renewed sense of hope and possibility for the future.

Summary

- The trauma or event may affect a single individual, such as a person with a history of childhood abuse, a child newly diagnosed with type 1 diabetes, or an adult with an acute coronary syndrome such as a myocardial infarction or unstable angina.
- Anxiety is a vague feeling of dread or apprehension' it is a response to external or internal stimuli that can have behavioral, emotional, cognitive, and physical symptoms. Anxiety is distinguished from fear, which is feeling afraid or threatened by a clearly identifiable external stimulus that represents danger to the person.
- Posttraumatic stress disorder (PTSD) is a disturbing pattern of behavior demonstrated by someone who has experienced, witnessed, or been confronted with a traumatic event such as a natural disaster, combat, or an assault.
- Reactive attachment disorder (RAD) and disinhibited social engagement disorder (DSED) occur before the age of 5 in response to the trauma of child abuse or neglect, called grossly pathogenic care.
- Dissociation is a subconscious defense mechanism that helps a person protect his or her emotional self from recognizing the full effects of some horrific or traumatic event by allowing the mind to forget or remove itself from the painful situation or memory.
- Moderate anxiety is the disturbing feeling that something is definitely wrong' the person becomes nervous or agitated. In moderate anxiety, the person can still process information, solve problems, and learn new things with assistance from others.
- Nurses encounter anxious clients and families in a wide variety of situations, such as before surgery and in emergency departments, intensive care units (ICUs), offices, and clinics.
- Stress-related illness is a broad term that covers a spectrum of illnesses that result from or worsen because of chronic, long-term, or unresolved stress. Chronic stress that is repressed can cause eating disorders, such as anorexia nervosa and bulimia.
- Anxiety disorders are diagnosed when anxiety no longer functions as a signal of danger or motivation for needed change but becomes chronic and permeates major portions of the person's life, resulting in maladaptive behaviors and emotional disability.
- Gamma-aminobutyric acid (GABA) is the amino acid neurotransmitter believed to be dysfunctional in anxiety disorders. GABA, an inhibitory neurotransmitter, functions as the body's natural antianxiety agent by reducing cell excitability, thus decreasing the rate of neuronal firing.
- Nurses encounter many people with anxiety disorders in community settings rather than in inpatient settings. Formal treatment for these clients usually occurs in community mental health clinics and in the offices of physicians, psychiatric clinical specialists, psychologists, or other mental health counselors.
- Panic disorder is composed of discrete episodes of panic attacks, that is, 15 to 30 minutes of rapid, intense, escalating anxiety in which the person experiences great emotional fear as well as physiological discomfort.
- A phobia is an illogical, intense, and persistent fear of a specific object or a social situation

that causes extreme distress and interferes with normal functioning. Phobias usually do not result from past negative experiences.

- Behavioral therapy works well. Behavioral therapists initially focus on teaching what anxiety is, helping the client identify anxiety responses, teaching relaxation techniques, setting goals, discussing methods to achieve those goals, and helping the client visualize phobic situations.

References

1. Bloch, E. (2017). Literature review and meta-analysis of risk factors for delayed posttraumatic stress disorder in older adults after a fall. *International Journal of Geriatric Psychiatry, 32*(2), 136–140.
2. Campbell, M., Decker, K. P., Kruk, K., & Deaver, S. P. (2016). Art therapy and cognitive processing therapy for combat-related PTSD: A randomized controlled trial. *Art Therapy, 33*(4), 169–177.
3. Carpenter, J. K., Andrews, L. A., Witcraft, S. M., Powers, M. B., Smits, J. A. J., & Hofmann, S. G. (2018). Cognitive behavioral therapy for anxiety and related disorders: A meta-analysis of randomized placebo-controlled trials. *Depression and Anxiety, 35*(6), 502–514.
4. Dan, A., Mondal, T., Chakraborty, K., Chaudhuri, A., & Biswas, A. (2017). Clinical course and treatment outcome of Koro: A follow-up study from a Koro epidemic reported from West Bengal, India. *Asian Journal of Psychiatry, 26*, 14–20.
5. De La Vega, D., Giner, L., & Courtet, P. (2018). Suicidality in subjects with anxiety or obsessive-compulsive and related disorders: Recent advances. *Current Psychiatry Reports, 20*(4), 26.
6. Feder, A., Costi, S., Iacoviello, B. M., Murrough, J. W., & Charney, D. S. (2017). Anxiety disorders: Neurobiology and neuroscience. In B. J. Sadock, V. A. Sadock, & P. Ruiz (Eds.), *Comprehensive Textbook of Psychiatry* (Vol. 1, 10th ed., pp. 1741–1751). Wolters Kluwer/Lippincott.
7. Freud, S. (1936). *The Problem of Anxiety*. W. W. Norton.
8. Friedman, M. J., & Bernardy, N. C. (2017). Considering future pharmacotherapy for PTSD. *Neuroscience Letters, 649*, 181–185.
9. Georgiadou, E., Morawa, E., & Erim, Y. (2017). High manifestations of mental distress in Arabic asylum seekers accommodated in collective centers for refugees in Germany. *International Journal of Environmental Research and Public Health, 14*(6), 612.
10. Gerlach, L. B., Wiechers, I. R., & Maust, D. T. (2018). Prescription benzodiazepine use among older adults: A critical review. *Harvard Review of Psychiatry, 26*(5), 264–273.
11. Greenbaum, M. A., Neylan, T. C., & Rosen, C. S. (2017). Symptom presentation and prescription of sleep medications for veterans with posttraumatic stress disorder. *Journal of Nervous and Mental Disease, 205*(2), 112–118.
12. Gutemann, J., Schwartzkopff, L., & Steil, R. (2017). Meta-analysis of the long-term treatment effects of psychological interventions in youth with PTSD symptoms. *Clinical Child and Family Psychology Review, 20*(4), 422–434.
13. Hauck, M. J., Gleason, M. M., & Zeanah, C. H. (2017). Reactive attachment disorder and disinhibited social engagement disorder. In B. J. Sadock, V. A. Sadock, & P. Ruiz (Eds.), *Comprehensive Textbook of Psychiatry* (Vol. 2, 10th ed., pp. 3662–3667). Wolters Kluwer/Lippincott, Williams, & Wilkins.

14. Hettema, J. M., & Otowa, T. (2017). Genetics of anxiety disorders. In B. J. Sadock, V. A. Sadock, & P. Ruiz (Eds.), *Comprehensive Textbook of Psychiatry* (Vol. 1, 10th ed., pp. 1737–1741). Wolters Kluwer/Lippincott.

15. Horesh, D., Qian, M., Freedman, S., & Shalev, A. (2017). Differential effect of exposure-based therapy and cognitive therapy on post-traumatic stress disorder symptom clusters: A randomized controlled trial. *Psychology and Psychotherapy, 90*(2), 235–243.

16. Huppert, J. D., & Foa, E. B. (2017). Anxiety disorders: Cognitive-behavioral therapy. In B. J. Sadock, V. A. Sadock, & P. Ruiz (Eds.), *Comprehensive Textbook of Psychiatry* (Vol. 1, 10th ed., pp. 1768–1778). Wolters Kluwer/Lippincott.

17. Jakel, R. J. (2018). Posttraumatic stress disorder in the elderly. *Psychiatric Clinics of North America, 41*(1), 165–175.

18. Katzman, J. W., & Geppert, C. M. A. (2017). Adjustment disorders. In B. J. Sadock, V. A. Sadock, & P. Ruiz (Eds.), *Comprehensive Textbook of Psychiatry* (Vol. 1, 10th ed., pp. 2116–2125). Wolters Kluwer/Lippincott, Williams, & Wilkins.

19. Kimmel, R. J., & Roy-Byrne, P. (2017). Clinical features of the anxiety disorders. In B. J. Sadock, V. A. Sadock, & P. Ruiz (Eds.), *Comprehensive Textbook of Psychiatry* (Vol. 1, 10th ed., pp. 1723–1730). Wolters Kluwer/Lippincott.

20. Levine, A. B., Levine, L. M., & Levine, T. B. (2014). Posttraumatic stress disorder and cardiometabolic disease. *Cardiology, 127*(1), 1–19.

21. Lies, J., Lau, S. T., Jones, L. E., Jensen, M. P., & Tan, G. (2017). Predictors and moderators of post-traumatic stress disorder: An investigation of anxiety sensitivity and resilience in individuals with chronic pain. *Annals of Academic Medicine, 46*(3), 102–110.

22. Lowenstein, R. J., Frewen, P., & Lewis-Fernandez, R. (2017). Dissociative disorders. In B. J. Sadock, V. A. Sadock, & P. Ruiz (Eds.), *Comprehensive Textbook of Psychiatry* (Vol. 1, 10th ed., pp. 1866–1952). Philadelphia, PA: Lippincott Williams & Wilkins/Wolters Kluwer.

23. Merikangas, K. R., & Eun, J. D. (2017). Epidemiology of anxiety disorders. In B. J. Sadock, V. A. Sadock, & P. Ruiz (Eds.), *Comprehensive Textbook of Psychiatry* (Vol. 1, 10th ed., pp. 1730–1737). Philadelphia, PA: Wolters Kluwer/Lippincott.

24. Morgan-Mullane, A. (2018). Trauma-focused behavioral therapy with children of incarcerated parents. *Clinical Social Work Journal, 46*(3), 200–201.

25. Peplau, H. (1952). *Interpersonal Relations*. Putnam.

26. Petkus, A. J., Wetherell, J. J., Stein, M. B., Chavira, D. A., Craske, M. G., Sherbourne, C., & Roy-Byrne, P. (2018). Age differences in death and suicidal ideation in anxious primary care patients. *Clinical Gerontologist, 41*(4), 271–281.

27. Ravindran, L., & Stein, M. B. (2017). Somatic therapies for anxiety disorders. In B. J. Sadock, V. A. Sadock, & P. Ruiz (Eds.), *Comprehensive Textbook of psychiatry* (Vol. 1, 10th ed., pp. 1778–1784). Philadelphia, PA: Wolters Kluwer/Lippincott.

28. Reinders, A. A., Willemsen, A. T., Vissia, E. M., Vos, H. P., den Boer, J. A., & Nijenhuis, E. R. (2016). The psychobiology of authentic and simulated dissociative personality states: The Full Monty. *Journal of Nervous and Mental Disease, 204*(6), 445–457.

29. Rosen, C., Jones, N., Longden, E., Chase, K. A., Shattell, M., Melbourne, J. K., & Sharma, R. P.

(2017). Exploring the intersections of trauma, structural adversity, and psychosis among a primarily African-American sample: A mixed methods analysis. *Frontiers in Psychiatry, 8*, 57.

30. Rozanov, V., & Carli, V. (2012). Suicide among war veterans. *International Journal of Environmental Research and Public Health, 9*(7), 2504–2519.
31. Sadock, V. A., Sadock, B. J., & Ruiz, P. (Eds.). (2017). *Comprehensive Textbook of Psychiatry* (Vol. 1, 10th ed., pp. 1778–1784). Philadelphia, PA: Wolters Kluwer/Lippincott.
32. Selye, H. (1956). *The Stress of Life*. McGraw-Hill.
33. Selye, H. (1974). *Stress Without Distress*. J. B. Lippincott.
34. Shalev, A. R., & Marmar, C. P. (2017). Posttraumatic stress disorder. In B. J. Sadock, V. A. Sadock, & P. Ruiz (Eds.), *Comprehensive Textbook of Psychiatry* (Vol. 1, 10th ed., pp. 1812–1826). Philadelphia, PA: Wolters Kluwer/Lippincott, Williams, & Wilkins.
35. Stayton, L. E., Dickstein, B. D., & Chard, K. M. (2018). Impact of self-blame on cognitive processing therapy: A comparison of treatment outcomes. *Journal of Traumatic Stress, 31*(3), 419–426.
36. Sullivan, H. S. (1952). *Interpersonal Theory of Psychiatry*. W. W. Norton.
37. Tanquay Bernard, M. M., & Luc, M. (2018). Patterns of benzodiazepine use in primary care adults with anxiety disorders. *Heliyon, 4*(7), e00688.
38. Tutus, D., Keller, F., Sachser, C., Pfeiffer, E., & Goldbeck, L. (2017). Change in parental depressive symptoms in trauma-focused cognitive-behavior therapy: Results from a randomized controlled trial. *Journal of Child and Adolescent Psychopharmacology, 27*(2), 200–205.
39. Yeterian, J. D., Berke, D. S., & Litz, B. T. (2017). Psychosocial rehabilitation after war trauma with adaptive disclosure: Design and rationale of a comparative efficacy trial. *Contemporary Clinical Trials, 61*, 10–15.

Chapter

SYMPTOMS OF MENTAL ILLNESS OR EMOTIONAL PROBLEMS

6

Contents

Introduction

Effective identification, diagnosis, and treatment of mental illness or emotional problems depend on an understanding of their symptoms. A wide range of conditions that impact people's thoughts, feelings, behaviors, and general well-being are collectively referred to as mental illnesses. Persistent mood swings that severely affect every day functioning and quality of life, such as protracted feelings of melancholy, hopelessness, or irritability, are among the classic signs of mental illness. These mood disorders can show up as a variety of symptoms, such as energy swings, irregular sleep or eating patterns, and a loss of interest in or enjoyment from previously enjoyed activities. Furthermore, cognitive symptoms are prevalent and can include anything from racing thoughts or persistent worries that interfere with daily tasks to problems with memory, concentration, or decision-making. Moreover, there could be behavioral shifts, like social disengagement, heightened agitation or impulsivity, or engaging in self-destructive activities like substance abuse or self-harm. The physical manifestations of stress or emotional distress can include headaches, stomachaches, and exhaustion. Interpersonal problems are frequently seen, such as relationship problems, communication or trust issues, and feelings of isolation or loneliness. It's critical to understand that symptoms of mental illness can differ greatly from person to person and that it can affect people of all ages, socioeconomic backgrounds, and lifestyles. Through early detection and comprehension of these indications, individuals, families, and medical professionals can promptly take action and offer suitable assistance and therapy to facilitate recuperation and enhance general health.

Orientation and Directional Terms

Term	Definition	Illustration
Autism	Autism is clinically regarded as a spectrum disorder, meaning that it can manifest very differently in each person.	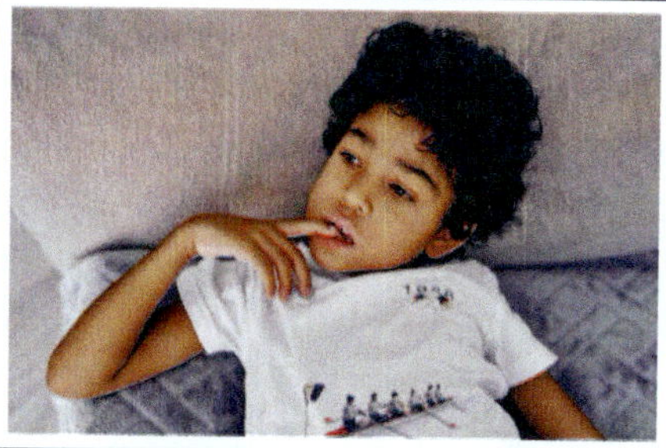
Schizophrenia	Schizophrenia is a serious mental illness that can affect a person's thoughts, feelings, and behaviors.	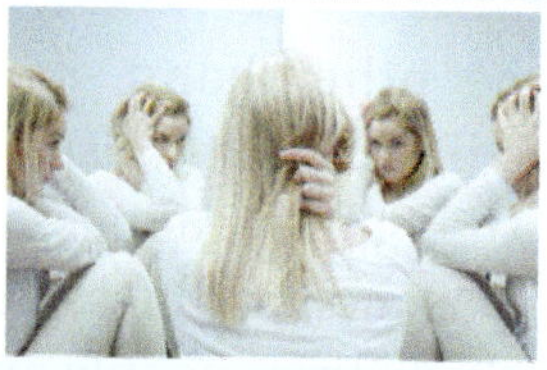
Depression	**Depression** (major **depressive** disorder) is a common and serious medical illness that negatively affects how you feel, the way you think and how you act.	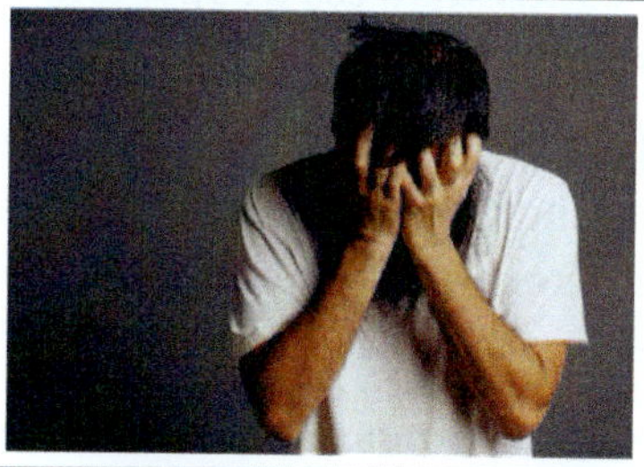
Obsessive compulsive disorder	Obsessive compulsive disorder (OCD) is a mental and behavioral disorder that causes people to have recurring, unwanted thoughts, ideas, or sensations (obsessions).	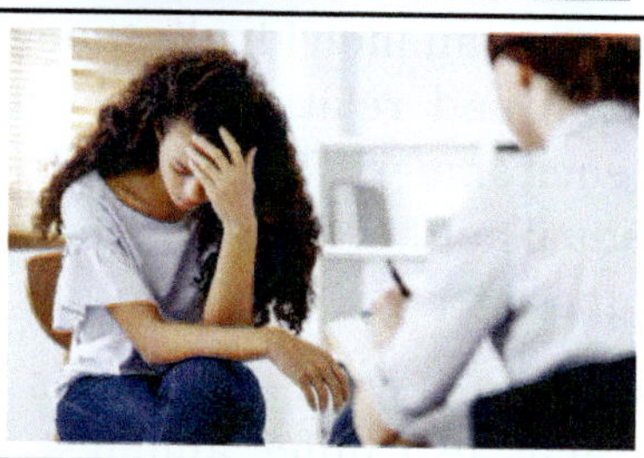
Anger	Anger is a normal emotion that can be useful when expressed appropriately. However, uncontrolled anger can have negative effects on your health and relationships.	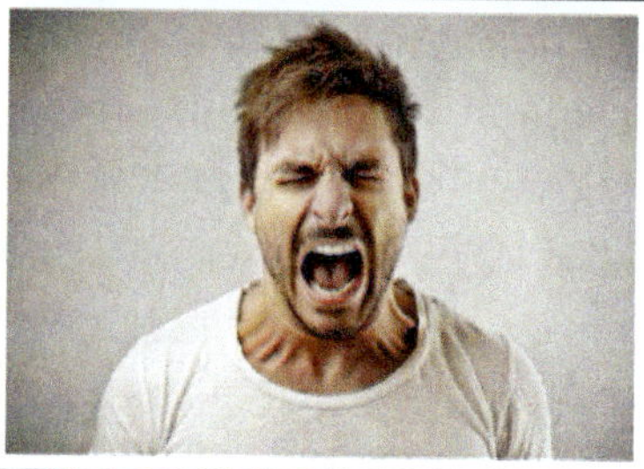

6.1. Mental Illness

Mental illness is defined by the American Psychiatric Association as a medical condition characterized by "changes in emotion, thinking, or behavior—or a combination of these.". It's critical to understand the distinctions between mental health and mental illness. Your capacity to carry out daily tasks, maintain positive relationships, and deal with challenges head-on are all considered indicators of your mental well-being.

On the other hand, diagnosable mental health conditions that cause noticeable changes in one's thoughts, feelings, and behavior are referred to as mental illnesses. These alterations significantly distress people and make it difficult to function.

There is no stigma associated with mental illness, and treatment and support are accessible, much like with other medical conditions like diabetes or heart disease.

Mental illnesses are disorders or diseases that impact an individual's thoughts, emotions, behavior, and relationships with others and their environment. They occur frequently. Many individuals either have one or know someone who does.

Mild to severe symptoms are possible. They may also differ amongst individuals. It often makes day-to-day living difficult. But you can frequently turn your life around when a specialist makes a diagnosis and assists with receiving treatment.

A mental illness is characterized as a medical condition that alters a person's thinking, feelings, or behavior—or all three—and results in distress and functional difficulties for the individual. Like many other illnesses, mental illness can range in severity from mild to severe. Even in cases where their condition is mild, people with mental illnesses don't always appear sick. Some people might exhibit more overt signs like agitation, disorientation, or withdrawal. There are numerous mental health conditions, such as schizophrenia, depression, autism, attention deficit hyperactivity disorder (ADHD), and obsessive compulsive disorder. Every illness affects a person differently in terms of their thoughts, feelings, and/or behaviors. We will talk about specific mental illnesses in this module at times, as well as general mental illnesses. Compared to other mental illnesses, depression, schizophrenia, and ADHD will be covered in more detail.

Not every brain disease falls under the mental illness category. Though they are classified as neurological diseases rather than mental illnesses, conditions like epilepsy, Parkinson's disease, and multiple sclerosis are still classified as brain disorders. It's interesting to note that there is some blurring of the distinctions between these other neurological or brain disorders and mental illnesses. As researchers continue to look into the brains of those who suffer from mental illnesses, they are discovering that these disorders do, in fact, have a biological basis and are linked to changes in the chemistry, structure, and function of the brain.

6.1.1. Mental Illness in the Population

Many people believe that mental illness is uncommon, that it only affects people in drastically different situations than their own, and that it will never touch them. Studies on the epidemiology of mental illness show how inaccurate this belief is. Indeed, according to the surgeon general, mental illnesses are so prevalent that few U.S. S. Families remain unaffected by them.

6.1.1.1. Mental Illness in Adults

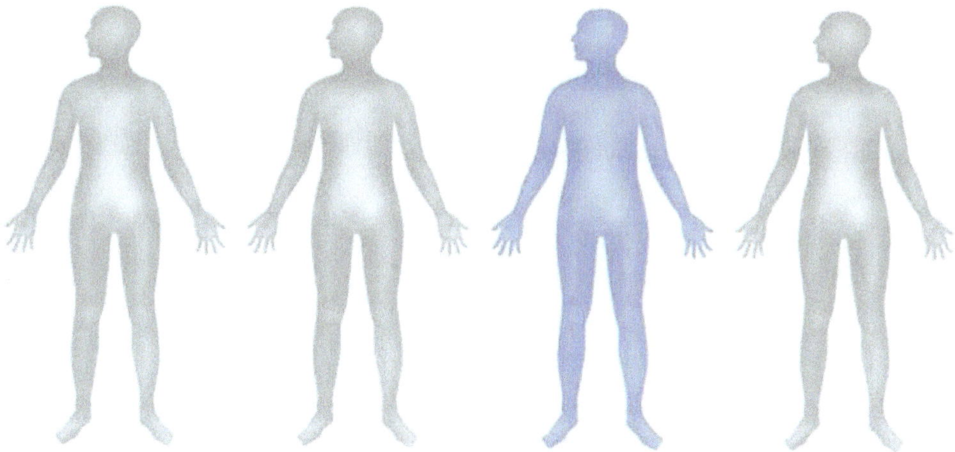

Figure 6.1. *Scientists estimate that one of every four people is affected by mental illness either directly or indirectly.*

Source: https://www.ncbi.nlm.nih.gov/books/NBK20369/bin/mentalhealthf1.jpg.

You have likely known someone who has dealt with mental illness, even if you or a family member have not personally experienced it. It is estimated that one in four individuals experience mental illness, either directly or indirectly. Consider the following statistics to get an idea of just how widespread the effects of mental illness are in society (Figure 6.1):

- According to recent estimates, approximately 20% of Americans, or about one in five people over the age of 18, suffer from a diagnosable mental disorder in a given year.
- Four of the 10 leading causes of disability—major depression, bipolar disorder, schizophrenia, and obsessive compulsive disorder—are mental illnesses.
- About 3% of the population have more than one mental illness at a time.
- About 5% of adults are affected so seriously by mental illness that it interferes with their ability to function in society. These severe and persistent mental illnesses include schizophrenia, bipolar disorder, other severe forms of depression, panic disorder, and obsessive compulsive disorder.
- Approximately 20% of doctor's appointments are related to anxiety disorders such as panic attacks.
- Eight million people have depression each year.
- Two million Americans have schizophrenia disorders, and 300,000 new cases are diagnosed each year.

6.1.1.2. Mental Illness in Children and Adolescents

Adolescents and children are not immune against mental illness. There are 12 million kids under 18 who suffer from mental illnesses. The National Mental Health Association has compiled some statistics about mental illness in children and adolescents which includes:

- Mental health problems affect one in every five young people at any given time.
- An estimated two-thirds of all young people with mental health problems are not receiving the help they need.
- Less than one-third of the children under age 18 who have a serious mental health problem receive any mental health services.
- As many as 1 in every 33 children may be depressed. Depression in adolescents may be as high as 1 in 8.
- Suicide is the third leading cause of death for 15- to 24-years-olds and the sixth leading cause of death for 5- to 15-year-olds.
- Schizophrenia is rare in children under age 12, but it occurs in about 3 of every 1,000 adolescents.
- Between 118,700 and 186,600 youths in the juvenile justice system have at least one mental illness.
- Of the 100,000 teenagers in juvenile detention, an estimated 60% have behavioral, cognitive, or emotional problems.

6.1.2. Warning Signs for Mental Illness

Each mental illness has its own characteristic symptoms. However, there are some general warning signs that might alert you that someone needs professional help. Some of these signs include:

- marked personality change;
- inability to cope with problems and daily activities;
- strange or grandiose ideas;
- excessive anxieties;
- prolonged depression and apathy;
- marked changes in eating or sleeping patterns;
- thinking or talking about suicide or harming oneself;
- extreme mood swings—high or low;
- abuse of alcohol or drugs; and
- excessive anger, hostility, or violent behavior.

6.2. Diagnosing Mental Illness

6.2.1. Mental Health Professionals

A person needs to be assessed by a licensed practitioner with experience in mental health in order to receive a diagnosis of mental illness. Psychiatric nurses, mental health counselors, psychiatrists, psychologists, and social workers are examples of mental health professionals. Pediatricians, internists, and family physicians are typically qualified to diagnose common mental illnesses like ADHD, anxiety disorders, and depression. A mental health professional who is not a psychiatrist will frequently refer a patient to one, depending on the patient and his or her symptoms. A physician (M.D.) is a psychiatrist. Who has taken additional courses in the study of mental diseases and mental health. Psychiatrists assess a patient's mental health alongside their physical health and are able to recommend medication. Just M.Ds and psychiatrists are able to prescribe drugs to treat mental health conditions.

6.2.2. Mental Illnesses Are Diagnosed by Symptoms

In contrast to other medical diagnoses, mental illness cannot be diagnosed by a blood test or by culture of certain microorganisms. In the interim, mental health practitioners will have to diagnose mental illnesses based on a patient's symptoms. Perhaps in the future, scientists will create distinct physiological tests for mental illnesses. It is common practice to base a diagnosis on a patient's symptoms rather than a quantitative medical test, such as a urinalysis, X-rays, throat swab, or blood chemistry test. Based solely on symptoms, doctors can diagnose a wide range of illnesses, such as Parkinson's disease, Alzheimer's disease, and migraines. Doctors use symptom analysis to gain a good idea of the nature of other diseases, like mononucleosis or asthma, and then perform a physiological test to confirm the diagnosis or provide more information.

When working with someone who may be experiencing mental health issues, a mental health professional will collaborate with the person to ascertain the symptoms, duration of the symptoms, and impact on the person's life. In order to get information, mental health providers frequently interview patients to learn about their symptoms, including how long they have been present and how severe they are. To get a more complete picture, the medical professional will frequently also speak with the patient's family members. The patient's medical history and a physical examination will probably be performed by a doctor to rule out additional health issues.

Experts in mental health assess symptoms in order to diagnose mental disease. To diagnose a particular mental illness, they use the criteria listed in the Diagnostic and Statistical Manual of Mental Disorders (DSM-IV' currently, the fourth edition), published by the American Psychiatric Association. The DSM-IV provides a general description and a list of typical symptoms for each mental illness. The DSM-IV is consulted by mental health practitioners to verify whether a patient's symptoms correspond to a particular mental disorder. Mental health professionals understand that while the DSM-IV offers useful information to aid in the diagnosis of mental illness, it is crucial to observe patients over an extended period of time to fully comprehend the patient's mental illness and its impact on their life.

6.3. Mental Illness and the Brain

The phrase "mental illness" makes it abundantly evident that there is a mental health issue. As scientists continue to look into mental illnesses and their causes, they are learning more and more about how the biological processes that make the brain function are altered when a person has a mental illness. But is it just the mind in an abstract sense, or is there a physical basis to mental illness?

6.3.1. The Basics of Brain Function

It's helpful to consider how the brain normally works before considering the issues that arise in the brain when someone has a mental illness. The brain is an extraordinarily intricate organ. Although it only accounts for 2% of our body weight, it uses up 20% of the oxygen we breathe and 20% of the energy we absorb. It regulates almost every aspect of human experience, including movement, perception of our surroundings, involuntary bodily functions like breathing, and emotional regulation. The brain undergoes hundreds of thousands of chemical reactions every second, which are the basis for the ideas, deeds, and behaviors we use to react to the stimuli around us. To put it briefly, the brain controls the bodily functions and tendencies that enable us to live (Figure 6.2).

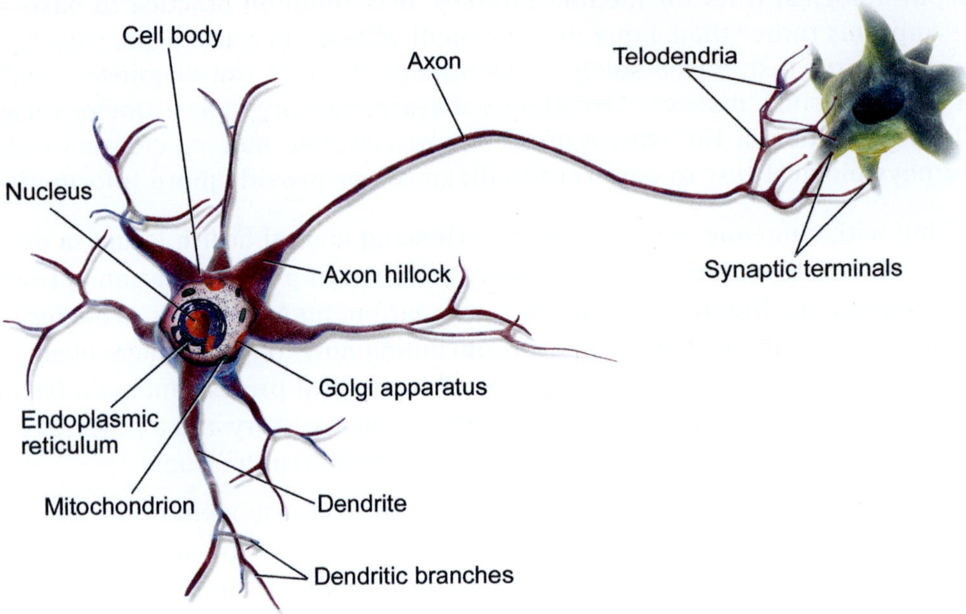

Figure 6.2. *The neuron, or nerve cell, is the functional unit of the nervous system. The neuron has processes called dendrites that receive signals and an axon that transmits signals to another neuron.*

Source: By BruceBlaus - Own work, CC BY 3.0, https://commons.wikimedia.org/w/index.php?curid=28761830.

The neuron is the basic functional unit of the brain' how does it process all this information and come up with a response? A neuron is a type of specialized cell with precise connections to muscle cells, other neurons, and sensory receptors that enable it to perform a variety of actions. Four anatomically and functionally distinct regions make up a typical neuron: the cell body, dendrites, axons, and axon terminals.

The neuron's metabolic core is located in the cell body. The majority of the cell's protein synthesis takes place in the nucleus, which is housed in the cell body.

A neuron's cell body normally contains a number of fibers called dendrites that extend from it. These functions, which resemble tree branches when they branch out, are the primary means of receiving information from other nerve cells.

The axon is also derived from the cell body. Axons can reach lengths of up to one meter' in most circumstances, they are significantly longer than dendrites. The portion of the neuron that is dedicated to transmitting signals to other cells and away from the cell body is called the axon. A fatty insulating substance known as myelin envelops some large axons, allowing electrical signals to move through them more quickly.

The axon splits into numerous fine branches near its end, each of which has a specialized swelling known as an axon terminal or presynaptic terminal. The dendrites of another neuron are close to where the axon terminals end. The message from the axon terminals of one neuron is received by the dendrites of that neuron (Figure 6.3).

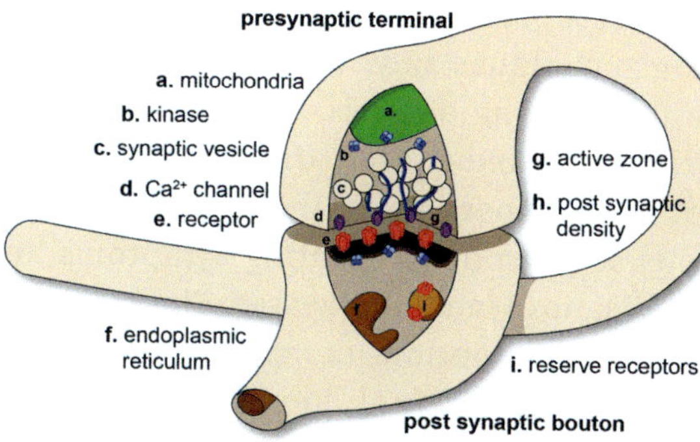

Figure 6.3. *Diagram of a synapse.*

Source: By Curtis Neveu - Own work, CC BY-SA 4.0, https://commons.wikimedia.org/w/index.php?curid=117410942.

The synapse is the location where an axon terminal ends up next to a receiving dendrite. The presynaptic neuron is the cell that transmits information, and the postsynaptic neuron is the cell that receives it. It is crucial to understand that there is no cytoplasmic connection between the two neurons at the synapse, nor is there a physical connection. The synaptic space, also known as the synaptic cleft, is the intercellular region that separates the presynaptic and postsynaptic neurons. An average neuron connects to other neurons through about 1,000 synapses. According to estimates, the human brain contains more synapses than stars in our galaxy. Moreover, synaptic connections change over time. In reaction to events in life, neurons create new synapses or fortify existing ones. Learning is based on this dynamic shift in neural connections (Figure 6.4).

Both chemical and electrical signals are used by neurons to communicate. A presynaptic neuron's axon carries information in the form of an electrical impulse away from the cell body of the neuron and toward the axon terminals. The electrical signal is unable to pass through the synaptic cleft or synaptic space once it reaches the presynaptic axon terminal. Rather, the postsynaptic cell is affected by chemical changes that are triggered by the electrical signal and can travel across the synapse. Vesicles, which are membrane sacs, travel toward the axon terminal membrane when an electrical impulse reaches the presynaptic axon terminal. The vesicles merge with the membrane upon reaching it, releasing their contents into the synaptic space. Neurotransmitters are chemical compounds that are present in the vesicles. Numerous neurotransmitter molecules are present in each vesicle. The released neurotransmitter molecules attach to unique proteins on the postsynaptic neuron known as receptors after drifting across the synaptic cleft. A molecule of a neurotransmitter will only attach to a particular type of receptor.

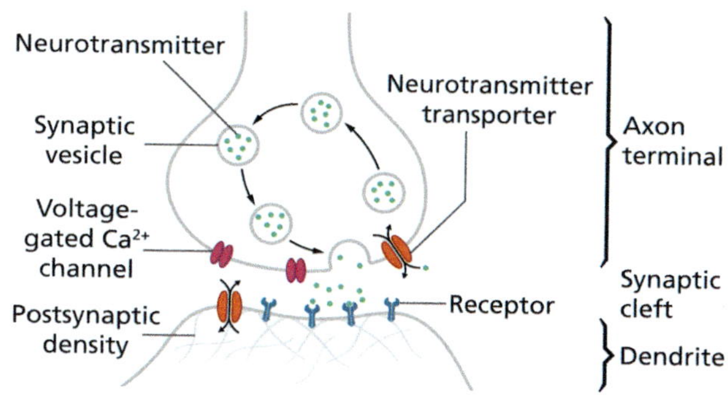

Figure 6.4. *Neurons relay their information using both electrical signals and chemical messages in a process called neurotransmission.*

Source: By Thomas Splettstoesser (www.scistyle.com) - Own work, CC BY-SA 4.0, https://commons.wikimedia.org/w/index.php?curid=41349083.

A neuron produces an electrical impulse when neurotransmitters bind to their receptors. The electrical impulse then travels toward the cell body from the dendritic ending. The neurotransmitter releases from the receptor and returns to the synaptic space after stimulating an electrical impulse in the postsynaptic neuron. The neurotransmitter is transported back into the presynaptic neuron by certain proteins known as transporters or reuptake pumps.

Repackaged into vesicles, the neurotransmitter molecules are ready for release the next time an electrical impulse reaches the presynaptic axon terminal. Neurotransmitter molecules that are not taken up again into the presynaptic neuron are broken down by synaptic space enzymes.

Although the nervous system makes use of a wide range of neurotransmitter molecules, each neuron is only capable of synthesizing and secreting one particular kind of neurotransmitter. The brain contains a variety of neurotransmitters, some of which are glutamate, GABA, serotonin, dopamine, and norepinephrine. A few of these names will come up in relation to specific mental illnesses, but the specifics of each neurotransmitter's distribution and function in the brain are outside the purview of this module.

6.3.2. Investigating Brain Function

The symptoms that an individual displays serve as the basis for the diagnosis and treatment of mental illness by mental health professionals. When these specialists treat a patient, their aim is to get rid of any symptoms that are making it difficult for the patient to live their life normally. Conversely, research scientists aim to achieve something different. They are interested in finding out what structural or chemical alterations take place in the brains of those suffering from mental illnesses. Scientists can create more effective treatments or discover a cure if they can figure out what exactly goes on in the brain (Figure 6.5).

Depending on the questions they want to answer, scientists employ different methods to study the brain. For some inquiries, researchers look into particular genes or proteins in the neurons using molecular or biochemical techniques. In order to better understand how the activity or structure of the brain changes, scientists are interested in visualizing changes in the brain. In the past, scientists could only study brains after a person had passed away, but new imaging techniques now allow them to study the brain in living animals, including humans. It's critical to understand that mental illness cannot be diagnosed using these brain imaging methods. A person's presenting symptoms are used to diagnose mental illnesses. The following paragraphs' descriptions of imaging techniques won't help the mental health practitioner diagnose or treat the patient more successfully. Additionally, some of the methods involve slight radiation exposure for the patients and are invasive. Typically, children and adolescents are not involved in research studies that employ these tests.

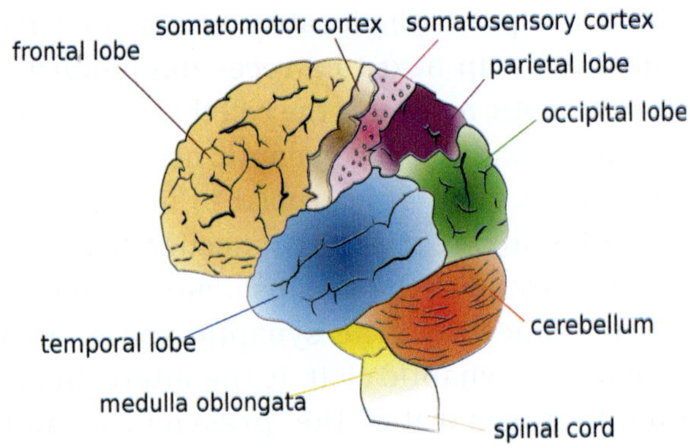

Figure 6.5. *Scientists use a variety of imaging techniques to investigate brain structure and function.*

Source: By vectorized by Jkwchui - http://training.seer.cancer.gov/module_anatomy/unit5_3_nerve_org1_cns.html, CC BY-SA 3.0, https://commons.wikimedia.org/w/index.php?curid=29055751.

Positron emission tomography (PET) is a widely used method to investigate brain activity and the ways in which mental illness alters the brain. PET scans track the movement and spatial distribution of a radioactive substance injected into living subjects' tissues. The method can be used to look into the connection between alterations in brain activity and behavioral and physiological effects while the patient is conscious. PET scans have a spatial resolution of roughly 4 millimeters and are capable of detecting very small (nanomolar) concentrations of tracer molecules. Furthermore, two or three dimensional reconstruction of images from a PET scan can be done by computers.

Compounds labeled with positron-emitting isotopes must be used for PET. An electron has a negative charge, whereas a positron has a positive charge. An electron and a positron have the same mass and spin. To create these isotopes, protons are accelerated into the nuclei of nitrogen, carbon, oxygen, or fluorine using a cyclotron. The isotope is unstable due to the extra proton. The proton needs to decay into a neutron and a positron in order to return to its stable state. The unstable positron dissipates energy as it moves away from the site of generation. When the positron and electron eventually collide, two gamma rays that are 180 degrees apart are released. When the gamma rays hit two detectors, the event is recorded. Because the detectors only react to simultaneous emissions, the source of the gamma rays can be precisely mapped by scientists. The radioactive substances utilized in PET have a very brief half-life. Depending on the particular compound, the half-life (or the amount of time it takes for half of the radioactive label to break down) of the widely used radioisotopes can vary from less than two hours to about two minutes. Humans can safely use this technique because a PET scan only needs a small amount of short-lived radioisotopes—a few micrograms—to perform.

Where the neurons are most active in the brain is one of the many questions about brain function that PET scans can address. Different radiolabeled compounds are used by scientists to look into various biological questions. Radiolabeled glucose, for instance, can be used to pinpoint the areas of the brain that light up in response to a particular stimulus. Compared to inactive neurons, active neurons consume more glucose. More positrons are released by active neurons, which appear on PET scans as red or yellow instead of blue or purple in regions where the neurons are not very active. (While various computer enhancement methods may employ a different color scheme, it is common to use a spectrum with blue denoting low activity and red denoting high activity. Researchers can use PET to track alterations in a patient's brain activity in particular regions when they suffer from a mental illness. Researchers can also look into how treatment affects the brains of those with mental illnesses.

Researchers employ a variety of methods to study how mental illness alters the brain, including PET imaging. Scientists receive different information from different techniques. Magnetic resonance imaging is an additional crucial method (MRI). MRI is used to look at structural changes in the brain, as opposed to PET, which shows changes in activity level. For instance, ventricles, or spaces within the brain, are larger in people with schizophrenia than they are in healthy people, according to MRI studies. Electroencephalography (EEG), functional magnetic resonance imaging (fMRI), and single photon emission computed tomography (SPECT) are additional methods that scientists use to study brain function in a living organism. Every method has benefits of its own and offers unique insights into the composition and operations of the brain.

6.4. The Causes of Mental Illnesses

Right now, scientists are still unsure of the exact causes of mental illnesses. It is hardly surprising that determining the causes of mental illnesses is a difficult task when you consider the structural and organizational complexity of the brain as well as the complexity of effects that mental illnesses have on thoughts, feelings, and behaviors. The relationships between people's behaviors, thoughts, and feelings and how their actions can occasionally spiral out of control are explored in different ways by the disciplines of neuroscience, psychiatry, and psychology. Scientists are attempting to determine the causes of mental illnesses with the help of this multidisciplinary research. Scientists can create new therapies or attempt to find a cure once they have identified the underlying causes of mental illnesses.

6.4.1. The Biology of Mental Illnesses

The majority of scientists think that issues with neurotransmission—the flow of information between brain neurons—are the cause of mental illnesses. For instance, people with depression have reduced levels of the neurotransmitter serotonin. This discovery prompted the creation of specific drugs to treat the condition. The mechanism of action of selective serotonin reuptake inhibitors (SSRIs) is to decrease the quantity of serotonin reabsorbed by presynaptic neurons. As a result, there is more serotonin in the synaptic space available to bind to the postsynaptic neuron's receptor. Depression may also be accompanied by changes in other neurotransmitters, in addition to serotonin, which complicates the underlying cause of the illness (Figure 6.6).

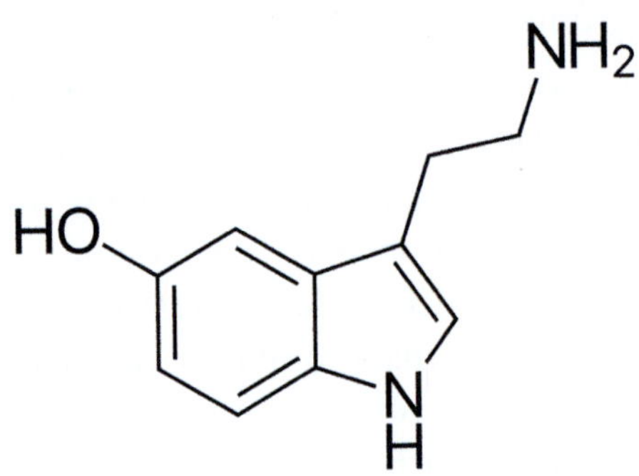

Figure 6.6. *Scientists understand that mental illnesses are associated with changes in neurochemicals. For example, in people who have depression, less of the neurotransmitter serotonin (small circles) is released into the synaptic space than in people who do not have depression. Certain medications called selective serotonin reuptake inhibitors (SSRIs) relieve symptoms of depression by causing an increase in the amount of serotonin in the synaptic space.*

Source: By CYL - Own work, Public Domain, https://commons.wikimedia.org/w/index.php?curid=18074053.

Dopamine, glutamate, and norepinephrine neurotransmitter abnormalities are thought to be present in schizophrenia patients. The fact that cocaine addicts occasionally exhibit schizophrenia-like symptoms is one clue that dopamine may play a significant role in the neurotransmitter disease. Cocaine stimulates dopamine-containing brain neurons to raise the concentration of dopamine in the synapses.

6.4.2. Risk Factors for Mental Illnesses

While the exact causes of mental illnesses are still unknown, scientists have discovered risk factors for people. These factors can be classified as social, genetic, or environmental. Indeed, the likelihood of someone developing mental illness is probably influenced by a combination of all these factors. The risk of developing mental illness is influenced by a combination of social, environmental, and genetic factors.

The chance of developing a mental illness can be raised by environmental factors such as head injuries, poor nutrition, and exposure to toxins like lead and tobacco smoke.

The likelihood that someone will experience mental illness is also influenced by their genes. The conditions that are most likely to have a genetic basis are ADHD, bipolar disorder, autism, and schizophrenia. One indication that genetics may play a part in determining an individual's susceptibility to ADHD is the finding that children with the disorder are significantly more likely to have a parent or sibling who also has the disorder. According to twin studies, identical twins are much more likely than fraternal twins to have ADHD. The same is true for depression and schizophrenia. Scientists believe that interactions between multiple genes may cause mental illnesses rather than changes in a single gene. Furthermore, the severity of a mental illness may depend on a confluence of social, environmental, and genetic factors.

Social factors also present risks and can harm an individual's, especially a child's, mental health. Social factors include

- severe parental discord;
- death of a family member or close friend;
- parent's mental illness;
- parent's criminality;
- overcrowding;
- economic hardship;
- abuse;
- neglect; and
- exposure to violence.

6.5. Treating Mental Illnesses

While the majority of mental illnesses are currently incurable, they can typically be managed well enough to reduce symptoms and restore the patient's ability to function in social, occupational, and educational settings. An individual must see a licensed mental health professional in order to start treatment. Speaking with the patient to learn more about the symptoms, their duration, and how they are affecting their life is the first step a doctor or other mental health specialist will take. A physical examination will also be performed by the doctor to rule out any further health issues. For instance, certain symptoms (like mood swings) may be brought on by hormonal or neurological issues linked to long-term conditions like heart disease, or they may be a side effect of specific drugs. The doctor will create a treatment plan after assessing the patient's general health and diagnosing the ailment. Depending on the illness and how severe it is, treatment options may include both medication and psychotherapy.

6.5.1. Medications

Mental illnesses are frequently treated with medications. We are learning more about those medications through magazine and television advertisements. Medication for mental illness must be taken for a few days or weeks in order for it to fully work. When a patient starts taking medication, it's critical for a physician to keep an eye on their health. The doctor may adjust the dosage or prescribe an alternative medication with fewer side effects if the medication is causing unwanted side effects. A different medication may be prescribed by the doctor if the current one does not relieve the symptoms (Figure 6.7).

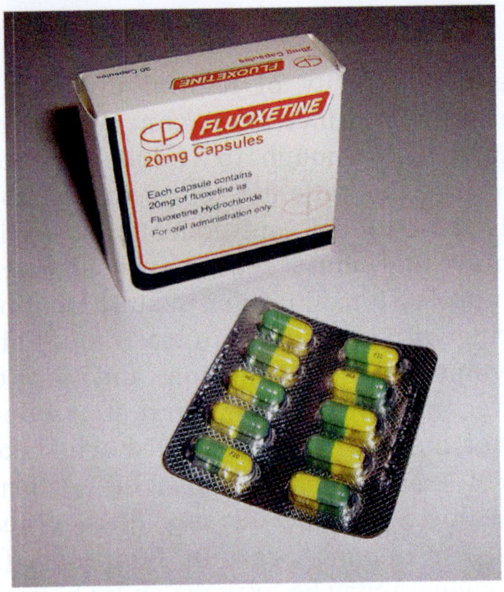

Figure 6.7. *Medicines are one part of an effective treatment plan for mental illnesses.*

Source: By Lanfear's Bane at English Wikipedia, CC BY-SA 3.0, https://commons.wikimedia.org/w/index.php?curid=5222497.

Because of the side effects, people with mental illnesses occasionally refuse to take their medications. It's critical to keep in mind that every medication has both advantages and disadvantages. Antibiotics, for instance, have completely changed how certain bacterial illnesses are treated. Antibiotics, however, frequently disrupt the good bacteria in the human body, resulting in adverse reactions like nausea and diarrhea. Like other medications, psychiatric drugs can lessen the symptoms of mental illness, but they can also have unintended side effects. When taking medication for a medical condition, be it mental health or another illness, patients should consult with their doctors to fully understand the prescription, its purpose, how to take it, and potential side effects.

From time to time, stories in the media link psychiatric medication side effects to potentially dangerous outcomes, like suicide. In these situations, it is typically very difficult to assess the relative contributions of the mental illness and the medication to the suicidal behavior. Like other medications, those used to treat mental illness may have side effects. To reduce side effects, the psychiatrist or doctor can typically change the medication or dose.

6.5.2. Psychotherapy

Psychotherapy is a type of treatment where the patient and a mental health professional—a psychologist, psychiatrist, or other mental health professional—discuss issues and feelings. Patients can identify solutions and comprehend the causes of their issues through this conversation. There are various forms of psychotherapy. The therapy can help patients

- change thought or behavior patterns;
- understand how past experiences influence current behaviors;
- solve other problems in specific ways; or
- learn illness self-management skills.

Psychotherapy can take place between a therapist and a patient, between a therapist and a patient's family, or between a therapist and a group. Psychotherapy and medication are often the most effective combination for treating mental illness. Medication eases the symptoms of severe mental illnesses, while psychotherapy assists patients in managing their condition.

Similar to how there are no drugs that can treat mental illnesses instantly, psychotherapy is a continuous process. Depending on the nature of the illness or issue, a person may attend psychotherapy for a few visits or several years. Psychotherapy should generally last longer the more serious the issue.

6.5.3. The Stigma of Mental Illness

"People with mental illnesses are crazy, insane, and wacky. "Those with mental illnesses are morally repugnant. "Those with mental illnesses ought to be permanently committed to an asylum because they are dangerous. "Those who suffer from mental illness require care from someone.". "We may even be guilty of saying things like these ourselves. How often have we heard remarks like these or seen these kinds of portrayals in films, TV series, or books? Are these depictions accurate, or are they just a result of our ignorance and fear? (Figure 6.8)

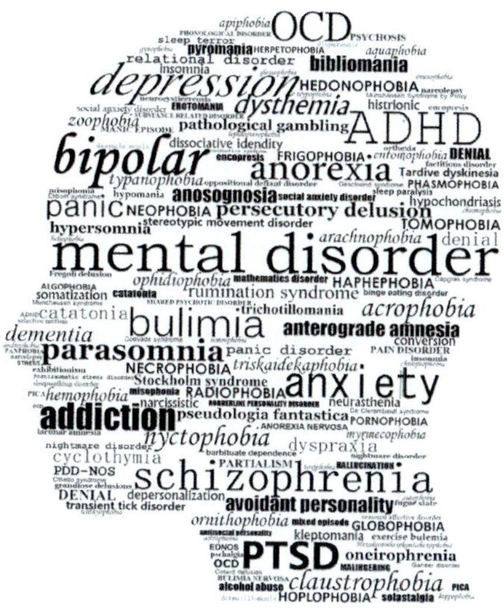

Figure 6.8. *Words can hurt. Many derogatory words and phrases are used in relation to mental illness. However, these words maintain the stereotyped image and not the reality about mental illness. Try not to use these words, and encourage students not to use them. It is more appropriate to refer to "a person who has a mental illness" when speaking about someone.*

Source: By Paget Michael Creelman - Own work, CC BY-SA 4.0, https://commons.wikimedia.org/w/index.php?curid=67346556.

Stigmas are negative stereotypes about groups of people. Common stigmas about people who are mentally ill are

- Individuals who have a mental illness are dangerous.
- Individuals who have a mental illness are irresponsible and can't make life decisions for themselves.
- People who have a mental illness are childlike and must be taken care of by parents or guardians.
- People who have a mental illness should just get over it.

All those stereotypes about those with mental illnesses are based on misinformation. There are very few dangerous mental illness sufferers in our society. Most are able to live freely, work, and go to school. No more so than a person with a different chronic illness like diabetes, asthma, or heart disease can someone with a mental illness just decide to get over it. Similar to other diseases, mental illness arises from a physical issue within the body.

Discrimination against individuals with mental illness results in unfair treatment in housing, employment, and education. Overcoming these stigmas is a tough challenge for those with mental illness, as the negative attitudes they face can be more disabling than the illness itself. The shame and guilt brought on by these stigmas lead to low self-esteem, dependence on others, and feelings of isolation and hopelessness. The fear of stigma also prevents many from seeking the treatment that could greatly improve their symptoms.

One effective method for reducing stigmas surrounding mental illness is by providing accurate information. Advocacy groups actively fight against the stereotypes placed on individuals with mental illnesses, urging the media to portray them more accurately and encouraging the public to stop believing negative misconceptions. A powerful way to combat these stereotypes is through personal interactions with individuals managing serious mental illnesses successfully, such as holding down jobs, supporting themselves, and actively participating in their communities. Interacting with those with mental illnesses can challenge and change a person's preconceived notions and attitudes towards mental illness.

Though there is still a long way to go before people acknowledge that mental illness is a disease with a biological basis, attitudes regarding mental illness are gradually shifting. According to a National Mental Health Association survey, 55% of those who have never had a depression diagnosis acknowledge that it is an illness and not something that people should "snap out of.". Compared to the 38% of survey participants in 1991 who identified depression as a disease, this represents a significant increase.

6.5.4. The Consequences of Not Treating Mental Illness

Many individuals seek medical treatment without hesitation for physical illnesses like bronchitis, asthma, diabetes, or heart disease. Unfortunately, the same cannot be said for those suffering from mental illnesses. Studies show that a large number of young people with mental health issues do not receive the necessary treatment, with estimates stating that two-thirds of them do not receive help. Similarly, less than one-third of children under 18 with serious mental health problems receive any form of mental health services. The problem of untreated mental illnesses extends to adults as well.

In September 2000, a conference on children's mental health was organized by the U.S. surgeon general. Dr. David Satcher, the former surgeon general, highlighted the significance of mental health in children, emphasizing that missed prevention opportunities, fragmented services, and limited resources were causing suffering for children and families. Dr. Satcher also addressed the stigma surrounding mental illness as a major concern. Mental illness in children and teenagers can have serious repercussions. A lot of mental health practitioners talk about the deficits that build up when children's mental illness goes untreated. Firstly, learning can be negatively impacted by mental illness in students. Teens with mental illnesses who do not receive prompt, aggressive treatment often find themselves falling further and further behind in their academics. When they grow up, they have a lower likelihood of becoming fully integrated members of society and a higher likelihood of dropping out of school. Furthermore, we now understand that young people with depressive disorders have an increased risk of illness as well as ongoing interpersonal and psychosocial challenges following their depressive episode. In addition, a large number of adults with mental illnesses have childhood-onset issues. Childhood depression may be a sign of more serious illness later in life. Once believed to only affect children and adolescents, attention deficit hyperactivity disorder may continue into adulthood and be linked to issues in the social, legal, and professional spheres.

The impact of mental illness on society is significant due to its high incidence. Employers lose more than $23 billion annually as a result of employee absenteeism and decreased productivity during depressions alone. Disability-adjusted life years, or DALYs, are units of measurement used by the World Health Organization to quantify the burden of all diseases. These years are lost due to premature death or disability. Mental illness was the cause of more than 15% of all DALYs. Over $69 billion was spent on the direct treatment of mental illnesses in the US in 1996. The United States lost $79 billion as a result of the indirect costs of mental illness resulting from lost productivity at work, in schools, or in homes. S. the 1990s economy. For patients, their families, and society as a whole, treatment—including psychotherapy and medication management—is reasonably priced. Benefits include decreased need for psychiatric hospitalization, fewer sick days and disability claims, less trips to other doctors' offices, diagnostic centers, and hospitals for physical ailments based on psychological distress, and more stable employment. On the other hand, failing to treat mental health issues can result in broken relationships, poor performance at work or loss of employment, mental anguish, substance misuse, needless medical procedures, psychiatric hospitalization, and suicide.

6.6. Common Mental Health Disorders

Diagnosing mental illness is a complex process that does not have a simple solution. Tests to determine if a person has a mental illness are not always accurate. Qualified healthcare professionals need to identify specific symptoms exhibited by the person in order to make a diagnosis. Each mental illness comes with its own set of signs and symptoms that are connected to biological dysfunction. The sections below outline the symptoms and effects of three highlighted mental illnesses in this curriculum supplement: depression, attention deficit hyperactivity disorder, and schizophrenia.

6.6.1. Depression

Depression, also known as depressive disorders, is one of the main causes of disability both domestically and internationally. In any given year, it is estimated to impact 90.5% of adult Americans. Depression affects almost twice as many women as men. According to epidemiological studies, up to 2% of children and 8% of adolescents in the US experience depression.

6.6.1.1. The Symptoms of Depression

Depression is more than just feeling depressed or unhappy. These emotions are common to everyone, but they do not always indicate depression. In actuality, there are three primary categories of depressive disorders, not just depression. They are

- major depressive disorder;
- dysthymia; and
- bipolar disorder (manic-depression).

While some depressive symptoms are typical during a transient "blue mood," major depressive disorder is identified when a person experiences five or more symptoms almost daily for two weeks. Symptoms of depression include

- a sad mood;
- a loss of interest in activities that one used to enjoy;
- a change in appetite or weight;
- oversleeping or difficulty sleeping;
- physical slowing or agitation;
- energy loss;
- feelings of worthlessness or inappropriate guilt;
- difficulty concentrating; and
- recurrent thoughts of death or suicide.

Depression can have a severe impact on people's lives, causing difficulties in functioning at work or school and a lack of interest in typical family and social activities. If left untreated, a major depressive episode in adults can last an average of nine months. Additionally, at least half of those who experience a major depressive episode are likely to have another episode in the future.

In children, depression lasts an average of seven to nine months with symptoms similar to those in adults.

Symptoms in children may include:

- sadness;
- loss of interest in activities they used to enjoy;
- self-criticism;
- feelings that they are unloved;
- hopelessness about the future;
- thoughts of suicide;
- irritability;
- indecisiveness;
- trouble concentrating; and
- lack of energy.

Headaches, stomachaches, and general aches and pains are more common in children and adolescents with depression than in adults. Major depressive disorder affects most children and adolescents, but most also suffer from anxiety disorders, substance abuse disorders, or disruptive or antisocial behavior. Adolescents and children with depression have a higher suicide risk than other young people. Depression episodes are likely to recur, just like in adults.

While more chronic, dysthymia is less severe than major depressive disorder. Dysthymia is characterized by a depressed mood that lasts for at least two years in adults, or one year in children or adolescents, along with at least two other symptoms of depression. While these symptoms might not be as incapacitating, they do prevent affected individuals from feeling well or functioning normally. Dysthymia frequently starts in early adulthood, adolescence, or childhood. In children and adolescents, dysthymia typically lasts four years without treatment.

Bipolar disorder, also known as manic-depression, is a third type of depressive disorder where individuals experience alternating episodes of major depression and mania, characterized by abnormally elevated mood or irritability. During manic periods, the person will also have three or more of the following symptoms:

- overly inflated self-esteem;
- decreased need for sleep;
- increased talkativeness;
- racing thoughts;
- distractibility;
- increased goal-directed activity or physical agitation; and
- excessive involvement in pleasurable activities that have a high potential for painful consequences.

Adolescents who are manic may do dangerous or careless things like speeding and having inappropriate sex.

Bipolar disorder typically emerges during the teenage years or early adulthood. In adults, episodes of mania and depression are distinct and occur every few years. However, children and teens with bipolar disorder may experience rapid mood swings between depression and mania multiple times a day. Diagnosing bipolar disorder in young individuals can be challenging as the symptoms can be similar to those of other mental disorders like ADHD, conduct disorder, or oppositional defiant disorder.

6.6.1.2. The Causes of Depression (Depressive Disorders)

Although the precise causes of depression are unknown, it is likely a result of a combination of biological, environmental, and social factors, much like other mental illnesses. For a long time, researchers believed that depression was caused by low brain concentrations of specific neurotransmitters, such as norepinephrine, serotonin, or dopamine. Scientists now think that depression is caused by a much more complex interplay of factors. Family studies have indicated that there may be genetic reasons for depression in children and adolescents, as evidenced by the fact that 20% to 50% of these individuals have a history of depression in their family and that children of depressed parents are more than three times more likely to suffer from a depressive disorder than children of nondepressed parents. Depression may be brought on by abnormal endocrine function, particularly of the hypothalamus or pituitary. Other risk factors for depressive disorders in youths include:

- stress;
- cigarette smoking;
- loss of a parent;
- the breakup of a romantic relationship;
- attention disorders;
- learning disorders;
- abuse;
- neglect; and
- other trauma including experiencing a natural disaster.

Although the precise causes of depression are unknown, it is likely a result of a combination of biological, environmental, and social factors, much like other mental illnesses.

Researchers have examined alterations in the brain linked to depression. PET imaging studies have revealed that while brain activity in some regions of the brain is significantly reduced in depressed individuals, activity in other regions of the brain increases when compared to the same individual following successful treatment. Additionally, depression has been linked to decreased neurotransmitter receptor binding potential in specific brain regions, according to PET imaging studies. Researchers examining the alterations in bipolar patients' brains discovered reductions in the size of the cerebellum (the area of the brain responsible for balance and coordinated movements), modifications in the metabolism of certain substances, and a drop in activity in particular brain regions (prefrontal cortex) during the depressive episode.

6.6.1.3. Treating Depression

Depression is treated with a range of antidepressant drugs and psychotherapies. For the majority of patients, a combination of medicine and psychotherapy is the most successful course of treatment.

We frequently see the advertisements for medications on television and in magazines, so we are aware that there are treatments for depressive disorders. Medication is an effective treatment for depression in up to 70% of cases. The neurotransmission pathway is often the target of medications used to treat depression disorders. For instance, certain drugs have an impact on the activity of neurotransmitters like norepinephrine and serotonin. Different pharmacological treatments are needed for different depressive disorders. For instance, people with bipolar disorder are frequently treated with a combination of mood-stabilizing and antidepressant medications during their depressive phase and a mood-stabilizing drug, such as lithium, during their manic phase.

Typically, medications can alleviate symptoms of depression within six to eight weeks. If one medication is ineffective, doctors can prescribe a different antidepressant. Like other mental health medications, patients are closely monitored by their doctors for symptoms and side effects. Patients who continue medication for at least six months after recovering from major depression have a 70% lower risk of relapse.

Patients who receive psychotherapy can learn more efficient coping mechanisms for the issues in their lives. Typically, these therapies require six to twenty weekly meetings. If within three or four months there is no improvement in the symptoms, these treatment plans should be adjusted.

Although doctors can use other techniques, the combination of medication and psychotherapy is the standard of care and is effective in most cases. When psychotherapy and antidepressants are ineffective, electroconvulsive therapy (ECT), also known as electroshock therapy, is a very successful treatment. ECT is not frequently administered to minors and young adults. The patient is put to sleep before receiving an electrical shock to particular brain regions during an ECT procedure. The shock is not felt by the patient consciously. Although ECT can produce dramatic and quick relief, its effects typically wear off rather quickly. People typically take antidepressants after electroconvulsive therapy (ECT).

The combination of medications and psychotherapy is effective in the majority of cases.

Several years back, the herbal remedy John's wort got a lot of attention when it came to over-the-counter treatments for mild to moderate depression. Nevertheless, a lot of the assertions lacked solid scientific support. The efficacy and security of St. John's wort are still unclear, and using it is generally discouraged.

6.6.1.4. Coping with Depression

Anxiety, worthlessness, powerlessness, and hopelessness are common feelings in people with depression (or other depressive disorders). Some individuals feel like giving up because of these depressing thoughts and emotions that come with the illness. As the treatment starts to work, these thoughts start to fade. Some strategies that can help a person waiting for treatment to take effect includes:

- setting realistic goals in light of the depression and assuming a reasonable amount of responsibility;
- breaking large tasks into small ones, setting some priorities, and doing what one can as one can;
- trying to be with other people and to confide in someone—it is usually better than being alone and secretive;
- participating in activities that may make one feel better;
- getting some mild exercise, going to a movie or a ball game, or participating in religious, social, or other activities;
- expecting one's mood to improve gradually, not immediately (feeling better takes time);
- postponing important decisions until the depression has lifted and discussing big decisions with family or friends who have a more objective view of the situation;
- remembering that positive thinking will replace the negative thinking that is part of the depression as one's depression responds to treatment; and
- letting one's family and friends help.

6.6.2. Suicide

Suicide is a tragically possible side effect of untreated depression. Suicide accounted for over 30,000 deaths in the US in 1997, and it was the third most common cause of death for those aged 10 to 24. More than 90% of these individuals suffered from a mental illness, most commonly from a substance-abuse disorder or a depressive disorder. According to data from the National Institute of Mental Health, up to 7% of teenagers with major depressive disorder go on to commit suicide.

Danger signs that a teen may be considering suicide include:

- undergoing dramatic personality change;
- giving away prized possessions;
- writing notes or poems about death;
- talking about suicide, even jokingly;
- making comments such as, "I can't take it anymore" or "I won't be a problem for you much longer";
- previously attempting suicide;
- running away from home; and
- having other symptoms or risk factors for depression, such as difficulty getting along with parents and friends, difficulty in school, or acting bored or withdrawn.

Suicidal children and teenagers describe feelings of worthlessness, hopelessness, rage, depression, and anxiety. They feel powerless to alter annoying situations or discover a fix for their issues. Family disputes and the suicide death of a friend, relative, or acquaintance are risk factors for child and adolescent suicide in addition to depression. Children and teenagers may require intervention in the event of another person's suicide in order to avoid social isolation, trauma, or guilt feelings. Programs designed to address these issues and which school professionals offer can be very beneficial in identifying grieving youth who may require assistance.

Establishing phone crisis hotlines, limiting access to suicide tools (such as guns), counseling the media to stop "copycat" suicides, testing teenagers for suicide risk factors, and educating medical professionals on better diagnosing and treating mood disorders are all examples of public health strategies to prevent suicide. The screening and training strategies are more beneficial than the other methods in preventing youth suicides, according to research on the efficacy of these approaches.

6.6.3. Attention Deficit Hyperactivity Disorder (ADHD)

The most often identified behavioral disorder in children is attention deficit hyperactivity disorder (ADHD). Approximately 41.1% of youths aged 9 to 17 are estimated to be affected by ADHD in any given six-month period. ADHD is two to three times more common in boys than in girls. Despite being most commonly linked to children, ADHD can still exist in adults. According to one researcher, up to two-thirds of the children he evaluated for ADHD still had the disorder in their twenties, and many of the individuals who no longer met the criteria for ADHD still experienced severe difficulties at work or in other social situations.

6.6.3.1. The Symptoms of ADHD

The three main signs of ADHD are an inability to control one's level of activity (hyperactivity), pay attention to tasks (inattention), and restrain one's behavior (impulsivity). ADHD sufferers may exhibit impulsive/hyperactive behavior most of the time, hyperactive/impulsive behavior most of the time, or a combination of the two. Children and adolescents with ADHD

- are often unpopular among their peers;
- have trouble in school;
- have higher injury rates than their peers;
- have difficulty paying attention to details;
- are easily distracted;
- find it difficult and unpleasant to finish their schoolwork;
- put off things that require continued mental effort;

- make careless mistakes;
- are disorganized;
- appear not to listen when spoken to; and
- fail to follow through on tasks.

Before diagnosing ADHD, the DSM-IV lists a number of conditions in addition to the symptoms mentioned above. For a diagnosis of ADHD, the behaviors must

- appear before age seven;
- continue for at least six months;
- be more frequent or severe than in other children of the same age' and
- cause dysfunction in at least two areas of life, such as school, home, work, or social settings.

Diagnostic interview techniques that have been tried and tested are a reliable way to diagnose ADHD. There isn't currently a reliable, independent test for ADHD, though.

ADHD commonly coexists with other behavioral, emotional, or learning issues in children, including depression, anxiety disorders, oppositional defiant disorder, and learning disabilities.

6.6.3.2. The Causes of ADHD

Although the precise causes of ADHD are unknown, research has shown that the disorder is not caused by factors that many people associate with its development. For instance, small head injuries, birth trauma, food allergies, excessive sugar intake, excessive television viewing, subpar education, or inadequate parenting do not contribute to ADHD. It is unknown what causes ADHD in one person. Instead, a number of important risk factors that have an impact on behavior expression and neurodevelopment have been linked. ADHD risk can be raised by factors like maternal alcohol and tobacco use that impact fetal brain development. Iron deficiency and other environmental pollutants have also been linked to brain damage.

Researchers have looked into how the neurotransmitter dopamine contributes to the development of ADHD because it is essential for controlling movement, boosting motivation and alertness, and causing sleeplessness. The finding that ADHD typically runs in families is compelling evidence in favor of a genetic component to the illness. At least one close relative suffers from ADHD, which is common among children with the disorder. According to one set of studies, a child's likelihood of developing ADHD is 11–18 times higher in identical twins than in nontwin siblings.

Studies on specific genes linked to ADHD have concentrated on two genes: the dopamine transporter gene (DAT1) on chromosome 5 and the dopamine receptor gene (DRD) on chromosome 11. Studies on the relationship between these genes and others and ADHD are still ongoing. The likelihood that someone has ADHD is most likely influenced by a number of genes as well as environmental variables.

According to imaging studies, boys with ADHD and boys without the disorder have different brain morphologies. Researchers discovered that boys with ADHD typically have smaller brains in specific regions. Research has indicated that the overall brain volume of girls with ADHD is smaller than that of control subjects' these findings are consistent with findings regarding the brains of boys with ADHD. The incapacity to suppress thoughts, a symptom of attention deficit hyperactivity disorder (ADHD), may be related to alterations in specific brain regions, according to scientific conjecture.

6.6.3.3. Treating ADHD

To treat ADHD, a range of drugs and behavioral therapies are employed. The most commonly used drugs are amphetamines, d-amphetamine, and methylphenidate (Ritalin). These medications act as stimulants, altering the amount of the neurotransmitter dopamine present at the synapses. When using one of these medications, nine out of ten kids get better.

These medications are thought to be fairly safe when taken as directed by licensed medical professionals. Diminished appetite and sleeplessness are side effects linked to moderate dosages. Usually starting early in the course of treatment, these side effects frequently go away over time. According to certain research, stimulants used to treat ADHD slow down growth rate without affecting final height.

Various interventions are utilized to treat ADHD, including cognitive-behavioral therapy, social skills training, support groups, and training for parents and educators. Combining medication with psychotherapy has been found to be more effective than either treatment alone in enhancing social skills, improving parent-child relationships, boosting reading achievement, and mitigating aggressive symptoms.

In order to improve social skills, parent-child relationships, reading achievement, and aggressive symptoms, treating ADHD with a combination of medication and psychotherapy is more effective than treating the disorder with either treatment alone.

Some parents and therapists have attempted a range of nutritional interventions in addition to the well-proven therapies mentioned above to treat ADHD. Some children respond well to these kinds of treatments, according to a few studies. However, no proven nutritional intervention has been demonstrated to be consistently effective in treating ADHD.

6.6.3.4. Coping with ADHD

ADHD interferes with a person's daily life, as the symptoms suggest. In addition to the treatment options available to help individuals and alleviate symptoms, the following basic strategies can also be helpful.

- Asking the teacher or boss to repeat instructions (rather than guessing what they were).
- Breaking large assignments or job tasks into small, simple tasks. Set a deadline for each task and give a reward as each one is completed.
- Making a list of what needs to be done each day. Plan the best order for doing each task. Then make a schedule for doing them. Use a calendar or daily planner to keep on track.
- Working in a quiet area. Do one thing at a time. Take short breaks.
- Writing things that need to be remembered in a notebook with dividers. Carry the book at all times.
- Posting notes as reminders of things to do.
- Storing similar things together.
- Creating a routine. Get ready for school or work at the same time, in the same way, every day.
- Exercising, eating a balanced diet, and getting enough sleep.

6.6.4. Schizophrenia

About 0.2 million Americans, or 1% of the population, suffer from schizophrenia. S. grownups. Both men and women are impacted equally. Most cases of the illness occur in young adults who are in their teens or twenties. Schizophrenia is rare until adolescence, even though it can strike children over five. In children, the illness typically progresses gradually and is frequently accompanied by delays in the development of speech or motor skills. Compared to adult-onset schizophrenia, childhood-onset schizophrenia typically has a worse prognosis and is more difficult to treat.

6.6.4.1. The Symptoms of Schizophrenia

There are a lot of false beliefs and myths regarding schizophrenia. People with schizophrenia are not multiple or split personalities, nor are they psychotic or incoherently insane all the time. While people with schizophrenia are frequently portrayed in the media as violent, in actuality, very few of these individuals pose a threat to others. Actually, rather than being violent themselves, people with schizophrenia are more likely to be victims of violence.

Schizophrenia has severe symptoms. A diagnosis of schizophrenia requires that at least two of the symptoms below be present during a significant portion of a one-month period:

- delusions (false beliefs such as conspiracies, mind control, or persecution);
- hallucinations (usually voices criticizing or commenting on the person's behavior);
- disorganized speech (incomprehensible or difficult to understand);
- grossly disorganized or catatonic behavior; and
- negative symptoms such as flat emotions, lack of facial expressions, and inattention to basic self-care needs such as bathing and eating.

However, if the delusions are particularly strange or if the hallucinations include one or more voices continuously commenting on the subject's actions or thoughts, the presence of any one of the first two symptoms is sufficient to diagnose schizophrenia.

- The DSM-IV specifies additional criteria for a diagnosis of schizophrenia are:
- social or occupational dysfunction;
- persistence of the disturbance for at least six months;
- exclusion of a mood disorder;
- exclusion of a substance-abuse or medical condition that causes similar symptoms; and
- consideration of a possible pervasive developmental disorder.

The majority of individuals with schizophrenia typically go through one or more relapses following their initial psychotic episode. Relapses are times when an illness's symptoms—such as hallucinations and delusions—are more severe. Negative symptoms pertaining to emotion or self-care are typically still present during remissions. 10% or so of patients never fully recover from their severe illnesses and never return to their pre-illness states. Up to one-third to one-half of those with schizophrenia experience significant improvement or even full recovery from their condition, according to several long-term studies.

6.6.4.2. The Causes of Schizophrenia

Similar to the other mental illnesses covered here, the cause of schizophrenia is still a mystery to scientists. The disease is most likely caused by a combination of genetic and environmental factors, just like other mental illnesses. Many research point to the involvement of imbalances in the brain's chemical neurotransmitter systems, such as those involving glutamate, norepinephrine,

GABA, and dopamine, in the development of schizophrenia.

Studies on adoption, twins, and families lend credence to the notion that genetics plays a significant part in the illness. For instance, compared to the general population, children of individuals with schizophrenia are 13 times more likely to develop the disorder, and identical twins are 48 times more likely. Researchers are still searching for genes that could contribute to schizophrenia. Researchers studying schizophrenia are interested in a gene that produces an enzyme that degrades dopamine at the synapses. The function of this and other genes is still being investigated.

Imaging studies have shown that the brain structure and function of people with schizophrenia differ from those of control subjects. According to research on brain imaging, the brains of young people with schizophrenia differ structurally from those of people without the disorder. Reduced amounts of gray matter, which makes up the majority of the brain and is primarily composed of neuron cell bodies and dendrites, enlarged brain ventricles—the cavities or spaces in the brain that are filled with cerebrospinal fluid—and other abnormalities are some of the changes that have occurred. The cerebrum, the upper portion of the brain that is divided into halves, has also shrunk in volume. The frontal lobes, or the front portion of the cerebral lobes, exhibit less brain activity in the identical twin with schizophrenia than in the twin without the disorder, according to PET scans of the twins. Over the course of five years, one team of researchers used MRI to periodically scan the brains of teenagers with childhood-onset schizophrenia and an age-matched control group. They found that teens with schizophrenia lose four times the amount of neurons in a specific region of the brain that teens in the control group lose.

6.6.4.3. Treating Schizophrenia

Schizophrenia cannot be cured, but there are effective treatments that help most affected individuals manage their condition. Antipsychotic medication in addition to various psychotherapeutic interventions is the ideal course of treatment.

Antipsychotic medications, such as chlorpromazine and haloperidol, have been prescribed by physicians since the 1950s to treat schizophrenia-related hallucinations and delusions. More recently, it has been shown that newer antipsychotic medications—also referred to as atypical—like risperidone and clozapine are more efficacious. Prompt and consistent therapy, incorporating antipsychotic medication, is crucial for enhancing the disease's trajectory in the long run. Patients who stop taking their medication run the risk of getting sick again.

The most successful schizophrenia patients combine psychosocial rehabilitation (training in life skills) with medication. Schizophrenic patients benefit from therapies that combine behavioral and cognitive skills, education, and support from their families and communities to address particular issues. These approaches enhance the quality of life and functioning of the patients.

6.7. Emotional Problems

For all of us, health is an essential and natural concern. It's a dynamic process that varies continuously. Being well is a blessing and a necessity. A healthy person can accomplish more work in less time and doesn't put off doing their tasks. He can complete tasks on time and with reasonable efficiency. His work gains vitality and strength from his good health. He also takes pleasure in his food and lives life to the fullest. We can manage job success, physical activity, emotional issues, and stress management if we take responsibility for our own wellbeing. Wellness is an improvement in quality of life with personal growth or positive behaviors and attitude.

Taking care of your health is a valuable asset. You can do this by engaging in regular physical exercise, going for early morning walks, playing, eating a balanced diet, getting enough rest, and managing your stress levels. Neglecting your health can lead to disorders, such as mental illness, which can impact your ability to learn and grow intellectually. Mental disorders affect a person's behavior, emotions, and mood. While it is normal to experience a range of emotions, if these feelings start to disrupt your life, you may be experiencing a mental or emotional disorder.

Disorders can start in childhood or adolescence and may remain undiagnosed or untreated for many years. Emotional turmoil can lead to a mental disorder, often caused by abnormalities in brain development or function. If your emotions and feelings are not functioning properly, it may be a psychological issue. Excessive emotional thinking and dramatic behavior can be clear signs of an emotional disorder.

Emotional disorders are not highly specialized' rather, there is a relationship between the disorders and specific circumstances such as physical abuse, poverty, neglect, parental stress, excessive expectations, rule changes, confusions, and so forth. Eight emotional issues that arise in daily life are defined here along with their corresponding solutions.

6.7.1. Anorexia and Bulimia

An eating disorder called anorexia causes unhealthful weight loss. Anorexics may have a skewed perception of their bodies, leading them to purge or restrict calories in an attempt to achieve unattainable weight targets. Meal skipping, reduced portion sizes, and a growing number of restricted food options are common effects of calorie restriction. Remorse over what you eat can cause you to purge through food, exercise, or prescription drugs like laxatives. Malnutrition can occur and may cause damage to normal development and growth.

Anorexia can affect anyone, even though it more commonly affects women. Any gender, race, ethnicity, age, social class, and economic status can develop anorexia.

Many times, people who develop anorexia begin with the very understandable desire to lead a healthier lifestyle. But eventually, compulsive ideas about working out, dieting, and losing weight take over. These result in excessive weight loss and unhealthy behaviors.

The child may become secretive about their eating habits and restrictions as a result of the eating disorder. Eating disorders can develop subtly, and parents and physicians frequently fail to identify them. Anorexics regulate their body weight. They may:

- Eat only a small number of "safe" foods, usually low in calories and fat;
- Avoid eating food on their plate by moving it around or cutting it up into tiny pieces;
- Not eat food they cook for others;
- Do things to keep their mind off their hunger, such as chewing gum or drinking large amounts of water;
- Exercise in excess.

Your child may also:

- Wear baggy clothes to hide their body;
- Spend more time alone and away from friends and family;
- Tire more quickly;
- Seem depressed or anxious;

- Be more emotional, or quick to cry or get angry.

Malnutrition can cause anorexia over time, which can impact the entire body. It most obviously affects the heart, brain, bones, reproductive, and digestive systems. A lack of food can cause both physical and mental changes in the body.

Physical changes with anorexia:

- Always feeling cold because the body has lost the fat it needs to keep warm.
- Dizziness, fainting, or near fainting.
- More noticeable bones because of a loss of normal fat layers and muscle.
- Hair loss.
- Brittle hair and fingernails.
- Dry and rough skin.
- Affected menstrual periods. If anorexia develops before a girl's first period, periods may not start. For girls developing anorexia later, periods may stop.
- Stomach pain, constipation and bloating.
- Stunted growth that could be permanent.
- Anemia (low count of red blood cells) causing tiredness, weakness and dizziness.

Mental changes with anorexia:

- Feeling depressed, anxious or irritable;
- Decreased concentration;
- Increased difficulty completing tasks, such as schoolwork.

When it comes to mental illnesses, anorexia has the highest death rate. Suicide or malnutrition (the body not getting enough nutrients) are two possible causes of death.

Bulimia is an eating disorder characterized by binge eating excessive amounts of food followed by an attempt to somehow neutralize the effects of the binge. Usually, the individual gets rid of (purges) the food they've consumed.

Bulimics frequently consume large quantities of food in a short period of time during a binge. A person's binge usually comes to an end when they run out of food, experience stomach pains after eating, or are distracted. Because the person experiencing the binge frequently feels helpless and out of control, binges are typically emotionally upsetting.

Bulimia sufferers often experience guilt and fear of gaining weight after bingeing. Through vomiting or other means, they rid their bodies of the food in an attempt to alleviate their guilt and fear. They might also resort to rigorous dieting or intense exercise. This "control" period continues until the subsequent binge. After then, the cycle resumes.

In contrast to bulimics, binge-eaters experience extreme guilt after consuming large amounts of food quickly, but they do not purge after a binge.

While bulimia is most commonly seen in teenage girls and young adult women, it can affect individuals regardless of gender, race, age, ethnicity, or social and economic background.

Individuals with bulimia experience dissatisfaction with their bodies, leading them to engage in bingeing behaviors as a response to anxiety and other emotions. Those with bulimia may exhibit underweight, overweight, or average weight.

People with bulimia have difficulty controlling their eating behavior. They may

- Become very secretive about binge eating;

- Spend a lot of time thinking about and planning the next binge. For example, they may;
- Set aside certain times to binge and purge:
  - Avoid social activities to binge and purge;
  - Steal food or hide it in different places, such as under their bed or in closets;
  - Exercise or use laxatives to "purge" their body of food consumed.

People with bulimia often face other problems as well, such as:

- Depression and thoughts of suicide;
- Substance use.

Bulimia harms a person's physical and mental health. For example,

- Teeth start to decay from contact with stomach acids during vomiting.
- Weight goes up and down.
- Menstrual periods may become irregular or stop.
- The face and throat may look puffy and swollen.
- Dizziness and fainting may occur.
- Dehydration caused by loss of body fluids occurs.
- Upset stomach, constipation, and sore throat.
- Damage to vital organs such as the liver and kidneys' heart problems.
- Death.

Eating disorders have no known cause. Still, there are a few things that could be involved. These include certain personality traits, environmental factors, and a family history of eating disorders or mood disorders. Recovery from an eating disorder is more likely the earlier it is identified. Therapy is based on numerous factors. These include the eating disorder's stage, the person's readiness to change, and the support of family members.

Treatment for eating disorders requires a team approach to be successful. Numerous medical professionals collaborate as a team. Every single one addresses a particular facet of the illness.

A pediatrician should be consulted before starting treatment so they can evaluate the physical effects of the eating disorder. In the event that the effects are severe, hospitalization may be required. Successful treatment of the eating disorder requires first restoring good nutrition and physical health.

The team assists a patient in returning to a healthy weight as part of their anorexia treatment. Regaining weight is essential to a full recovery. A person may require hospital admission for nourishment if they refuse to eat.

When treating bulimia, the medical team may decide to admit the patient to the hospital in order to address comorbid conditions like electrolyte imbalance or dehydration, or to break the binge-purge cycle.

6.7.2. Antisocial Personality Disorder

Although the official diagnosis of true antisocial personality disorder cannot be made until the adolescent is eighteen, most teens with this disorder have shown this pattern of behavior since before the age of fifteen. Without expert assistance and a loving family, they might develop into immature, careless adults with a startling lack of morality as adults.

6.7.2.1. Signs of Antisocial Personality Disorder

- Irritability and aggressiveness;
- Frequent fighting;
- Lying, cheating and other deceitful behavior;
- Impulsivity;
- Reckless disregard for personal safety or the safety of others;
- Lack of remorse for hurtful acts;
- Failure to apply oneself in school;
- History of truancy, delinquency, vandalism, theft, unlawful acts.

6.7.3. Bipolar Disorder

You might wonder if your child's extreme mood swings are a normal part of growing up or if there's something more serious going on if they also show significant changes in how they interact with friends, family, and school.

Recently, there has been much discussion about mental health, and almost all parents and caregivers are worried about it. Many of us believe that our children will manage somehow if they are loved and understood. In addition, we are aware that 1 in 6 youth suffer from a mental illness that is incurable without medical attention.

Approximately 1% to 2% of all U. S. Children under the age of eighteen suffer from bipolar disorder, a condition marked by sporadic changes in behavior and mood. Here are some things to consider about bipolar disorder and how to recognize symptoms in your child. Children and teenagers with bipolar disorder can eventually get better with treatment.

Bipolar disorder, formerly known as manic depression, is a brain illness that results in abrupt mood swings. Individuals diagnosed with bipolar disorder (bipolar I, bipolar II, or cyclothymia) experience manic episodes characterized by heightened mood, irritability, and high energy levels. Sometimes, they might also experience depressive episodes where they feel down, discouraged, and hopeless. Even during acute manic or depressive episodes, children and adolescents are more prone to experience mood swings.

Children who have bipolar disorder may also exhibit symptoms that are eerily similar to those of other common childhood disorders, including major depressive disorder, anxiety disorders, conduct disorders, and substance use disorders, as well as attention deficit hyperactivity disorder (ADHD) and disruptive mood dysregulation disorder (DMDD). Additionally, childhood trauma is very important for mental health. These are just a few of the explanations for why, even in cases where children exhibit multiple symptoms suggestive of bipolar disorder, medical professionals frequently struggle to reach a definitive diagnosis.

Children who suffer from bipolar disorder experience abrupt and severe swings in their sleep, mood, and energy levels, which can interfere with their ability to think clearly and interact socially.

When a child is experiencing mania, they might:

- Act incredibly happy, silly or even giddy;
- Feel more irritable or impatient than usual;
- Talk rapidly, hopping from subject to subject;
- Need much less sleep than usual without feeling tired;
- Struggle to stay focused on one task or topic;
- Show strong interest in dangerous/ risky activities;

- Make snap decisions that seem out of character;
- Lose or break things they value (mobile phones, bikes, jewelry, etc.);
- Experience more conflicts or misunderstandings with others.

When they're in a depressed mood, kids with bipolar disorder might:

- Feel sad, discouraged or hopeless;
- Show more anger and irritability than usual;
- Complain of pain, such as stomach troubles or headaches;
- Sleep much more than usual—or have trouble getting to sleep;
- Experience "brain fog" that makes it hard for them to concentrate;
- Have much less energy than normal for them;
- Turn away from friends, family and activities they usually love;
- Eat too much or too little;
- Talk or think about death or suicide.

6.7.4. Emotional Eating

Beyond sating hunger and meeting nutritional needs, food is used by both adults and children for other purposes. Actually, a lot of the time, kids who are obese eat because it fulfills them.

Think about if your own parents in your home relied on food for comfort. This is a typical occurrence that starts at birth. Breast milk or infant formula is usually given to a crying or agitated baby, and feeding him becomes a means of soothing and quieting him. Children are frequently given cookies or other desserts at birthdays and holidays when they are surrounded by family and feel loved' these treats then come to represent this love and caring. These days, your own child may turn to food as a comfort when he is feeling anxious, possibly because of an impending math test or because he is being teased at school. On the other hand, children may eat for a variety of other reasons besides comfort.

Youngsters sometimes reach for food when he's experiencing any of the following

- Boredom;
- Insecurity;
- Anger;
- Depression;
- Loneliness;
- Happiness;
- Stress;
- Fatigue;
- Frustration;
- Resentment.

Your child may come to enjoy food, but the results might not be exactly what he was hoping for. Ironically, he might feel worse after a food binge knowing that it can exacerbate his weight problem if he overeats to ease feelings of insecurity or depression, for example, or maybe because he is stressed about giving an oral report at school. He may feel guilty or ashamed even before the food has had a chance to break down.

Determining whether your child is eating for the correct reasons is actually one of your biggest parenting challenges. Consider the following: Does he eat outside of regular mealtimes and snacks? Does he constantly munch? What possible causes of his overeating exist that require your intervention?

When parents reward their kids with food—does getting an A on an exam sometimes mean going to the ice cream shop?—they unintentionally contribute to their kids' obesity. Praise and rewards can be given in healthier ways. Consider rewarding a young child with a few stickers or planning a shopping trip to purchase a new pair of shoes or a toy.

Don't undervalue the significance of verbal affirmation. Inform your child when he is acting appropriately. Observe how encouraging remarks can help him feel better about himself and be inspired to keep choosing the best course of action for his weight and health. Look for alternative methods to express gratitude, even if he's struggling to stick to his diet ("You walked more than half a mile today, that's so great!"). Don't bother him or give him the impression that he failed when he regresses. Encourage him to press on, regardless of his occasional complaints ("I want a soft drink, not ice water"), and to persevere through the situation. Give him all of the assistance he requires and merits.

6.7.5. Disruptive Behavior Disorders

Of all the coexisting conditions, disruptive behavior disorders are among the easiest to recognize because they involve actions that are easy to observe, like throwing tantrums, physically attacking other children, arguing excessively, stealing, and other acts of defiance or resistance to authority. These disorders, which include CD and ODD, usually become noticeable when they affect peer and family relationships or academic performance, and they often get worse over time.

Disruptive behavior disorders (DBD), ODD, and CD are all regarded as distinct conditions that can occur separately. However, behaviors characteristic of DBD can closely resemble ADHD—particularly when impulsivity and hyperactivity are involved. Coexisting ODD and CD are present in up to one-third of children with ADHD and up to 25% of children with CD, respectively. Because their defiant behavior causes so many conflicts with adults and other people they interact with, children with both conditions typically lead more difficult lives than those with ADHD alone. On the other hand, your child's chances of learning to control these behaviors may increase with early detection and treatment.

6.7.5.1. Oppositional Defiant Disorder

Many kids with ADHD occasionally act in an oppositional manner. The Diagnostic and Statistical Manual of Mental Disorders, Fourth Edition (DSM-IV) published by the American Psychiatric Association defines oppositional defiant disorder as characterized by recurrent episodes of "negativistic, defiant, disobedient, and hostile behaviors toward authority figures.". In addition to arguing with adults frequently, losing his temper easily, disobeying rules, blaming others for his own mistakes, purposefully upsetting others, and acting in other ways that are angry, resentful, and vindictive, a child with ODD may also exhibit these behaviors. He will probably run into disciplinary issues and social conflicts at school on a regular basis. Many times, these symptoms get worse over time, sometimes to the point where a conduct disorder diagnosis is made, especially in the absence of early diagnosis and treatment.

6.7.5.2. Conduct Disorder

Conduct disorder is a more severe condition than ODD. It is characterized by a repetitive and persistent pattern of behavior that involves violating the basic rights of others or major age-appropriate social rules. Symptoms of CD may include serious aggression towards people, harm to animals, destruction of property, stealing, running away from home, skipping school, or breaking social rules without consequences. Many children with CD may have previously been diagnosed with ODD, especially if they were physically aggressive at a younger age. Children with CD often continue to exhibit symptoms of ODD, such as argumentativeness and resistance. These behaviors, combined with impulsivity and hyperactivity of ADHD, may lead to these children being perceived as delinquent. They are more likely to be suspended from school and have more police contact compared to children with ADHD alone or ADHD with ODD.

Compared to adults with ADHD alone or ADHD plus ODD, children with ADHD whose CD symptoms began early also typically have worse outcomes as adults, especially when it comes to delinquency, criminal activity, and drug abuse.

Behavioral strategies tailored to the needs of children with ADHD and disruptive behavior disorders can be used both at home and in the classroom. These strategies usually involve teaching your child to recognize his own anger cues and to use them as cues to start different coping mechanisms, such as "Take five deep breaths and consider the three best options for how to respond before lashing out at a teacher."), and give himself praise (saying to himself, "Well done, you saw the cue and applied your tactics!"), for exercising self-control. In the meantime, you and your child's teachers can learn how to better handle ODD or CD-type behavior by bargaining, making concessions, working through problems with your child, anticipating and averting potentially explosive situations, and setting priorities so that less critical issues are put off until more critical ones have been resolved. Professional behavior therapists or other mental health specialists recommended by your child's pediatrician, school psychologist, or other family-related professionals can teach these extremely specific techniques.

It might be decided to put your child in a special classroom at school that is designed for more rigorous behavior management if he has a diagnosis of coexisting ODD or CD and well-planned classroom behavioral techniques in his mainstream classroom have not worked. Still, schools are required to educate your child in a mainstream classroom whenever feasible and to revisit your child's education plan on a regular basis to determine whether or not it is still the best fit for him.

An increasing body of research suggests that the stimulant drugs used to treat core ADHD symptoms may also benefit coexisting CD and ODD. It has been demonstrated that stimulants can lessen stealing, vandalism, hostile peer interactions, and physical and verbal aggression. Stimulant drugs may lessen the aggression that prevents kids from forming relationships with people their own age, even though they don't teach them new skills like recognizing and responding to others' social cues. Because of this, when it comes to medication treatment for children who have both ADHD and a co-occurring disruptive behavior disorder, stimulants are typically the first option.

Introducing stimulants to address coexisting ODD or CD at an early stage is highly beneficial. If a child with disruptive behavior disorder does not receive treatment for their aggressive behavior, they may gravitate towards others who also exhibit discipline issues. As they enter adolescence, they may reject treatment that could assist in changing their behavior, potentially causing them to be excluded by these peers. By this point, they may have become accustomed to their defiant nature and feel out of place when stimulants curb their reckless behavior. Treating these behaviors during elementary school or earlier can greatly reduce the chances of your child developing a negative self-image.

Your child's pediatrician may decide to reassess the situation and substitute other medications for the stimulant if your child has received treatment with two or more types of stimulants and his aggressive symptoms remain the same or worse. His pediatrician may continue to prescribe stimulants in combination with one of these other agents if the stimulant medication alone produced some but not enough improvement.

6.7.6. Fears and Phobias

Fears are common as children develop and learn about the world around them, often encountering new situations and obstacles.

One common childhood fear is the fear of being alone in the dark. A fear of animals, like big barking dogs, is also included. Certain kids have a fear of thunderstorms, high places, and fires. Others worry about terrorism or war because they are aware of the images in the media. They might start worrying about the well-being of people around them if there has been a recent serious illness or death in the family.

The fears in your child may come and go. Most phobias in childhood are small. However, even when they worsen, they usually go away on their own with time, comfort, and support. However, there are instances when fears can turn into phobias because they are so intense, enduring, and narrowly focused.

Strong, illogical fears are known as phobias, and they can seriously disrupt a child's regular daily activities. For instance, a 6-year-old who has a dog phobia may become so anxious about potential dog encounters that they won't venture outside at all. A 10-year-old child may insist on spending the night with his parents due to fear stemming from news reports about a serial killer.

6.7.6.1. Social Phobias

Some kids get phobias related to the people they come into contact with on a daily basis. Their extreme shyness may prevent them from relating to most adults, especially strangers, and from forming friends at school. They might purposefully stay away from social events like club meetings, birthday celebrations, and sporting events. They might find it awkward to converse with anyone outside of their close family.

In children, separation anxiety is also prevalent. This anxiety can occasionally get worse when the family transfers to a new neighborhood or daycare. These kids might develop anxiety related to attending school or summer camp. They may experience physical symptoms from their phobias, such as headaches or stomachaches.

6.7.6.2. Treatment for Childhood Fears & Phobias

Thankfully, the majority of phobias are easily treated. If your child's anxiety keeps getting in the way of their enjoyment of life, they may benefit from seeing a child psychologist or psychiatrist who treats phobias.

6.7.6.3. Behavioral Therapy

Many therapists recommend exposing your child to the source of their anxiety in small, nonthreatening doses as part of a phobia treatment plan.

A child who is afraid of dogs may start by talking about this fear and by watching pictures or videos of dogs, under the supervision of a therapist. After that, they might observe a neighborhood dog from the protection of a window. Then, they might spend a few minutes in the same room as a kind, amiable puppy with a parent or therapist by their side. They will eventually be able to stroke the dog. They will gradually become more comfortable around bigger, stranger dogs.

This process, known as desensitization, involves your child becoming less sensitive to their fear each time they face it. Eventually, they will no longer feel the need to avoid the situation that triggers their phobia. Psychotherapy can occasionally aid in children's development of greater confidence and decreased fear. Children can benefit from breathing techniques and relaxation exercises when they are under stress.

Phobias are treated initially with behavior therapy. Your child's doctor may suggest medication as part of the treatment plan in rare instances where behavioral therapy isn't providing enough assistance. This would serve as an additional therapeutic tool rather than behavioral therapy as the only one. Among these medications are antidepressants, which work to lessen the anxiety and panic that frequently accompany these issues.

6.7.7. Fecal Soiling

Boys are more likely than girls to experience fecal soiling, which is referred to medically as encopresis in children over the age of four. It affects approximately 10.5% of young schoolchildren. Although less common than inadvertent urination or small leaks, it can cause greater distress for both parents and children. Not only is the smell more overpowering and unsettling, but in our culture, even two-year-olds are expected to "know better" than to sully their pants.

Fecal soiling, however, is typically not a choice' rather, it happens when a child resists having bowel movements due to emotional stress, resistance to toilet training, or physical pain. Constipation results from this resistance, or stool retention, and when the pressure builds up, it causes involuntary leakage or soiling. If this keeps happening, the child may find it more difficult to feel the urge to urinate because the muscles involved in ejecting stool may start to stretch and local nerve sensations may decrease. The intestines might become less able to contract, which would make bowel movements even more difficult and increased likelihood of fecal soiling.

Most of the time, treating the underlying issue that is making your child resisting a bowel movement is the best course of action when it comes to dealing with the problem of fecal soiling caused by constipation. If you support him while he defecates or lessen the pressure to use the potty, for example, he might stop holding onto his stool. Additionally, if his bowel movements become more regular, his fecal soiling may go away.

But make sure to schedule a visit with your child's pediatrician if the issue persists after one or two mishaps. He will look over your child's medical history to see if the soiling is due to a physical condition instead of stool retention. Accidental soiling can occasionally result from allergies, ulcerative colitis, congenital megacolon or Hirschsprung's disease (a congenital condition that prevents a child from feeling the sensation of having a full bowel), or even from a diet that contains an excessive amount of dairy products or high-fat foods.

Emotional or psychological causes should be taken into consideration if the physical causes have also been ruled out. Fecal soiling can happen when a child experiences anxiety or emotional distress related to an uncontrollable aspect of their life, like family disputes, academic setbacks, or social interaction issues. If soiling persists, it might also be necessary to take into account sexual and physical abuse.

Of course, it's not out of the question for any young child to experience an incident like this once or twice. Whatever the reason, your child needs to understand that he is not to blame for what happened, and that you are aware of it as well.

Similar to bedwetting, the best course of action is to tidy up right away, try to minimize feelings of shame and embarrassment, and give him the knowledge he needs to better regulate his bowel movements and maintain clean clothes. After ensuring that your child's feelings are safeguarded, you can move forward with determining the root cause, keeping in mind that a solution might not be available right away.

A Closer Look

Agitation

Agitation is a common and distressing symptom characterized by a state of heightened arousal, restlessness, and emotional tension. It can manifest in various ways, ranging from pacing, fidgeting, and hand-wringing to verbal outbursts, aggression, and hostility. Agitation often accompanies underlying medical or psychiatric conditions and can significantly impair an individual's ability to function and interact with others.

Agitation can arise from a wide range of factors, including medical conditions, psychiatric disorders, substance use, environmental stressors, and medication side effects. Common medical causes include pain, infection, dehydration, metabolic imbalances, and neurological conditions such as dementia, traumatic brain injury, or stroke. Psychiatric disorders such as anxiety, depression, bipolar disorder, and psychosis may also present with agitation as a prominent symptom.

The symptoms of agitation can vary widely but often include physical restlessness, pacing, hand-wringing, or tapping. Individuals may exhibit verbal agitation through yelling, cursing, or screaming, or they may display aggressive behaviors such as hitting, pushing, or throwing objects. Emotional symptoms may include heightened irritability, anxiety, or fear, as well as emotional lability or mood swings. In severe cases, agitation can lead to self-injurious behaviors or harm to others.

Managing agitation requires a comprehensive approach tailored to the underlying cause and individual needs. Non-pharmacological interventions such as providing a calm and structured environment, reducing sensory stimuli, using distraction techniques, or engaging in therapeutic activities (e.g., music, relaxation exercises) can help de-escalate agitation. Pharmacological interventions, including antipsychotic medications, benzodiazepines, or sedatives, may be necessary in cases of severe agitation or when non-pharmacological measures are ineffective or contraindicated. However, the use of medications should be carefully considered, weighing potential risks and benefits, and monitored closely to minimize adverse effects.

Summary

- Mental illnesses are diseases or conditions that affect how you think, feel, act, or relate to other people or to your surroundings.
- Many people feel that mental illness is rare, something that only happens to people with life situations very different from their own, and that it will never affect them.
- Suicide is the third leading cause of death for 15- to 24-year-olds and the sixth leading cause of death for 5- to 15-year-olds.
- Schizophrenia is rare in children under age 12, but it occurs in about 3 of every 1,000 adolescents.
- Some of the predominant neurotransmitters in the brain include glutamate, GABA, serotonin, dopamine, and norepinephrine.
- PET measures the spatial distribution and movement of a radioactive chemical injected into the tissues of living subjects.
- Genetic, environmental, and social factors interact to influence whether someone becomes mentally ill.
- Medications are often used to treat mental illnesses. Through television commercials and magazine advertisements, we are becoming more aware of those medications.
- Depression is more than just being in a bad mood or feeling sad. Everyone experiences these feelings on occasion, but that does not constitute depression.
- Children and adolescents who are suicidal report feelings of depression, anger, anxiety, hopelessness, and worthlessness.
- Attention deficit hyperactivity disorder (ADHD) is the most commonly diagnosed behavioral disorder of childhood. In any six-month period, ADHD affects an estimated 4.1% of youths ages 9 to 17.
- Schizophrenia is not a multiple or split personality, nor are individuals who have this illness constantly incoherent or psychotic.

References

1. Agency for Healthcare Policy and Research. (1999). *Treatment of Depression—Newer Pharmacotherapies*. Summary, Evidence Report/Technology Assessment, Number 7. Retrieved from: http://www.ahcpr.gov/clinic/deprsumm.htm (accessed on 7 September 2024).
2. American Psychiatric Association. (2000). *Diagnostic and Statistical Manual of Mental Disorders* (4th ed., text rev.). Washington, DC: American Psychiatric Press.
3. Castellanos, F. X., Giedd, J. N., Berquin, P. C., Walter, J. M., Sharp, W., Tran, T., Vaituzis, A. C., Blumenthal, J. D., Nelson, J., Bastain, T. M., Zijdenbos, A., Evans, A. C., & Rapoport, J. L. (2001). Quantitative brain magnetic resonance imaging in girls with attention-deficit/hyperactivity disorder. *Archives of General Psychiatry, 58*, 289–295.
4. Castellanos, F. X., Giedd, J. N., Marsh, W. L., Hamburger, S. D., Vaituzis, A. C., Dickstein, D. P., Sarfatti, S. E., Vauss, Y. C., Snell, J. W., Lange, N., Kaysen, D., Krain, A. L., Ritchie, G. F.,

Rajapakse, J. C., & Rapoport, J. L. (1996). Quantitative brain magnetic resonance imaging in attention-deficit hyperactivity disorder. *Archives of General Psychiatry, 53*, 607–616.

5. Commission on Behavioral and Social Sciences Education, National Research Council. (2000). *How People Learn: Brain, Mind, Experience, and School*. Washington, DC: National Academies Press.
6. Corrigan, P., & Lundin, R. (2001). *Don't Call Me Nuts*. Tinley Park, IL: Recovery Press.
7. Egan, M. F., Goldberg, T. E., Koachana, B. S., Callicott, J. H., Mazzanti, C. M., Straub, R. E., Goldman, D., & Weinberger, D. R. (2001). Effect of COMT Val 108/158 Met genotype on frontal lobe function and risk for schizophrenia. *Proceedings of the National Academy of Sciences USA, 98*, 6917–6922.
8. Jaska, P. (1998). *Fact Sheet on Attention Deficit Hyperactivity Disorder (ADHD/ADD)*. Retrieved from: http://www.add.org/content/abc/factsheet.htm (accessed on 7 September 2024).
9. Joint Committee on National Health Education Standards. (1995). *National Health Education Standards: Achieving Health Literacy*. Atlanta, GA: American Cancer Society.
10. Loucks-Horsley, S., Love, N., Hewson, P. W., & Stiles, K. E. (1998). *Designing Professional Development for Teachers of Science and Mathematics*. Thousand Oaks, CA: Corwin Press.
11. National Alliance for the Mentally Ill. (2001). *Schizophrenia*. Retrieved from: http://www.nami.org/helpline/schizophrenia.html (accessed on 7 September 2024).
12. National Institute of Mental Health. (1996). *Attention Deficit Hyperactivity Disorder*. Retrieved from: http://www.nimh.nih.gov/publicat/adhd.cfm (accessed on 7 September 2024).
13. National Institute of Mental Health. (1999a). *Schizophrenia*. Retrieved from: http://www.nimh.nih.gov/publicat/schizoph.cfm (accessed on 7 September 2024).
14. Pearlson, G. D. (2000). Neurobiology of schizophrenia. *Annals of Neurology, 48*, 556–566.
15. Rapoport, J. L., Castellanos, F. X., Gogate, N., Janson, K., Kohler, S., & Nelson, P. (2001). Imaging normal and abnormal brain development: New perspectives for child psychiatry. *Australian and New Zealand Journal of Psychiatry, 35*, 272–281.
16. Rapoport, J. L., Giedd, J., Kumra, S., Jacobsen, L., Smith, A., Lee, P., Nelson, J., & Hamburger, S. (1997). Childhood-onset schizophrenia: Progressive ventricular change during adolescence. *Archives of General Psychiatry, 54*, 897–903.
17. Sowell, E. R., Toga, A. W., & Asarnow, R. (2000). Brain abnormalities observed in childhood-onset schizophrenia: A review of the structural magnetic resonance imaging literature. *Mental Retardation and Developmental Disabilities Research Review, 6*, 180–185.
18. Stoll, A. L., Renshaw, P. F., Yurgelun-Todd, D. A., & Cohen, B. M. (2000). Neuroimaging in bipolar disorder: What have we learned? *Biological Psychiatry, 15*, 505–517.
19. Thompson, P. M., Vidal, C., Giedd, J. N., Gochman, P., Blumenthal, J., Nicolson, R., Toga, A. W., & Rapoport, J. L. (2001). Mapping adolescent brain change reveals dynamic wave of accelerated gray matter loss in very early-onset schizophrenia. *Proceedings of the National Academy of Sciences USA, 98*, 11650–11655.
20. U.S. Public Health Service. (2000). *Report of the Surgeon General's Conference on Children's Mental Health: A National Action Agenda*. Retrieved from: http://www.surgeongeneral.gov/cmh/childreport.htm (accessed on 7 September 2024).

21. Yatham, L. N., Liddle, P. F., Shiah, I. S., Scarrow, G., Lam, R. W., Adam, M. J., Zis, A. P., & Ruth, T. J. (2000). Brain serotonin2 receptors in major depression: A positron emission tomography study. *Archives of General Psychiatry, 57*, 850–858.

Chapter

7

OBSESSIVE – COMPULSIVE, RELATED DISORDERS, AND PERSONALITY DISORDERS

Contents

Introduction

The extreme anxiety that some people experience led to the previous classification of obsessive compulsive disorder (OCD) as an anxiety disorder. But there are some key distinctions between it and other anxiety disorders. A spectrum of obsessive compulsive disorders can be used to describe certain disorders, like OCD, that are marked by recurrent thoughts and/or behaviors. The spectrum approach covers a wide range of repetitive behaviors, including hoarding, kleptomania, pyromania, or oniomania' disorders of body appearance or function, such as body dysmorphic disorder (BDD)' and self-soothing behaviors, such as trichotillomania, dermatillomania, or onychophagia. Several conditions included in the obsessive compulsive spectrum are not recognized as official diagnoses by the American Psychiatric Association. Psychiatrists are still engaged in scholarly debate over whether various behavioral clusters are symptoms of a distinct disorder or should be included in a different diagnosis based on their identification and analysis. As in the instance of dissociative identity disorder, also referred to as multiple personality disorder, discussions and debates can rage for years without reaching a consensus. Diagnostic criteria for OCD, BDD, trichotillomania (hair pulling), excoriation (skin picking), hoarding disorder, and disorders resulting from substance abuse, medication, or other sources are listed in the Diagnostic and Statistical Manual of Mental Disorders, Fifth Edition (DSM5).

Orientation and Directional Terms

Term	Definition	Illustration
Obsessive-compulsive disorder (OCD)	Obsessive-compulsive disorder (OCD) is a disorder in which people have recurring, unwanted thoughts, ideas or sensations (obsessions). To get rid of the thoughts, they feel driven to do something repetitively (compulsions). The repetitive behaviors, such as hand washing/cleaning, checking on things, and mental acts like (counting) or other activities, can significantly interfere with a person's daily activities and social interactions.	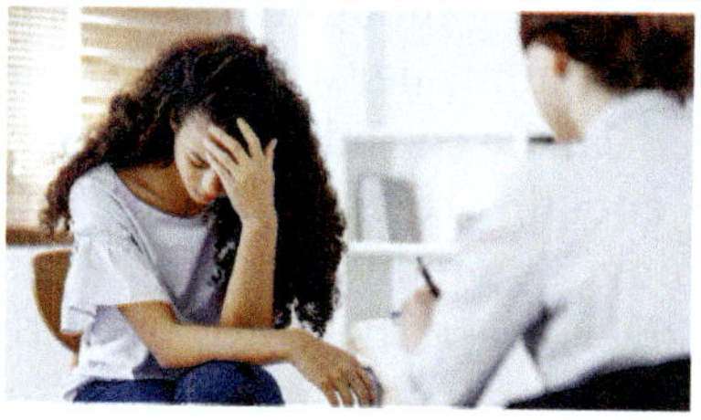
Body dysmorphic disorder (BDD)	Body dysmorphic disorder is a mental health condition that disrupts how you see and feel about your own body and appearance. People commonly experience negative thoughts and emotions about how they look, which can cause severe disruptions in their life and undermine their mental and physical well-being.	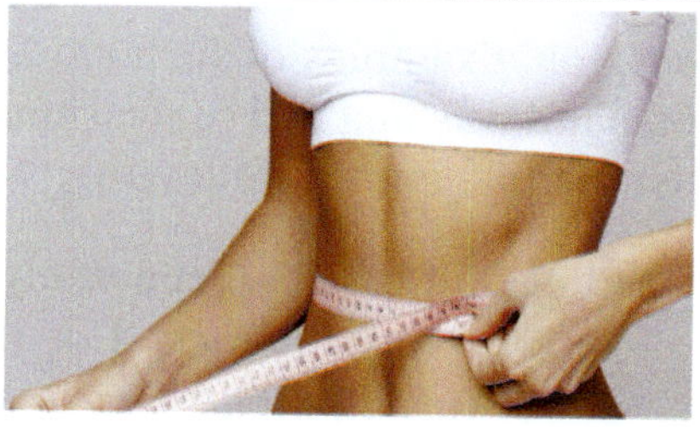
Trichotillomania	Trichotillomania is a mental disorder characterized by a long-term urge that results in the pulling out of one's own hair.	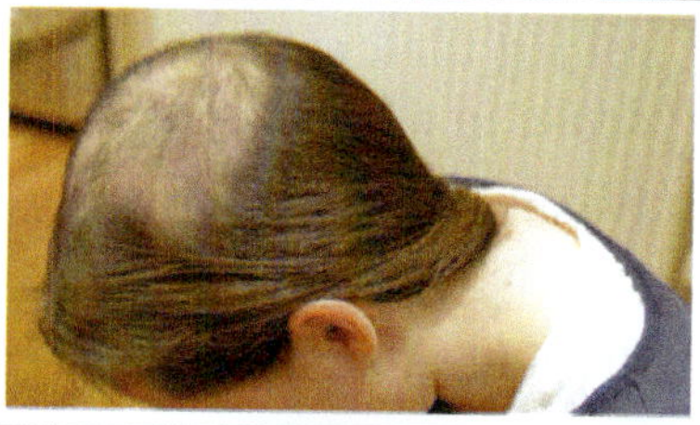
Selective serotonin reuptake inhibitors	Selective serotonin reuptake inhibitors are a class of drugs that are typically used as antidepressants in the treatment of major depressive disorder, anxiety disorders, and other psychological conditions.	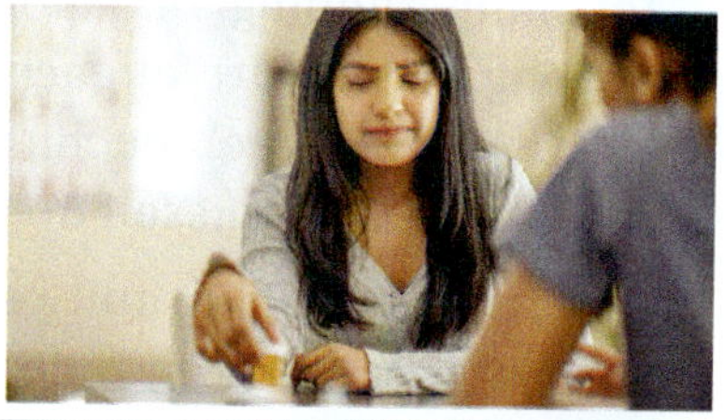
Personality disorders	Personality disorders are a class of mental disorders characterized by enduring maladaptive patterns of behavior, cognition, and inner experience, exhibited across many contexts and deviating from those accepted by the individual's culture.	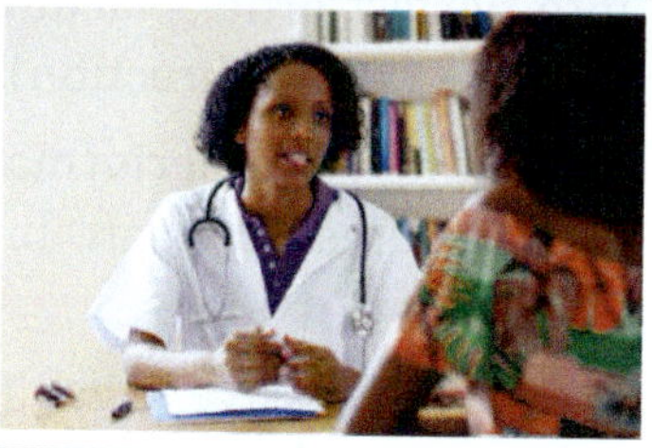

7.1. Obsessive Compulsive Disorder

Anxiety-inducing thoughts, images, or impulses that are frequent, persistent, bothersome, and unwanted can be considered an obsession if they impede social, professional, or interpersonal functioning. The individual thinks they have no control over these thoughts, even though they are excessive or irrational. In an effort to offset anxiety, some people develop compulsions, which are ritualistic, repetitive actions or thoughts. When someone is obsessed with contamination, for example, or with blasphemous thoughts, it is common for the ritual's theme to be linked to the obsession. Examples of such rituals include repeated hand washing and confession. Common compulsions include the following:

- Checking rituals (repeatedly making sure the door is locked or the coffee pot is turned off);
- Counting rituals (each step taken, ceiling tiles, concrete blocks, or desks in a classroom);
- Washing and scrubbing until the skin is raw;
- Praying or chanting;
- Touching, rubbing, or tapping (feeling the texture of each material in a clothing store' touching people, doors, walls, or oneself);
- Ordering (arranging and rearranging furniture or items on a desk or shelf into perfect order' vacuuming the rug pile in one direction);
- Exhibiting rigid performance (getting dressed in an unvarying pattern);
- Having aggressive urges (for instance, to throw one's child against a wall).

A person is only diagnosed with OCD when their thoughts, images, and impulses overwhelm them, or when they feel driven to act out the behaviors to the point where it interferes with their ability to function in social, professional, and personal domains. Examples include a woman who feels obligated to wash her hands after touching any object or person, or a man who is unable to work because he spends most of his day aligning and realigning everything in his apartment. A wide range of repetitive, pointless, and challenging to overcome behaviors are indicative of OCD. The individual feels compelled to carry out these rituals, even though they are strange and unreasonable, in order to reduce anxiety or stop bad thoughts. Compulsions and obsessions cause the person great distress and embarrassment, and they may even go to considerable measures to conceal them.

OCD can develop in childhood, particularly in men. It usually starts in the 20s in females. The distribution of the sexes is equal overall. Symptoms usually begin in late adolescence and fluctuate throughout life, with periods of increased and decreased severity. There may be times when a person functions reasonably well and has few symptoms. At times, they encounter a heightened intensity of symptoms that could be associated with stress. A small percentage of patients experience either total symptom remission or a progressive, worsening course of the illness. There are various differences between people with early-onset OCD (average age of 11) and late-onset OCD (average age of 23). Males are more likely to experience early onset, which is associated with more severe symptoms, comorbid diagnoses, and a higher chance of a family history of OCD.

7.1.1. Related Disorders

The following are DSM-5 diagnoses. They are included in the diagnostic classification by the American Psychiatric Association.

7.1.1.1. Excoriation Disorder

Excoriation disorder, or skin-picking disorder, also called dermatillomania, is classified as a self-soothing behavior. This means that individuals engage in the behavior in an effort to calm or comfort themselves, rather than because the act of picking is inherently pleasant. Eventually, the behavior may cause the person great distress, and it may also result in health issues and a loss of ability to perform one's job. On the treatment team, it might be required to include psychiatry, medicine, surgery, and/or plastic surgery. When incorporated into the treatment plan, complementary therapies like yoga, acupuncture, and biofeedback can be beneficial.

7.1.1.2. Trichotillomania

Trichotillomania, a self-soothing behavior that can lead to distress and functional impairment, is the chronic repetitive pulling of hair. While childhood is the most common time for it to start, anxiety and depression can also persist into adulthood. In comparison to men, it affects women more frequently. Behavioral therapy is a successful treatment for trichotillomania, though long-term outcomes are not well-documented and results are inconsistent. BDD is an obsession with an imagined or slight physical flaw that causes the sufferer great distress and makes it difficult for them to go about their daily lives normally. The individual dwells on the flaw and worries excessively about it, frequently attributing all of life's difficulties to his or her "flawed" appearance—that is, the reason for feelings of unhappiness, failures at work or in relationships, and so on—as a result of the appearance. People frequently seek out elective cosmetic surgery in an attempt to "fix the flaw," but either after the procedure they become even less satisfied or discover new flaws in their appearance. It turns into an endless loop. BDD and other diagnoses like anxiety, depression, social anxiety disorder, and excoriation disorder share a great deal of similarities. Relapse prevention has been demonstrated by the use of selective serotonin reuptake inhibitors (SSRIs) in treatment.

7.1.1.3. Hoarding Disorder

Hoarding disorder is a compulsive, progressive, and crippling condition that was only recently identified on its own. Although hoarding was once considered an OCD symptom, it is very different from OCD. The most common age range for diagnosis is 20 to 30 years old. Age-related increases in the disorder's prevalence and severity are observed in 2–5% of the population. According to Dozier, Porter, and Ayers (2016), it is more prevalent in females who have a parent or first-degree relative who also hoards. Excessive acquisition of animals or objects that seem pointless, cluttered living spaces that become uninhabitable, and severe distress or impairment for the hoarder are all signs of hoarding. A person's quality of life may be severely compromised by hoarding, and it may even pose a risk to one's own health, safety, or the public's health. Medication, cognitive-behavioral therapy (CBT), self-help groups, or assistance from outside community agencies are some possible forms of treatment and interventions. At this point, not much is known about how well these strategies have worked. The following conditions—repetitive, compulsive behavior that may be harmful to the individual—are occasionally thought to be connected to OCD. Some see them as behavioral addictions, marked by an inability to control the impulse to do something that could be dangerous.

7.1.1.4. Onychophagia

Chronic nail biting, or onychophagia, is a self-soothing behavior. Childhood is usually the onset age, and by the age of 18, behavior has decreased. But some people continue to bite their nails into adulthood. It may result in issues with the nails and oral cavity, as well as psychological issues. Onychophagia can be effectively treated with SSRIs. Compulsive stealing, also known as kleptomania, is a behavior driven by rewards. The thrill of stealing something and escaping detection is the real prize, not the stolen item. The theft of necessities for survival—like when a parent takes food from a hungry child—is not the same as kleptomania. Females who frequently have co-occurring diagnoses of depression and substance abuse are more likely to experience kleptomania. It has serious legal ramifications attached to it. Although there is no set course of treatment for kleptomania, it appears that longer-term counseling may be necessary rather than just a few short sessions (10 or 12).

7.1.1.5. Oniomania

The acquisition form of rewards-seeking behavior is called omnimania, or compulsive buying. More enjoyable than any later enjoyment of using the purchased item is the process of obtaining it. Frequently, a person's spending habits are out of control and far above their means. Furthermore, the item might be used sporadically or never after it is acquired. In the early 20s, compulsive buying behavior first appears in about 80% of females' college students are particularly susceptible to it. A strong comorbidity between substance abuse and depression runs in the family, as does compulsive shopping.

7.1.1.6. Body Identity Integrity Disorder (BIID)

The term used to describe people who feel "overcomplete" or alienated from a part of their body and wish to have it amputated is body identity integrity disorder (BIID). Amputation love, also referred to as apotemnophilia or amputee identity disorder, is another name for this illness. There is dispute over the existence of the ailment, and this diagnosis is not formally recognized by the APA. After an amputation, people report feeling "natural, like they were intended to be" and describe feelings of anguish and distress with their intact bodies. Few surgeons will amputate a limb merely at a patient's request because of ethical concerns. Individuals suffering from BIID often take to packing their affected limb in dry ice until the damage gets so bad that amputation is required by medical professionals. In other instances, non-medical individuals even use power tools to perform amputations, leaving a doctor to save the patient's life and lessen the damage.

7.1.2. Etiology: Obsessive–Compulsive Disorder

Numerous angles are being used to study the etiology of OCD. Though promising, various studies have not yet provided a clear explanation for how or why individuals develop OCD. The cognitive approach to emotional disorders developed by Aaron Beck gives rise to cognitive models of OCD. This has long been recognized as a possible explanation for OCD, especially in light of the fact that CBT is an effective treatment. The cognitive model characterizes the individual's thinking as follows: (1) an excessive sense of personal responsibility stemming from a strict moral or religious upbringing' (2) perfectionism and an intolerance of uncertainty' and (3) an overestimation of the threat posed by one's thoughts due to an overly important belief that "If I think it, it will happen" and the consequent need to control those thoughts. The cognitive model concentrates on early life experiences and growing up in one's surroundings. That being said, OCD does not only develop as a result of environmental factors.

It's critical to keep in mind that the client is attempting to manage strong impulses and feelings, including anxiety. Even the client may find the compulsive behavior to be senseless and without purpose. However, it is the client's effort to prevent dreaded outcomes or control/reduce intense emotions that are spiraling out of control. It is impossible to tell the patient to just stop or to reason with them. Studies based on populations have shown that OCD has a significant heritability. Variations that may be involved in OCD pathology have been found by genome-wide and candidate gene association studies, which lend credence to the theory that a complex network of multiple genes may contribute to the genetic risk for OCD. Most people believe that OCD is fairly common or universal across national boundaries. Numerous studies discovered that while the diagnosis of OCD was universal across cultural boundaries, there were differences in the ways that symptoms were expressed or perceived. Extremely religious people—Muslims and Christians alike—may feel more guilty about their symptoms and think they should be in charge of limiting disturbing, unwanted thoughts. Among those who suffer from OCD and disorders related to OCD, shame and guilt are common emotions. Patients with OCD who come from cultures where there is a belief in a supernatural cause are far more likely to seek assistance from a faith healer.

The kinds of OCD symptoms or beliefs that people experience can also vary by ethnicity. Some have higher levels of obsessional beliefs, while others report more OCD symptoms related to contamination. This may suggest that treatment plans need to be modified to account for these variations when they occur. Even though OCD is a condition that affects everyone, there are significant differences in pharmacologic treatment. The percentage of people who used SSRIs ranged from 59% to 96% in seven distinct countries. These authors made the case for the necessity of researching these variations and contrasting them with treatment results.

7.1.3. Treatment

Medication and behavioral therapy are combined to provide the best treatment for OCD. First-line options for SSRI antidepressants include fluvoxamine (Luvox) and sertraline (Zoloft). Venlafaxine (Effexor) is the next best option. Second-generation antipsychotics like olanzapine (Zyprexa), quetiapine (Seroquel), and risperidone (Risperdal) may help treat OCD that is resistant to treatment. Even in cases where symptoms are unresponsive to treatment, behavioral therapy and SSRI antidepressants are effective treatments for OCD in children and adolescents. Specifically, response prevention and exposure are a part of behavioral therapy. Helping the client consciously face the stimuli and situations they typically avoid is known as exposure. The main goal of response prevention is to postpone or forgo ritual performance. The individual gains the ability to accept the thoughts and the anxiety and to understand that they will pass without having the terrible outcomes they had feared. The individual may also benefit from additional methods like deep breathing and relaxation to help them tolerate and ultimately control their anxiety (Albano and Pimentel, 2017' Casale et al., 2018).

7.2. Nursing Care Plan: OCD

7.2.1. Nursing Diagnosis

7.2.1.1. Ineffective Coping

Inability to form a valid appraisal of stressor, inadequate choices of practiced responses, and/or inability to use available resources

7.2.1.2. Assessment Data

- Ambivalence regarding decisions or choices;
- Disturbances in normal functioning due to obsessive thoughts or compulsive behaviors (loss of job, loss of/or alienation of family members, etc.);
- Inability to tolerate deviations from standards;
- Rumination;
- Low self-esteem;
- Feelings of worthlessness;
- Lack of insight;
- Difficulty or slowness completing daily living activities because of ritualistic behavior.

7.2.2. Expected Outcomes

7.2.2.1. Immediate

The client will

- Talk with staff and identify stresses, anxieties, and conflicts within 2 to 3 days.
- Verbalize realistic self-evaluation' for example, make a list of strengths and abilities and review list with staff within 3 to 4 days.
- Establish adequate nutrition, hydration, and elimination within 4 to 5 days.
- Establish a balance of rest, sleep, and activity' for example, sleep at least 4 hours per night.

7.2.2.2. Stabilization

The client will

- Identify alternative methods of dealing with stress and anxiety.
- Complete daily routine without staff assistance or prompting by a specified date.
- Verbalize knowledge of illness, treatment plan, and safe use of medications, if any.

7.2.2.3. Community

The client will

- Demonstrate a decrease in obsessive thoughts or ritualistic behaviors to a level at which the client can function independently.
- Demonstrate alternative ways of dealing with stress, anxiety, and life situations.
- Maintain adequate physiological functioning, including activity, sleep, and rest.
- Follow through with continued therapy if needed' for example, identify a therapist and make a follow-up appointment before discharge.

7.2.2.4. Implementation

Nursing Interventions	Rationale
Observe the client's eating, drinking, and elimination patterns, and assist the client as necessary.	The client may be unaware of physical needs or may ignore feelings of hunger, thirst, or the urge to defecate, and so forth.
Assess and monitor the client's sleep patterns, and prepare him or her for bedtime by decreasing stimuli and providing comfort measures or medication.	Limiting noise and other stimuli will encourage rest and sleep. Comfort measures and sleep medications will enhance the client's ability to relax and sleep.
You may need to allow extra time, or the client may need to be verbally directed to accomplish activities of daily living (personal hygiene, preparation for sleep, and so forth).	The client's thoughts or ritualistic behaviors may interfere with or lengthen the time necessary to perform tasks.
Encourage the client to try to gradually decrease the frequency of compulsive behaviors. Work with the client to identify a baseline frequency and keep a record of the decrease.	Gradually reducing the frequency of compulsive behaviors will diminish the client's anxiety and encourage success.
As the client's anxiety decreases and as a trust relationship builds, talk with the client about his or her thoughts and behavior and the client's feelings about them. Help the client identify alternative methods for dealing with anxiety.	The client may need to learn ways to manage anxiety so that he or she can deal with it directly. This will increase the client's confidence in managing anxiety and other feelings.
Convey honest interest in and concern for the client. Do not flatter or be otherwise dishonest.	Your presence and interest in the client convey your acceptance of the client. Clients do not benefit from flattery or undue praise, but genuine praise that the client has earned can foster self-esteem.
Provide opportunities for the client to participate in activities that are easily accomplished or enjoyed by the client' support the client for participation.	The client may be limited in his or her ability to deal with complex activities or in relating to others. Activities that the client can accomplish and enjoy can enhance self-esteem.
Teach the client social skills, such as appropriate conversation topics and active listening. Encourage him or her to practice these skills with staff members and other clients, and give the client feedback regarding interactions.	The client may feel embarrassed by his or her OCD behaviors and may have had limited social contact. He or she may have limited social skills and confidence, which may contribute to the client's anxiety.
Teach the client and family or significant others about the client's illness, treatment, or medications, if any.	The client and family or significant others may have little or no knowledge about these.
Encourage the client to participate in follow-up therapy, if indicated. Help the client identify supportive resources in the community or on the internet.	Clients often experience long-term difficulties in dealing with obsessive thoughts.

Source: Adapted from Schultz, J. M., & Videbeck, S. L. (2013). Lippincott's manual of psychiatric nursing care plans (9th ed.). Philadelphia, PA: Lippincott Williams & Wilkins.

7.2.3. Application of the Nursing Process

The client often doesn't seek treatment until obsessions become too much to handle or until compulsions get in the way of daily activities (like going to work, preparing meals, or spending time with friends and family), or until both occur. Only when a patient is totally unable to perform their daily activities are they admitted to the hospital. The majority of care is provided outside of a hospital. The client frequently states that rituals started years ago—some even as early as childhood. As the client ages and assumes greater responsibility, the more the rituals obstruct their capacity to carry out those obligations.

7.2.3.1. General Appearance and Motor Behavior

The client's behavior and appearance are evaluated by the nurse. OCD sufferers frequently project tension, anxiety, worry, and fretfulness. They might find it embarrassing to describe their symptoms. They don't have a particularly striking appearance, and nothing about them seems "out of the ordinary.". The client who is virtually immobilized by thoughts and the anxiety they cause is the exception.

7.2.3.2. Mood and Affect

Clients report persistent, overwhelming feelings of anxiety in response to the compulsive thoughts, images, or urges during mood and affect assessment. They can appear depressed and uneasy.

7.2.3.3. Thought Processes and Content

The nurse investigates the client's ideas and content. Numerous clients state that the obsessions appear out of nowhere in the middle of everyday activities. The thought or image gets more intense the harder the client tries to stop it. The client explains that these obsessions are not what they want to think about and that they would never voluntarily come up with such thoughts or pictures. Evaluation indicates that intellectual functioning is unharmed. When obsessions are strong, the client may report having trouble focusing or paying attention. Memory or sensory functioning are unaffected.

7.2.3.4. Judgment and Insight

The nurse assesses the client's discernment and judgment. Although the client is aware that the obsessions are unreasonable, they are uncontrollable. He or she is unable to act on sound judgments, such as "I know the house is safe". When the client's anxiety gets too much, they still act ritualistically.

7.2.3.5. Self-Concept

When exploring their self-concept, the client expresses fear that they are "going crazy". Low self-esteem is a result of feeling helpless to stop one's obsessions or compulsions. The client might think that he or she could manage these thoughts and behaviors if only they were "stronger" or possessed more willpower.

7.2.3.6. Roles and Relationships

The impact of OCD on the client's roles and relationships must be evaluated by the nurse. The client's capacity to successfully carry out their responsibilities in life declines as ritual performance time rises. Friends and family become weary of the client's habitual behavior and become less available to them as a result of the client's increased anxiety and ritualistic behavior, which further damages relationships.

7.2.3.7. Physiological and Self-Care Considerations

The nurse investigates how physiology and self-care are affected by OCD. OCD patients may experience difficulty sleeping, just like those with other anxiety disorders. Following rituals can keep one from sleeping for a longer period of time, or anxiety can make it difficult to fall asleep and wake up feeling rested. Additionally, clients may report unintended weight loss or an appetite loss. In extreme situations, personal hygiene may deteriorate as a result of the client's inability to finish necessary tasks.

7.2.4. Data Analysis

Depending on the particular obsession and its accompanying compulsions, clients have varying symptoms. Nursing diagnoses can include:

- Anxiety;
- Ineffective coping;
- Fatigue;
- Situational low self-esteem;
- Impaired skin integrity (if scrubbing or washing rituals).

7.2.4.1. Outcome Identification

Outcomes for clients with OCD include:

- The client will complete daily routine activities within a realistic time frame.
- The client will demonstrate effective use of relaxation techniques.
- The client will discuss feelings with another person.
- The client will demonstrate effective use of behavioral therapy techniques.
- The client will spend less time performing rituals.

7.2.5. Intervention

7.2.5.1. Using Therapeutic Communication

It's crucial to support and encourage the client to assist them in controlling their anxiety reactions. The nurse can affirm the client's intense emotions while expressing hope that the client will be able to make the necessary adjustments and take back control of their life. The nurse supports the patient in discussing their emotions and providing as much detail as they are comfortable with. Speaking with the nurse about these ideas, actions, and ensuing emotions is crucial since many clients attempt to conceal their rituals and obsessions. By doing this, the client who has been keeping some of the "burden" to themselves may start to feel less alone.

7.2.5.2. Teaching Relaxation and Behavioral Techniques

The client can learn relaxation techniques from the nurse, including progressive muscle relaxation, guided imagery, and deep breathing. For the client to benefit from this intervention and learn more efficiently, it should occur when the client is less anxious. The nurse can first show the client how to use the techniques and practice them together. Once the client feels confident using these methods on their own, the nurse advises them to be practiced. When the client's anxiety starts to rise, he or she can start using relaxation techniques that they have learned. Apart from reducing anxiety, the client experiences a boost in control that may result in enhanced self-worth. A baseline of duration and frequency is required to manage ritualistic behaviors and anxiety. To document obsession-triggering events, anxiety levels, ritual execution time, and avoidance behaviors, the client may choose to maintain a journal. Both the client and the nurse can clearly see this record. The client can then start using behavioral techniques for exposure and response prevention. When feeling anxious, the client can initially shorten the ritual's duration or postpone it. The ritualistic response can eventually be completely eliminated by the client or greatly reduced to the point where it barely interferes with day-to-day activities. In order to help them control and tolerate their anxiety, clients can learn relaxation techniques. It is crucial to remember that the client needs to be open to participating in response prevention and exposure. It is not possible to impose these methods on the client.

7.2.5.3. Completing a Daily Routine

The client may initially need more time to accommodate rituals in order to complete tasks effectively. The nurse must schedule that time into the client's schedule, for instance, if breakfast is at 8 AM and the client has a 45-minute ritual before eating. The nurse must avoid trying to stop the ritual or to interrupt it because doing so will cause the client's anxiety to skyrocket. One more time, the client needs to be prepared to modify their behavior. A strategy to reduce the amount of time spent on rituals can be agreed upon by the nurse and the client. They may choose to gradually shorten the morning ritual at a pace that the client can handle, starting at 40 minutes, then 35, and so on. The client must then perform the required activity after finishing the ritual or after the allotted amount of time has elapsed. The client can utilize stress-reduction and relaxation techniques during this potentially anxious time. The client can maintain a daily routine or written schedule that aids in task completion and responsibilities fulfilled while they are at home.

7.2.6. Nursing Interventions

For OCD:

- Offer encouragement, support, and compassion.
- Be clear with the client that you believe he or she can change.
- Encourage the client to talk about feelings, obsessions, and rituals in detail.
- Gradually decrease the time for the client to carry out ritualistic behaviors.
- Assist the client in using exposure and response prevention behavioral techniques.
- Encourage the client to use techniques to manage and tolerate anxiety responses.
- Assist the client in completing daily routine and activities within agreed-upon time limits.
- Encourage the client to develop and follow a written schedule with specified times and activities.

7.2.6.1. Providing Client and Family Education

It's critical that the client and their family are educated about OCD. Instead of the obsessions being a reflection of some "dark side" to the client's personality, they are frequently relieved to learn that the client is not "going crazy" and that they are unwanted. By assisting the client and family in having an honest conversation about the obsessions, anxiety, and rituals, the client is freed from the need to bear the guilt and keep these things hidden. If family members are properly informed, they can also provide the client with the emotional support that they need. To combat OCD, it is crucial to educate people about the significance of medication compliance. Until the client experiences a satisfactory response, it might be necessary to try various medications. When a client takes medication and practices behavior modification, the likelihood of improved OCD symptoms increases.

7.2.7. Evaluation

When a client's OCD symptoms no longer prevent them from performing their duties, the treatment has been successful. The client handles the anxiety that arises from obsessions without resorting to laborious or time-consuming rituals. He or she claims to have reclaimed control over their lives and to be able to tolerate and deal with anxiety with little difficulty.

7.3. Personality Disorders

The Greek term persona is where the word personality originates. Originally, it was used to refer to the theatrical mask that certain dramatic actors of the era were wearing. As time went on, the meaning of pretense and illusion faded, and it began to stand for the "real" person—the one hiding behind the mask. Features that a person is born with or acquires early in life are known as personality traits. They are fairly stable over time and have an impact on how he or she views and interacts with the world. When these characteristics become unyielding and unbending and lead to maladaptive behavioral patterns or functional impairments, personality disorders arise. Almost everyone occasionally displays some of the behaviors linked to the different personality disorders. As mentioned earlier, a person is considered to have a personality disorder only if they exhibit significant functional impairment in response to these personality traits. Development of personality happens in reaction to various biological and psychological factors. These factors include temperament, social interaction, experiential learning, and heredity, among others. Many theorists have made an effort to share knowledge regarding personality development. The majority propose that it happens in a systematic, phased manner. However, because maturation happens at varying rates in different people, these stages overlap. There was a presentation of the theories of Mahler (Mahler, Pine, and Bergman, 1975), Erikson (1963), and Sullivan (1953). The nurse should first learn about what is deemed maladaptive so that she can comprehend "normal" personality development (Table 7.1).

The epidemiological and historical dimensions of personality disorders. The following are risk factors that have been linked to the development of personality disorders. To give background information for evaluating clients with personality disorders, symptomatology is explained. Acute care settings do not frequently treat individuals with personality disorders for which the disorder is the primary psychiatric diagnosis. Nonetheless, personality disorder symptoms are present in a large number of patients with other medical and psychiatric diagnoses. In all healthcare settings, nurses are likely to come across clients who exhibit these personality traits on a regular basis. It is common for nurses working in psychiatric settings to come across patients who exhibit antisocial and borderline personality traits. Due to attempts at self-harm, patients with borderline personality disorder frequently need to be hospitalized due to their extremely unstable behavior. A court-ordered evaluation may lead the client with antisocial personality disorder into the psychiatric setting. If psychiatric intervention is thought to have potential benefits, it could be used as a substitute for incarceration in cases of antisocial behavior. Within the framework of nursing practice, providing nursing care to clients who suffer from antisocial or borderline personality disorders. Numerous medical approaches to treating personality disorders are examined.

Table 7.1. *Comparison of Personality Development—Sullivan, Erikson, and Mahler*

MAJOR DEVELOPMENTAL TASKS AND DESIGNATED AGES		
SULLIVAN	**ERIKSON**	**MAHLER**
Birth to 18 months: Relief from anxiety through oral gratification of needs.	Birth to 18 months: To develop a basic trust in the mothering figure and be able to generalize it to others.	Birth to 1 month: Fulfillment of basic needs for survival and comfort.
18 months to 6 years: Learning to experience a delay in personal gratification without undue anxiety.	18 months to 3 years: To gain some self-control and independence within the environment.	1 to 5 months: Developing awareness of external source of need fulfillment.
6 to 9 years: Learning to form satisfactory peer relationships.	3 to 6 years: To develop a sense of purpose and the ability to initiate and direct own activities.	5 to 10 months: Commencement of a primary recognition of separateness from the mothering figure.
9 to 12 years: Learning to form satisfactory relationships with persons of the same gender; the initiation of feelings of affection for another person.	6 to 12 years: To achieve a sense of self-confidence by learning, competing, performing successfully, and receiving recognition from significant others, peers, and acquaintances.	10 to 16 months: Increased independence through locomotor functioning; increased sense of separateness of self.
12 to 14 years: Learning to form satisfactory relationships with persons of the opposite gender; developing a sense of identity.	12 to 20 years: To integrate the tasks mastered in the previous stages into a secure sense of self.	16 to 24 months: Acute awareness of separateness of self; learning to seek "emotional refueling" from mothering figure to maintain feeling of security.
14 to 21 years: Establishing self-identity; experiences satisfying relationships; working to develop a lasting, intimate opposite-gender relationship.	20 to 30 years: To form an intense, lasting relationship or a commitment to another person, a cause, an institution, or a creative effort.	24 to 36 months: Sense of separateness established; on the way to object constancy: able to internalize a sustained image of loved object/person when it is out of sight; resolution of separation anxiety.
	30 to 65 years: To achieve the life goals established for oneself, while also considering the welfare of future generations.	
	65 years to death: To review one's life and derive meaning from both positive and negative events, while achieving a positive sense of self-worth.	

Source: https://repository.poltekkes-kaltim.ac.id/625/1/Psychiatric%20Mental%20Health%20Nursing%20Concepts%20of%20Care%20in%20Evidence-Based%20Practice%20by%20Mary%20C.%20Townsend%20DSN%20%20PMHCNS-BC%20(z-lib.org).pdf.

7.3.1. Historical Aspects

According to Skodal and Gunderson (2008), there have been descriptions of personality disorders for thousands of years. Hippocrates came to the conclusion in the fourth century BC that malady resulted from an excess or imbalance of the four body humors (blood, phlegm, yellow and black bile, and both). Hippocrates distinguished four basic personality types, all of which he concluded resulted from excesses in the four humors: the overly sanguine and extraverted sanguine (blood)' the pessimistic melancholic (black bile)' the apathetic phlegmatic (phlegm)' and the irritable and hostile choleric (yellow bile). Recognizing that an individual can behave irrationally even when their intellectual faculties are intact, the medical profession began to take personality disorders seriously in 1801, separate from psychosis. The term moral insanity, which defines what we now refer to as personality disorders, was adopted by psychiatrists in the 19th century. Persons suffering from personality disorders have traditionally been stigmatized as "bad" or "immoral" and classified as deviants from the norm regarding various aspects of personality. Personality pathology arises from intricate and challenging to decipher events and sequences. For this intricate behavioral phenomenon to be better understood, more research is required.

The classification of personality disorders has proven to be a significant challenge for psychiatrists. The Diagnostic and Statistical Manual of Mental Disorders, Fifth Edition (DSM-5) (American Psychiatric Association [APA], 2013) lists ten distinct categories of personality disorders. To specifically identify impairments in personality functioning related to the dimensions of self and interpersonal relations as well as personality trait domains and facets, the American Psychological Association has proposed a sophisticated diagnostic system. The symptoms that may vary not only between personality disorders but also between people with the same disorder are addressed by this highly specific diagnostic system. The DSM-5 describes this trait-specific diagnostic methodology as a substitute for personality disorder diagnosis and suggests more research in this area.

The current diagnostic system classifies the personality disorders into three clusters according to description of personality traits. These include the following:

- **Cluster A:** Behaviors described as odd or eccentric.
  - Paranoid personality disorder;
  - Schizoid personality disorder;
  - Schizotypal personality disorder.
- **Cluster B:** Behaviors described as dramatic, emotional, or erratic.
  - Antisocial personality disorder;
  - Borderline personality disorder;
  - Histrionic personality disorder;
  - Narcissistic personality disorder.
- **Cluster C:** Behaviors described as anxious or fearful.
  - Avoidant personality disorder;
  - Dependent personality disorder;
  - Obsessive compulsive personality disorder (American Psychological Association).

7.4. Types of Personality Disorders

7.4.1. Paranoid Personality Disorder

7.4.1.1. Definition and Epidemiological Statistics

"A pervasive, persistent, and inappropriate mistrust of others" is define paranoid personality disorder. People suffering from this disorder tend to be suspicious of other people's intentions and believe that others are trying to take advantage of, hurt, or trick them. Estimates of the prevalence of paranoid personality disorder range from 1% to 4% in the general population, and the condition is frequently only identified after a person seeks treatment for an anxiety or mood disorder (Black and Andreasen, 2011). Males are diagnosed with the disorder more often than females.

7.4.1.2. Clinical Picture

Paranoid personality disorder sufferers are always alert, hypervigilant, and prepared for any threat, imagined or real. They look strained and agitated. They no longer seem to care about other people's feelings and have instead grown a hard exterior. To prevent having to give up some of their own power, they steer clear of social interactions. People have a persistent sense that people are only there to exploit them. Being highly sensitive, they often misread and magnify small cues from their surroundings, turning them into ideas of deceit and trickery. They "test" other people's honesty all the time because they don't trust anyone. Almost everybody they come into contact with feels intimidated and enraged by them. By placing the blame for their flaws on other people, people with paranoid personality disorder preserve their sense of self. They assign others' behaviors and emotions to themselves rather than taking ownership of them. When it comes to extremely successful people, they are jealous and hostile, thinking that their lack of success is solely due to unfair treatment. Anxious and defensive all the time, paranoid people are highly vulnerable. Alienation and rage, fed by old grudges, can be unleashed by any perceived or actual threat. A potential loss of control could lead to aggression and violence because the desire for vengeance and vindication is so strong. Typically, these episodes of intense behavior are short-lived, as the paranoid individual quickly reclaims control over their surroundings, justifies their actions, and reassembles the fundamental barriers that contribute to their personality type.

7.4.1.3. Predisposing Factors

According to research, paranoid personality disorder may have a genetic component. Studies have shown that relatives of clients with schizophrenia have a higher incidence of paranoid personality disorder than do control subjects (Sadock and Sadock, 2007). Parental hostility and harassment can have a psychosocial impact on individuals with paranoid personality disorder. They progressively gave up on any chance of love and acceptance and probably became scapegoats for their parents' bullying. They discovered that the outside world was cruel and unforgiving, requiring distrust and protective awareness. With a "chip-on-the-shoulder" mentality, they faced numerous rejections and snubs from people when they first arrived. Being paranoid meant that they would always attack first, expecting others to humiliate them or betray them.

7.4.2. Schizoid Personality Disorder

7.4.2.1. Definition and Epidemiological Statistics

A severe impairment in one's capacity to build relationships or meaningfully interact with others is the main characteristic of schizoid personality disorder (Black and Andreasen, 2011). These people have a consistent pattern of social disengagement throughout their lives, and it's clear they find social interaction uncomfortable. Between 3% and 7.5% of the general population is thought to suffer from schizoid personality disorder. A sizable portion of those suffering from the illness are never seen in a clinical context. Although it is more commonly diagnosed in men, the disorder's gender ratio is unknown.

7.4.2.2. Clinical Picture

Schizoid personality disorder patients come across as distant, icy, and uncaring toward other people. They are aloof and prefer to work alone' they have little need or desire for emotional connections. They have the capacity to devote a great deal of affective energy to intellectual endeavors. When they are around other people, they seem bashful, nervous, or uneasy. They have a hard time acting lightheartedly and take everything far too seriously. They are not very spontaneous in their behavior or conversation. They usually have a bland, constrained effect and are incapable of experiencing pleasure.

7.4.2.3. Predisposing Factors

Extraversion seems to be a highly inheritable trait, even though the exact role of heredity in the etiology of schizoid personality disorder is unknown. It is necessary to conduct additional research before making firm conclusions. Early interactional patterns that the person found cold and unsatisfying likely had a psychosocial influence on the development of schizoid personality. Numerous people have described these people's childhoods as desolate, unfriendly, and conspicuously devoid of empathy and guidance. A child raised with this kind of parenting may grow up to be schizoid if they have an introverted, shy, and nervous temperament.

Skodol and Gunderson (2008) state:

- Clinicians have observed that adults with schizoid personality disorder often had cold, uncaring, and unsatisfying relationships as early childhood experiences. This has caused these individuals to believe that relationships are unimportant and not worth pursuing.

7.4.3. Schizotypal Personality Disorder

7.4.3.1. Definition and Epidemiological Statistics

It used to be said that people with schizotypal personality disorder were "latent schizophrenics". They exhibit strange and eccentric behavior, but not to the extent of schizophrenia. A more severe variation of the pathologically less severe schizoid personality pattern is called schizotypal personality. Research suggests that between 1% and 2% of people suffer from schizotypal personality disorder (Black and Andreasen, 2011).

7.4.3.2. Clinical Picture

People who suffer from schizotypal personality disorder exhibit cold, solitary behaviors as well as bland, uninteresting attitudes. They live in a world where depersonalization, delusions, magical thinking, and concepts of reference are commonplace. Superstition, faith in telepathy, clairvoyance, or a "sixth sense," and convictions that "others can feel my feelings" are a few examples. "The speech pattern can occasionally be strange. Individuals who suffer from this disorder frequently struggle to organize their thoughts logically, getting bogged down in irrelevant personal tangents and digressions that don't seem to be related to the main point at hand. This aspect of their character just makes them seem more unlikeable to other people. These people may decompensate and exhibit psychotic symptoms under duress, such as delusional thoughts, hallucinations, or strange behaviors, but these episodes are typically transient (Sadock and Sadock, 2007). They seem to be "living in their own world" because they frequently talk or gesture to themselves. Their behavior is uninteresting or improper' for example, they laugh at their own troubles or at something that most people would find depressing.

7.4.3.3. Predisposing Factors

There is evidence to suggest that first-degree biological relatives of individuals with schizophrenia are more likely than the general population to suffer from schizotypal personality disorder. It is currently thought to be a component of the schizophrenia genetic spectrum (APA, 2013). Other biogenic factors that may play a role in the development of this disorder are hypothesized to include neurochemical dysfunctions or anatomical deficits that lead to reduced activation, reduced sensitivity to pleasure pain, and impaired cognitive functions. Skodol and Gunderson (2008) classified schizotypal personality disorder with schizophrenia instead of with the personality disorders in the International Classification of Diseases (ICD-10), taking into account these biological etiological factors that support the close relationship between schizotypal personality disorder and schizophrenia. The schizotypal personality disorder sufferer may have grown up in a family where formality, impassivity, or apathy were the norm, which resulted in a pattern of discomfort around intimacy and personal affection. Their early affective deficiencies rendered them undesirable and unsatisfying as social partners. They most likely experienced rejection, humiliation, disdain, and rejection from others, which left them with low self-esteem and a strong mistrust of social interactions. After experiencing repeated failures to deal with these hardships, they started to distance themselves and cut down on interactions with people and circumstances that made them feel depressed and ashamed. Their existence in their new inner world was more meaningful and possibly fulfilling than their life outside of it.

7.4.4. Antisocial Personality Disorder

7.4.4.1. Definition and Epidemiological Statistics

A pattern of socially irresponsible, exploitative, and guiltless behavior that displays a general disregard for other people's rights is known as antisocial personality disorder. These people don't care about following the law' instead, they take advantage of and manipulate others for their own gain. They struggle to maintain steady employment and form enduring relationships. Included in every edition of the Diagnostic and Statistical Manual of Mental Disorders, it is one of the most well-researched and ancient personality disorders. According to Black and Andreasen (2011), prevalence estimates in the US vary from 2% to 4% for men to roughly 1% for women. The disorder is more prevalent in lower socioeconomic groups, especially among highly mobile residents of urban poverty. Dissocial personality disorder is the ICD -10 diagnosis for this condition.

7.4.5. Borderline Personality Disorder

7.4.5.1. Definition and Epidemiological Statistics

A pattern of intense and chaotic relationships, along with affective instability and shifting attitudes toward other people, are characteristics of borderline personality disorder. These people lack a strong sense of self, act impulsively, and both directly and indirectly harm themselves. 1% to 2% of people are thought to have a borderline personality. According to estimates, the female-to-male ratio can reach up to 4 to

1, meaning that it is more common in women than in men (Lubit, 2011). This disorder is classified as emotionally unstable personality disorder by the ICD-10.

7.4.6. Histrionic Personality Disorder

7.4.6.1. Definition and Epidemiological Statistics

Exuberant, emotional people with histrionic personality disorder tend to be colorful, dramatic, and extroverted in their behavior. Long-term relationships are hard for them to maintain, even though they need others to constantly validate their acceptance and approval. The disorder is more common in women than in men, with a prevalence estimated to be between 2% and 3%.

7.4.6.2. Clinical Picture

Individuals suffering from histrionic personality disorder are often charming, attention-seeking, self-dramatizing, and excessively gregarious. They demand to be the center of attention by engaging in exhibitionistic and manipulative behaviors. People who suffer from histrionic personality disorder frequently exhibit traits that our society values in its members—namely, being liked, successful, popular, extroverted, attractive, and gregarious—in a mildly pathological way. Beneath these outward traits, though, lies a driven quality—a compulsive need for acceptance and a desperate attempt to stand out, arouse affection, or garner attention at any costs. Feelings of hopelessness and anxiety are frequently the outcome of not getting the attention and approval they desire. People who suffer from this disorder are naturally flighty and highly distractible. They struggle to focus on minute details. They are able to project a dual persona: one of carefree sophistication and the other of inhibition and naivety. They are frequently very impressionable, suggestible, and susceptible to outside influence. They rely on each other heavily. Human connections are transient and surface-level. Histrionic personality disorder sufferers are unable to truly sustain affection for another person because they have never been able to cultivate the depth of their own emotions and lack resources. These people frequently experience somatic complaints, and brief psychotic episodes may happen when they are under a lot of stress.

7.4.6.3. Predisposing Factors

The propensity for histrionic personality disorder has been linked to neurological factors. Coccaro and Siever (2000) have established a correlation between increased noradrenergic activity and the traits of enhanced sensitivity and reactivity to environmental stimuli in individuals with histrionic personality disorder. They proposed that impulsivity could be linked to a reduction in serotonergic activity. The disorder appears to be more common among first-degree biological relatives of individuals with the disorder than in the general population, suggesting that heredity may also play a role in this. According to Skodol and Gunderson's (2008) research, there may be a genetic component to the temperament that determines the behavioral traits of histrionic personality disorder. Histrionic personality disorder would result from "an extreme variation of temperamental disposition," according to this theory. Psychologically speaking, learning experiences could play a role in the emergence of histrionic personality disorder. The child might have come to understand that receiving positive reinforcement depended on exhibiting actions that their parents valued and approved of. The child most likely didn't get feedback very often, either positive or negative. Only when the behaviors matched the expectations of the parents did the parents show their approval and acceptance. According to Millon (2004), these children feel frustrated by their inability to consistently get their parents' attention. As a result, they exaggerate behaviors that are typical of their gender to get attention and affection. If not, people overlook them. These kids are practically ravenous for love and attention when they reach puberty.

7.4.7. Narcissistic Personality Disorder

7.4.7.1. Definition and Epidemiological Statistics

An inflated sense of self-worth characterizes those suffering from narcissistic personality disorder. They have little empathy and are extremely sensitive to other people's opinions. They think that their desire is enough reason to obtain what they want, and that they have the unalienable right to special treatment. The third edition of the Diagnostic and Statistical Manual of Mental Disorders included this diagnosis for the first time. But the 19th century is when the idea of narcissism first emerged. It was considered a typical stage of psychosexual development by early psychoanalysts. According to estimates by Black and Andreasen (2011), the prevalence of narcissistic personality disorder is approximately 6%. Men receive the diagnosis more frequently than women.

7.4.7.2. Clinical Picture

Narcissistic personality disorder sufferers exhibit a lack of humility, excessive self-centeredness, and exploitation of others in order to satisfy their own needs. Frequently, they don't think of their actions as improper or objectionable. They feel they should have particular rights and benefits because they consider themselves to be "superior" beings. Their attitude is typically upbeat, laid-back, joyful, and carefree, despite the fact that it is frequently based on grandiose distortions of reality. But because of their brittle self-esteem, this mood is easily manipulated. They could react with fury, shame, humiliation, or dejection if they don't get the positive reinforcement they expect from others, don't live up to their own expectations, or receive criticism from others. They might withdraw within themselves and imagine justifications that help them believe in their own superiority and perfection. Interpersonal relationships suffer when someone uses others for their own gain. When it comes to dating, narcissistic people usually go for someone who will give them the validation and encouragement they need and who won't ask for much in return.

7.4.7.3. Predisposing Factors

There are numerous psychodynamic theories explaining the narcissistic personality disorder propensity. Skodol and Gunderson (2008) posit that these people experienced rejection, contempt, or neglect as children in response to their fears, mistakes, or needs for dependence. They can never see others as sources of consolation and support because they are raised to despise these behaviors in both themselves and others. Their inability to feel deeply is a result of their projection of an image of self-sufficiency and invulnerability, which hides their true sense of emptiness. Martinez-Lewi (2008) makes the argument that narcissistic parents frequently exhibit narcissistic traits themselves. The child was subjected to unreasonable demands from her parents, who were critical, exacting, and demanding. Children take after their parents' conduct, which allows the adult narcissist to take over. According to certain clinicians, there is a possibility that the child was physically or emotionally abused or neglected by the parents. An environment where parents try to live their lives through their child may also contribute to the development of narcissism. It is their expectation that the child will accomplish what they were unable to accomplish, own what they were lacking, and lead a simpler and more pleasant life than their own. Because they are not subjected to the constraints and demands that may have dominated their parents' lives, the child grows up thinking they are exempt from obligations that apply to everyone else.

According to Bosson and Prewitt-Freilino (2007), there are parents who overindulge and pamper their children in ways that teach them that everything they ask for can be obtained without providing for others, that they can get attention without even trying hard, and that they should be in the spotlight. As a result, these children come to associate their identity with positive affect and form highly positive implicit self-representations. Nevertheless, in many cases of parental overindulgence, reality eventually steps in—in the form of personal failures, humiliations, weaknesses, and the like—and erodes the individual's explicit self-esteem because the world outside of the home will not be as kind and accepting. According to this viewpoint, the narcissistic traits of entitlement and exploitativeness are a reflection of the exaggerated implicit expectations that their parents instilled in them, and the shame-proneness is a reflection of their persistent belief that they are not good enough.

7.4.8. Avoidant Personality Disorder

7.4.8.1. Definition and Epidemiological Statistics

Because they are so sensitive to rejection, people with avoidant personality disorder often lead very socially isolated lives. It's not that he or she is asocial—instead, there might be a great desire to be with someone. However, excessive shyness and rejection anxiety lead to a need for exceptionally strong guarantees of acceptance without conditions. About 2% of the general population has the disorder, and both men and women seem to have it at the same rate (APA, 2013).

7.4.8.2. Clinical Picture

People who suffer from this disorder find it difficult to socialize and feel comfortable. Others may view them as shy, reserved, or even strange and frigid from a distance. However, those who are in closer relationships with them quickly discover their mistrust worthiness, evasiveness, touchiness, and sensitivities. Their speech is typically sluggish and restricted, with a lot of hesitations, disjointed thought processes, and sporadic irrelevant and confused asides. They frequently express feelings of loneliness and unwelcomeness. They consider others to be demeaning, treacherous, and critical. Although they would like to be in close relationships, they steer clear of them out of fear of rejection. Common emotions include depression, anxiety, and self-righteous rage at not being able to form social relationships.

7.4.8.3. Predisposing Factors

The cause of avoidant personality disorder is unclear. The most likely combination of biological, genetic, and psychosocial influences are contributing factors. There is a chance that some infants with characteristics like hyperirritability, crankiness, tension, and withdrawal may have a temperament that leans toward an avoidant pattern. Parental rejection and censure, which are frequently reinforced by peers, are the main psychosocial factors that predispose people to avoidant personality disorder (Millon, 2004). These kids are frequently raised in homes where they are ridiculed, rejected, and blamed, which stifles any innate optimism and replaces it with emotions of social disconnection and low self-worth. They acquire a suspicious mindset and perceive the outside world as unfriendly and hazardous.

7.4.9. Dependent Personality Disorder

7.4.9.1. Definition and Epidemiological Statistics

"A pattern of relying excessively on others for emotional support" is a characteristic of dependent personality disorder (Black and

Andreasen, 2011). This type of behavior is demonstrated by the propensity to delegate decision-making authority to others, to act weak and submit to others' needs, to act submissively, to put others' needs ahead of one's own, to put up with mistreatment from others, to minimize oneself in order to be accepted, and to perform inadequately in circumstances that call for assertive or dominant behavior. The illness is comparatively prevalent. Sadock and Sadock (2007) talk about the findings of a study on personality disorders that found that 2.5% of the participants had a dependent personality disorder diagnosis. It affects women more frequently than men, and it affects a family's youngest members more frequently.

7.4.9.2. Clinical Picture

Dependent personality disorder sufferers frequently exhibit a marked lack of confidence in their body language, speech pattern, and mannerisms. Usually, they are submissive and yield to the wishes of others. They downplay their own accomplishments and attractiveness while being unduly considerate and giving. Even though they could seem to "see the world through rose-colored glasses" to others, when they're by themselves, they could experience pessimism, discouragement, and depression. Others "struggle" in silence, unaware that others are feeling these things as well. Dependent personality disorder patients behave passively and submissively in interpersonal interactions. They are prepared to delegate major decision-making authority to others. Because they don't think they can take care of themselves, they feel scared and exposed should the dependent relationship end. They might try quickly and carelessly to build a new relationship with someone they think can give them the support and direction they require. When put in positions of authority, they shy away from them and get nervous. They feel inadequate and are easily offended by criticism and disapproval. They will go to great lengths to gain acceptance from others, even if it means doing something unpleasant or degrading.

7.4.9.3. Predisposing Factors

An infant may have a dependent temperament due to genetic predispositions. Identical twins exhibit a stronger correlation than fraternal twins in twin studies that assess submissiveness. Psychosocial dependence develops in infants when they receive their only source of stimulation and care. A newborn develops an attachment to one source at the expense of all others. This exclusive bond nurtures dependency if it persists in the child's development. When parents discourage their children from being independent and become overly protective, it can be problematic. When parents overly simplify new experiences for their children and prevent them from learning through trial and error, they are encouraging their child to give up on gaining independence. In this setting, the child may learn to fear losing the parental figure's love or attachment if they try independent activities because dependent behaviors may be subtly rewarded.

7.4.10. Obsessive compulsive Personality Disorder

7.4.10.1. Definition and Epidemiological Statistics

People who suffer from obsessive compulsive personality disorder are extremely serious, formal, and unable to communicate their feelings. They are extremely rule-focused, perfectionistic, and disciplined. They have an inflexible approach to the way things should be done and prioritize productivity over leisure time. Having a severe fear of making mistakes causes trouble making decisions. This is a rather common disorder that affects men more frequently than women. The oldest children in the family constellation seem to have it the most.

7.4.10.2. Clinical Picture

Obsessive compulsive personality disorder sufferers lack spontaneity and are rigid. When it comes to tasks that call for precision and self-control, they are meticulous and work hard and patiently. Their primary concerns are efficiency and organization, and they have a tendency to be strict and unyielding when it comes to policies and guidelines. Social conduct is typically courteous and formal. They exhibit behaviors that are more in line with those of "superiors" than those of "inferiors," suggesting that they are highly "rank conscious". They usually approach authority figures with great solicitude and ingratiation. However, the compulsive individual can become extremely authoritarian and judgmental with subordinates, frequently coming across as haughty and self-righteous. The "bureaucratic personality," or "company man," is typified by those suffering from obsessive compulsive personality disorder. They despise those whose actions they perceive to be frivolous and impetuous and regard as responsible, dependable, conscientious, and loyal. It is deemed immature and careless to exhibit emotional behavior. These people may seem composed and in control on the outside, but beneath there is a great deal of conflict, animosity, and ambivalence. The defensive mechanism of reaction formation is frequently employed by those suffering from this disorder. They withhold their true feelings of defiance and anger so strongly that the opposite feelings emerge because they dare not show them. Additionally, frequently seen are the defenses of undoing, intellectualization, rationalization, and isolation.

7.4.10.3. Predisposing Factors

The overcontrolling parenting style that produced the person with obsessive compulsive personality disorder is the perspective held by psychoanalytic theory. These parents condemn their children for not adhering to the standards of behavior they have set for them and expect them to live up to them. The youngster receives praise for good behavior far less frequently than they do for bad behavior. People in this setting become experts at knowing what they must not do in order to escape punishment and condemnation, as opposed to what they can do to get attention and recognition. They get used to following strict guidelines and regulations. Their parents are expected to point out rules violations and transgressions' positive accomplishments are expected, taken for granted, and only rarely acknowledged by them.

7.5. Application of the Nursing Process

7.5.1. Borderline Personality Disorder (Background Assessment Data)

In the past, there was a subset of patients who did not fit neatly into the neuroses or psychoses classification schemes. The term "borderline" was coined to describe these customers who appeared to be in between the two categories. The terms ambulatory schizophrenia, pseudoneurotic schizophrenia, and emotionally unstable personality have also been used in an effort to characterize this illness. When the DSM's third edition included the term "borderline," some psychiatrists expressed concern that it would be applied as a "wastebasket" diagnosis to patients who were difficult to treat. But a precise set of standards has been developed in order to diagnose what has been called "a consistent and stable course of unstable behavior".

7.5.1.1. Clinical Picture

People who have borderline personalities frequently appear to be experiencing a crisis. They have a highly intense affect, and their behavior is frequently erratic. Days, hours, or even minutes may pass before these changes take place. These people often display a single dominant affective tone, like depression, which can occasionally give way to anxious agitation or inappropriate outbursts of anger.

Chronic Depression

Due to the high prevalence of depression among those with this disorder, many of them were diagnosed with depressive disorder prior to the inclusion of borderline personality disorder in the DSM. Early childhood experiences of feeling abandoned by the mother can lead to depression (see "Predisposing Factors"). Anger, sometimes directed both outward on the surroundings and inward on oneself, is the root cause of depression. Rarely, until much later in long-term therapy, does the patient realize the true cause of these emotions.

Inability to Be Alone

Clients with borderline personality disorder have a low threshold for solitude due to their ongoing fear of being abandoned. Rather than sitting around feeling empty, lonely, and bored, they would rather engage in a frantic search for companionship, no matter how unsatisfactory (Sadock and Sadock, 2007).

7.5.1.2. Patterns of Interaction

Clinging and Distancing

Clinging and distancing behaviors characterize the pattern of interaction that the client with borderline personality disorder typically displays with others. Clients who are clinging to someone else may behave in a dependent, helpless, or even childlike manner. They overly romanticize a single person who they wish to spend all of their time, who they feel the need to speak to frequently, or who they look to for comfort all the time. They may act out or even commit self-harm if they are unable to be with this special someone. Distancing behaviors, which stem from a discomfort with closeness, are typified by hostility, anger, and devaluation of others. Distancing behaviors can also be a reaction to conflicts, separations, or efforts to restrict specific behaviors. When someone devalues another, it shows through casting doubt on their accomplishments and value as individuals.

Splitting

A common ego defense mechanism used by those with borderline personality disorder is splitting. It is a result of their failure to attain object constancy and shows up as an incapacity to accept and integrate both happy and sad emotions. They believe that everything in life, including themselves, can be classified as either good or bad. A caring caregiver is idealized, for instance, if they are encouraging and nurturing. Is there any way that the nurturing relationship could be endangered?, the caregiver has to relocate due to work obligations), the person is all of a sudden devalued, and the idealized portrayal shifts from that of a kind and helpful caregiver to one of an evil and brutal persecutor.

Manipulation

Clients with this disorder become skilled manipulators as they attempt to avoid the separation they so desperately fear. Almost any behavior can be used to achieve the desired outcome, which is the alleviation of separation anxiety. One common tactic to allay these fears of abandonment is to pit one person against the other.

Self-Destructive Behaviors

Frequent, self-destructive actions are well-known signs of borderline personality disorder.

Even though these behaviors can be lethal, they are typically deceptive actions meant to provoke significant others to come to their aid. Suicide attempts are not uncommon and are frequently brought on by feelings of abandonment after a significant relationship ends. Though the undertaking is frequently undertaken, adding a level of "safety" to the plan (e.g. ingesting pills in a place where others will undoubtedly find them' or ingesting pills and calling someone to report the action). Destructive behaviors can also involve burning, scratching, and cutting. There are many different theories explaining why these people can cause themselves pain. According to one theory, they might have bodies that contain more endorphins than the average person, which would increase their pain threshold. An additional theory pertains to the disturbance of the person's personal identity. It suggests that the individual does not initially feel the pain because many self-mutilating behaviors occur when they are in a state of depersonalization and derealization. The mutilation keeps going until pain is experienced in an effort to offset the surrealistic feelings. It has been stated by some clients with borderline personality disorder that "it is better to feel pain than nothing at all. The suffering confirms their existence.

Impulsivity

Primary process functioning indicates that impulse control is poor in people with borderline personality disorder. Gambling, substance abuse, promiscuity, careless driving, bingeing, and purging are examples of impulsive behaviors linked to borderline personality disorder. These overreactions to abandonment are frequently the result of actual or imagined feelings of abandonment.

7.5.1.3. Predisposing Factors to Borderline Personality Disorder

Biological Influences

- **Biochemical:** Clients with borderline personality disorder may have a serotonergic defect, according to Cummings and Mega (2003). Through the use of -[11C] methyl-L-tryptophan (-[11C]MTrp) in positron emission tomography, which measures serotonergic synthesis capability, patients with borderline personality showed significantly lower levels of -[11C]MTrp in the striatal, superior temporal, and medial frontal regions of the brain. Cummings and Mega (2003) state that a medial and orbitofrontal abnormality that may encourage the impulsive aggression exhibited by borderline personality disorder patients is supported by these functional imaging studies.
    - **Genetic:** Borderline personality disorder may have genetic roots related to serotonin deficiency. According to Sadock and Sadock (2007), clients with borderline personality disorder frequently have depression in their family histories. They say that people with borderline personality disorder frequently also have mood disorders, and these patients have more relatives with mood disorders than do control groups.

Psychosocial Influences

- **Childhood Trauma:** According to studies, a large number of people who suffer from borderline personality disorder grew up in households that were chaotic. According to Lubit (2011), "Family environments characterized by trauma, neglect, and/or separation' exposure to sexual and physical abuse' and serious parental psychopathology, such as substance abuse and antisocial personality disorder, are risk factors [for borderline personality disorder]". According to Gunderson (2011), 70% of people with borderline personality disorder report having experienced physical or sexual abuse in the past. This disorder has occasionally been compared to posttraumatic stress disorder, which is a reaction to maltreatment and trauma during childhood. According to Oldham et al. (2006), patients with borderline personality disorder may exhibit symptoms similar to PTSD even in the absence of all the criteria for comorbid PTSD. For instance, during psychotherapy, symptoms like intrusion, avoidance, and hyperarousal may surface. Understanding the trauma-related origins of these symptoms can help with symptom relief efforts involving both psychotherapy and medication.
- Developmental Factors
  - **Theory of Object Relations:** According to Mahler's theory of object relations (Mahler et al., 1975), the infant passes through six phases from birth to 36 months, when a sense of separateness from the parenting figure is finally established.

These phases include the following:

- **Phase 1 (Birth to 1 Month), Autistic Phase:** During this period, the baby spends most of his or her time in a half-waking, half-sleeping state. The main goal is fulfillment of needs for survival and comfort.
- **Phase 2 (1 to 5 Months), Symbiotic Phase:** At this time, there is a type of psychic fusion of mother and child. The child views the self as an extension of the parenting figure, although there is a developing awareness of external sources of need fulfillment.
- Phase 3 (5 to 10 Months), Differentiation Phase. The child is beginning to recognize that there is a separateness between the self and the parenting figure.
- **Phase 4 (10 to 16 Months), Practicing Phase:** This phase is characterized by increased locomotor functioning and the ability to explore the environment independently. A sense of separateness of the self is increased.
- **Phase 5 (16 to 24 Months), Rapprochement Phase:** Awareness of separateness of the self becomes acute. This is frightening to the child, who wants to regain some lost closeness but not return to symbiosis. The child wants the mother there as needed for "emotional refueling" and to maintain feelings of security.

- **Phase 6 (24 to 36 Months):** On the Way to Object Constancy Phase. In this phase, the child completes the individuation process and learns to relate to objects in an effective, constant manner. A sense of separateness is established, and the child is able to internalize a sustained image of the loved object or person when out of sight. Separation anxiety is resolved.

During the rapprochement phase of development, the person with borderline personality disorder becomes fixed. This happens when the child exhibits growing independence and separation. When the child is dependent, the mother feels safe in the relationship' however, as the child grows more independent, the mother starts to feel threatened. It's possible that the mother is going through her own abandonment fears. The mother withholds the emotional support, or "refueling," that the child so desperately needs during this stage in order to feel safe in response to separation behaviors. Rather, the mother encourages dependent, clinging behaviors while punishing independent, self-sufficient behaviors by not providing emotional support. The child learns to act in a way that fulfills the wishes of his or her parents because it feels like their emotional survival is on the line. The child experiences an internal conflict stemming from their fear of being abandoned. He or she desires the independence typical of this developmental stage, but they are afraid that if they do, their mother will stop providing emotional support. The child carries this unresolved fear of abandonment into adulthood. The depression that is so common in those with borderline personality disorder is a manifestation of internalized rage stemming from unresolved grief for the nurturing they did not receive.

7.5.2. Diagnosis/Outcome Identification

Nursing diagnoses are developed using the information acquired during the assessment stage as well as prior understanding of the disorder's risk factors. Care plans for clients with borderline personality disorder can be formulated using the list of client behaviors in Table 7.2 and the corresponding NANDA nursing diagnoses.

7.5.2.1. Outcome Criteria

The following criteria may be used for the measurement of outcomes in the care of clients with borderline personality disorder.

The client:

- Has not harmed self.
- Seeks out staff when desire for self-mutilation is strong.
- Can identify the true source of anger.
- Expresses anger appropriately.
- Relates to more than one staff member.
- Completes activities of daily living independently.
- Does not manipulate one staff member against the other in order to fulfill own desires.

7.5.3. Planning/Implementation

A selection of nursing diagnoses that are typical for clients with borderline personality disorder are shown in the following section, along with nursing interventions and short- and long-term goals for each.

Table 7.2. *Assigning Nursing Diagnoses to Behaviors Commonly Associated With Borderline Personality Disorder*

BEHAVIORS	NURSING DIAGNOSES
Risk factors: History of self-injurious behavior; history of inability to plan solutions; impulsivity; irresistible urge to damage self; feels threatened with loss of significant relationship	Risk for self-mutilation
Risk factors: History of suicide attempts; suicidal ideation; suicidal plan; impulsiveness; childhood abuse; fears of abandonment; internalized rage	Risk for self-directed violence; Risk for suicide
Risk factors: Body language (e.g., rigid posture, clenching of fists and jaw, hyperactivity, pacing, breathlessness, threatening stances); history of childhood abuse; impulsivity; transient psychotic symptomatology	Risk for other-directed violence
Depression; persistent emotional distress; rumination; separation distress; traumatic distress; verbalizes feeling empty; inappropriate expression of anger	Complicated grieving
Alternating clinging and distancing behaviors; staff splitting; manipulation	Impaired social interaction
Feelings of depersonalization and derealization	Disturbed personal identity
Transient psychotic symptoms (disorganized thinking; misinterpretation of the environment); increased tension; decreased perceptual field	Anxiety (severe to panic)
Dependent on others; excessively seeks reassurance; manipulation of others; inability to tolerate being alone	Chronic low self-esteem

Source. https://repository.poltekkes-kaltim.ac.id/625/1/Psychiatric%20Mental%20Health%20Nursing%20Concepts%20of%20Care%20in%20Evidence-Based%20Practice%20by%20Mary%20C.%20Townsend%20DSN%20%20PMHCNS-BC%20(z-lib.org).pdf.

7.5.3.1. Risk for Self-Mutilation/Risk for Self-Directed or Other Directed Violence

In order to achieve nonfatal injury and relieve tension, one must be "at risk for deliberate self-injurious behavior causing tissue damage" (NANDA International [NANDA-I], 2012). This definition includes the possibility of self-mutilation. According to NANDA-I (2012), "at risk for behaviors in which an individual demonstrates that he or she can be physically, emotionally, and/or sexually harmful to self or others" is the definition of risk for self-aggravated or other-directed violence.

Client Goals

- Outcome criteria include short- and long-term goals. Timelines are individually determined.

Short-Term Goals

- The client will seek out staff member if feelings of harming self or others emerge.

Long-Term Goal

- The client will not harm self or others.

Interventions

- Observe the client's behavior frequently. Do this through routine activities and interactions' avoid appearing watchful and suspicious. Close observation is required so that intervention can occur if required to ensure client's (and others') safety.
- Secure a verbal contract from the client that he or she will seek out a staff member when the urge for self-mutilation is experienced. Discussing feelings of self-harm with a trusted individual provides some relief to the client. A contract gets the subject out in the open and places some of the responsibility for his or her safety with the client. An attitude of acceptance of the client as a worthwhile individual is conveyed.
- If self-mutilation occurs, care for the client's wounds in a matter-of-fact manner. Do not give positive reinforcement to this behavior by offering sympathy or additional attention. Lack of attention to the maladaptive behavior may decrease repetition of its use.
- Encourage the client to talk about feelings he or she was having just before this behavior occurred. To problem-solve the situation with the client, knowledge of the precipitating factors is important.
- Act as a role model for the appropriate expression of angry feelings, and give positive reinforcement to the client when attempts to conform are made. It is vital that the client expresses angry feelings because suicide and other self-destructive behaviors are often viewed as a result of anger turned inward on the self.
- Remove all dangerous objects from the client's environment so that he or she may not purposefully or inadvertently use them to inflict harm self or others.
- Try to redirect violent behavior with physical outlets for the client's anxiety (e.g., punching bag, jogging). Physical exercise is a safe and effective way of relieving pent-up tension.
- Have sufficient staff available to indicate a show of strength to the client if it becomes necessary. This conveys to the client evidence of control over the situation and provides some physical security for staff.
- Administer tranquilizing medications as ordered by the physician or obtain an order if necessary. Monitor the client for effectiveness of the medication and for the appearance of adverse side effects. Tranquilizing medications such as anxiolytics or antipsychotics may have a calming effect on the client and may prevent aggressive behaviors.
- If client is not calmed by "talking down" or by medication, use of mechanical restraints may be necessary. The avenue of the "least restrictive alternative" must be selected when planning interventions for a violent client. Restraints should be used only as a last resort, after all other interventions have been

unsuccessful, and the client is clearly at risk of harm to self or others.

- If restraint is deemed necessary, ensure that sufficient staff is available to assist. Follow protocol established by the institution. The Joint Commission requires that an in-person evaluation by a physician or other licensed independent practitioner (LIP) be conducted within 1 hour of the initiation of the restraint or seclusion (The Joint Commission, 2010). The physician or LIP must reissue a new order for restraints every 4 hours for adults and every 1 to 2 hours for children and adolescents.
- The Joint Commission requires that the client in restraints be observed at least every 15 minutes to ensure that circulation to extremities is not compromised (check temperature, color, pulses)' to assist the client with needs related to nutrition, hydration, and elimination' and to position the client so that comfort is facilitated and aspiration is prevented. Some institutions may require continuous one-to-one monitoring of restrained clients, particularly those who are highly agitated, and for whom there is a high risk of self- or accidental injury.
- As agitation decreases, assess the client's readiness for restraint removal or reduction. Remove one restraint at a time while assessing the client's response. This minimizes the risk of injury to client and staff.
- If warranted by high acuity of the situation, staff may need to be assigned on a one-to-one basis. Because of their extreme fear of abandonment, clients with borderline personality disorder should not be left alone at a stressful time as it may cause an acute rise in anxiety and agitation levels.

7.5.3.2. Complicated Grieving

"A disorder that occurs after the death of a significant other [or any other loss of significance to the individual], in which the experience of distress accompanying bereavement fails to follow normative expectations and manifests in functional impairment" is the definition of complicated grieving (NANDA-I, 2012).

7.5.4. Antisocial Personality Disorder (Background Assessment Data)

Antisocial behavior was defined as a "sociopathic or psychopathic" reaction in the DSM-I, which could indicate any of a number of underlying personality disorders. It was depicted as a distinct personality type in the DSM-II, and this differentiation has persisted in later editions. Most clinical settings rarely see people with antisocial personality disorder, and when they do, it's usually as a means of avoiding legal repercussions. On occasion, a court order is used to admit them into the medical system so they can undergo psychological testing. But the majority of the time, you can find these people in jails, prisons, and rehabilitation centers.

7.5.4.1. Clinical Picture

Antisocial personality disorder is characterized by a pattern of exploitative, remorseless, and socially irresponsible behavior that shows a general disregard for the rights of others. These individuals are more concerned with taking advantage of and manipulating others for their own gain than they are with abiding by the law. They find it difficult to keep a stable job and build long-lasting relationships. Their harsh and aggressive demeanor often intimidates others, giving off the impression that they are heartless and aloof. They frequently argue and can be spiteful and malevolent. They lack compassion and warmth and are frequently wary of these traits in other people.

People with antisocial personalities act impulsively, have very little patience for waiting for satisfaction, and are unable to control their gratification. They are restless and easily bored' they frequently take risks and look for excitement, acting as though they are impervious to harm. People with this disorder behave cheerfully, even graciously and charmingly, when things go their way. This pleasant exterior can change very quickly due to their low threshold for frustration. They are prone to become enraged and vengeful when their current desires are threatened. They are easily agitated and have a tendency to dominate and denigrate others. They treat the weak and disadvantaged with disdain and hold the view that "good guys come in last". They take advantage of other people to satisfy their own needs and never feel guilty or ashamed of what they have done. The main ego defense mechanism used by people with antisocial personalities is projection, which leads them to perceive themselves as victims. They refuse to take accountability for the results of their actions. According to Gorman and Sultan (2008), manipulative people have come to believe that any institution or person could attempt to control them, leaving them defenseless and open to harm. This view serves as justification for their evil deeds in their own minds, protecting them from unfair criticism and animosity from others. People with antisocial personalities have learned to trust no one but themselves, which makes it impossible for them to maintain satisfying interpersonal relationships. According to their "it's every man for himself" mentality, one should do whatever it takes to keep from falling prey to deceit. The propensity to defy authority figures and norms is one of the most defining traits of people with antisocial personalities. They behave as though they are exempt from accepted social norms and rules about cooperation and self-control. Their blatant disregard for the law and other people's rights is evident.

7.5.4.2. Predisposing Factors to Antisocial Personality Disorder

Biological Influences

First-degree biological relatives of people with the disorder are more likely than the general population to exhibit antisocial personality (Tharp, 2009). Genetics may play a part in antisocial personality disorder, according to twin and adoptive studies (Skodol and Gunderson, 2008). Studies conducted on the families of those who have the disorder reveal a greater prevalence of relatives who suffer from alcoholism or antisocial personality disorder than is typical in the general population. Research has also indicated that children raised by people free of antisocial personality disorder are more likely to be diagnosed with antisocial personality disorder than children of parents who exhibit antisocial behavior, even if the children are taken from their biological parents at birth. Temperament traits in the baby may play a major role in the likelihood of developing antisocial personality disorder. When parents bring their children to clinics with behavior disorders, they frequently report that their child had tantrums since they were infants and would get upset when they were waiting for a bottle or to have their diaper changed. These kids grow up and frequently adopt a bullying mindset toward other kids. Parents claim that their children are generally very uncontrollable and unfazed by punishment. They seem unaffected by pain, and their willingness to risk bodily harm is bold and reckless. Antisocial personality disorder is predisposed to by conduct disorder and attention-deficit/hyperactivity disorder during childhood and adolescence, according to Fischer, Barkley, Smallish, and Fletcher (2002).

Despite the possibility that these biogenetic influences could explain a family pattern in the emergence of antisocial personality disorder, no fundamental pathological process has been identified as an etiological factor as of yet. Serotonergic dysregulation in the septohippocampal system may be the mediating factor for low levels of behavioral inhibition, according to Bienenfeld (2013). Antisocial personality disorder may also be associated with reduced autonomic activity and abnormalities in prefrontal brain systems, either acquired or developmental. This could be the cause of the low arousal, inadequate fear conditioning, and impaired decision-making that are associated with antisocial personality disorder.

Family Dynamics

A chaotic home life is often the root cause of antisocial personality disorder. Antisocial personality disorder development appears to be significantly predisposed to by parental deprivation during the first five years of life. Parental loss from other causes is not as strongly correlated with the disorder as separation brought on by parental delinquency. The most detrimental effect on the environment is not the death of a consistent parent, but rather the existence or sporadic appearance of inconsistent, impulsive parents. According to studies, people who suffer from antisocial personality disorder frequently experienced severe physical abuse as children. There are various ways in which abuse influences the emergence of antisocial behavior. It offers a behavior model first. Second, it might cause harm to the child's central nervous system, which would make it harder for them to operate normally. Ultimately, it makes the victimized child angry, which they then project onto other people and things around them.

Several factors associated with disordered family functioning have been implicated in the development of antisocial personality (Hill, 2003' Skodol & Gunderson, 2008' Ramsland, 2013). The following circumstances may influence the predisposition to antisocial personality disorder:

- Absence of parental discipline;
- Extreme poverty;
- Removal from the home;
- Growing up without parental figures of both genders;
- Erratic and inconsistent methods of discipline;
- Being "rescued" each time they are in trouble (never having to suffer the consequences of one's own behavior);
- Maternal deprivation.

7.5.5. Diagnosis/Outcome Identification

Nursing diagnoses are developed using the information acquired during the assessment stage as well as prior understanding of the disorder's risk factors. Care plans for clients with antisocial personality disorder can be formulated using the list of client behaviors in Table 7.3 and the corresponding NANDA nursing diagnoses.

7.5.5.1. Outcome Criteria

The following criteria may be used for measurement of outcomes in the care of the client with antisocial personality disorder.

The client:

- Discusses angry feelings with staff and in group sessions.
- Has not harmed self or others.
- Can rechannel hostility into socially acceptable behaviors.
- Follows rules and regulations of the therapy environment.
- Can verbalize which of his or her behaviors are not acceptable.
- Shows regard for the rights of others by delaying gratification of own desires when appropriate.
- Does not manipulate others in an attempt to increase feelings of self-worth.
- Verbalizes understanding of knowledge required to maintain basic health needs.

7.5.6. Planning/Implementation

A selection of nursing diagnoses that are typical for clients with antisocial personality disorder are shown in the section that follows, along with nursing interventions and short- and long-term goals for each.

Table 7.3. *Assigning Nursing Diagnoses to Behaviors Commonly Associated With Antisocial Personality Disorder*

BEHAVIORS	NURSING DIAGNOSES
Risk factors: Body language (e.g., rigid posture, clenching of fists and jaw, hyperactivity, pacing, breathlessness, threatening stances); cruelty to animals; rage reactions; history of childhood abuse; history of violence against others; impulsivity; substance abuse; negative role-modeling; inability to tolerate frustration	Risk for other-directed violence
Disregard for societal norms and laws; absence of guilty feelings; inability to delay gratification; denial of obvious problems; grandiosity; hostile laughter; projection of blame and responsibility; ridicule of others; superior attitude toward others	Defensive coping
Manipulation of others to fulfill own desires; inability to form close, personal relationships; frequent lack of success in life events; passive-aggressiveness; overt aggressiveness (hiding feelings of low self-esteem)	Chronic low self-esteem
Inability to form a satisfactory, enduring, intimate relationship with another; dysfunctional interaction with others; use of unsuccessful social interaction behaviors	Impaired social interaction
Demonstration of inability to take responsibility for meeting basic health practices; history of lack of health-seeking behavior; demonstrated lack of knowledge regarding basic health practices; lack of expressed interest in improving health behaviors	Ineffective health maintenance

Source: https://repository.poltekkes-kaltim.ac.id/625/1/Psychiatric%20Mental%20Health%20Nursing%20Concepts%20of%20Care%20in%20Evidence-Based%20Practice%20by%20Mary%20C.%20Townsend%20DSN%20%20PMHCNS-BC%20(z-lib.org).pdf.

7.5.6.1. Risk for Other-Directed Violence

The definition of "at risk for behaviors in which an individual demonstrates that he or she can be physically, emotionally, and/or sexually harmful to others" is "at risk for other-directed violence" (NANDA-I, 2012).

Client Goals

Outcome criteria include short- and long-term goals. Timelines are individually determined.

Short-Term Goals

- Within 3 days, the client will discuss angry feelings and situations that precipitate hostility.
- The client will not harm others.

Long-Term Goal

- The client will not harm others.

Interventions

- Show this customer that you are accepting of them. He or she has definitely experienced rejection before. Concentrate on building trust. Tell the client that it is not them, but the behavior that is unacceptable. Be truthful, and honor all of your commitments. Feelings of self-worth are enhanced by an accepting attitude. A therapeutic relationship is built on trust.
- Maintain a low level of stimuli in the client's environment (low lighting, few people, simple decor, low noise level). A stimulating environment may increase agitation and promote aggressive behavior.
- Observe the client's behavior frequently. Do this through routine activities and interactions' avoid appearing watchful and suspicious. Close observation is required so that intervention can occur if needed to ensure the client's (and others') safety.
- Remove all dangerous objects from the client's environment so that he or she may not purposefully or inadvertently use them to inflict harm on self or others.
- Help the client identify the true object of his or her hostility (e.g., "You seem to be upset with . . ."). Because of weak ego development, the client may be misusing the defense mechanism of displacement. Helping him or her recognize this in a nonthreatening manner may help reveal unresolved issues so that they may be confronted.
- Encourage the client to gradually verbalize hostile feelings. Verbalization of feelings in a nonthreatening environment may help client come to terms with unresolved issues.
- Explore with the client alternative ways of handling frustration (e.g., large motor skills that channel hostile energy into socially acceptable behavior). Physically demanding activities help to relieve pentup tension.

- The staff should maintain and convey a calm attitude toward the client. Anxiety is contagious and can be transferred from staff to client. A calm attitude provides the client with a feeling of safety and security.
- Have sufficient staff available to present a show of strength to the client if necessary. This conveys to the client evidence of control over the situation and provides some physical security for the staff.
- Administer tranquilizing medications as ordered by the physician or obtain an order if necessary. Monitor the client for effectiveness of the medication as well as for appearance of adverse side effects. Antianxiety agents (e.g., lorazepam, chlordiazepoxide, oxazepam) produce a calming effect and may help to allay hostile behaviors. (NOTE: Medications are not often prescribed for clients with antisocial personality disorder because of these individuals' strong susceptibility to addictions.)
- The use of mechanical restraints may be required if "talking down" or medication fails to calm the client. When designing interventions for a violent client, the "least restrictive alternative" must be chosen. Only in extreme cases, when no other interventions have worked and the client is obviously in danger of hurting themselves or others, should restraints be applied.
- If it is decided that restraint is required, make sure there is enough personnel on hand to help. Observe the guidelines set forth by the organization. Within one hour of the start of the restraint or seclusion, The Joint Commission mandates that an in-person evaluation be performed by a doctor or other licensed independent practitioner (LIP) (The Joint Commission, 2010). For adults, a new order for restraints must be issued by the doctor or LIP every 4 hours, and for children and adolescents, it must be issued every 1 to 2 hours.
- To ensure that circulation to the extremities is not compromised (check temperature, color, and pulses), to assist the client with needs related to nutrition, hydration, and elimination, and to position the client so aspiration is prevented, the Joint Commission mandates that the client in restraints be observed at least every 15 minutes. Certain establishments might necessitate ongoing individualized supervision of restrained patients, especially those who exhibit extreme agitation and a high potential for self-harm or unintentional injury.
- Evaluate the client's readiness to remove or reduce restraints when their agitation subsides. One constraint at a time, remove it while gauging the client's reaction. This reduces the possibility of staff and client injuries.

7.5.6.2. Defensive Coping

To defend against underlying perceived threats to positive self-regard, defensive coping is defined as "repeated projection of falsely positive self-evaluation based on a self-protective pattern" (NANDA-I, 2012).

Client Goals

Outcome criteria include short- and long-term goals. Timelines are individually determined.

Short-Term Goals

- Within 24 hours after admission, client will verbalize understanding of treatment setting rules and regulations and the consequences for violation of them.
- The client will verbalize personal responsibility for difficulties experienced in interpersonal relationships within (time period reasonable for client).

Long-Term Goals

- By the time of discharge from treatment, the client will be able to cope more adaptively by delaying gratification of own desires and following rules and regulations of the treatment setting.
- By the time of discharge from treatment, the client will demonstrate ability to interact with others without becoming defensive, rationalizing behaviors, or expressing grandiose ideas.

Interventions

- It is important to let the client know right away what behaviors are appropriate and inappropriate. Describe the repercussions for exceeding the boundaries. Something valuable for the client must be involved in the consequence. Enforcing these limits requires consistency from the entire staff. A matter-of-fact approach should be taken to administer consequences as soon as possible after the infraction. Staff members must define and enforce boundaries for maladaptive behaviors because the client cannot or will not set boundaries for themselves. Unfavorable outcomes could aid in reducing the likelihood that these actions will be repeated.
- The ideal goal would be for this client to eventually internalize societal norms, beginning with a step-by-step, "either/or" approach on the unit (either you do [don't do] this, or this will occur). Explanations must be concise, concrete, and clear, with little or no capacity for misinterpretation.
- Provide positive feedback or reward for acceptable behaviors. Positive reinforcement enhances self-esteem and encourages the repetition of desirable behaviors.
- Start extending the amount of time needed for appropriate behavior to receive the reward to help the client postpone gratification. One day of acceptable behavior for a therapeutic bowling activity, two hours for a phone call, four hours for two hours of television, and five days for a weekend pass, for instance, are all examples of acceptable behavior exchanges.
- A milieu unit creates the right setting for clients with antisocial personalities. Utilizing a democratic approach with clear guidelines, community meetings, and group therapy sessions mirrors the structure of society to help clients adapt. Peer feedback is often

more impactful than authoritative discipline. By adhering to group rules, clients take a positive step towards understanding and internalizing societal norms.

- Assist the client in understanding how they behave themselves. These people frequently justify their actions to the point where they contest the inappropriateness of what they are doing. Statements like "The owner of this store has so much money, he'll never miss the little bit I take" are an example of how thinking can be expressed. I have nothing, and he has everything. I should be able to share in some of his possessions' it's unfair. The client needs to be made aware of the fact that some behaviors are unacceptable in society and that disobedient individuals will face harsh penalties. Before the client can receive assistance, they must desire to contribute to society.
- Discuss previous actions with the client. Talk about the behaviors that are and are not acceptable under societal norms. Assist the client in recognizing the instances in which they have abused other people. Urge the client to consider what emotions they might experience in the opposite situation. To help the client gain insight into his or her own behavior, an attempt may be made to raise self-awareness and enlighten the client about the sensitivity of others.
- Keep up the mindset that "Your behavior, not you, is unacceptable" throughout your interaction with the client. Acceptance fosters a sense of worth and dignity in oneself.

7.6. Treatment Modalities

Treatment for personality disorders is challenging and, in certain cases, may even seem unattainable, but few would contest this. Characteristics of a personality are acquired very early in life and may even be inherited. Thus, it is not unexpected that it could take years for these ingrained behavioral patterns to alter, assuming they do at all. As stated by Skodol and Gunderson (2008), personality disorders have historically been associated with extreme resistance to change because it has been assumed that they are comprised of deeply rooted attitudes and behavior patterns that solidify during development and persist into early adulthood. Furthermore, patients with personality disorders often fail to identify their maladaptive personality traits as undesirable or in need of modification, which further complicates treatment efforts. The majority of clinicians think that minimizing the rigidity of the maladaptive traits and their disruption of daily activities and significant interpersonal relationships is the optimal goal. The choice of the most suitable therapy for treating personality disorders is not well supported by research. The most dysfunctional area, such as behavior, affect, cognition, or interpersonal relationships, is usually taken into consideration when choosing an intervention. The different types of therapy and the disorders they are typically used for are briefly described below.

7.6.1. Interpersonal Psychotherapy

Interpersonal psychotherapy for personality disorders can be short-term, time-limited, or involve long-term exploratory psychotherapy, depending on the therapeutic goals. Given that interpersonal style issues are often reflected in personality disorders, interpersonal psychotherapy may be especially useful. The goal of long-term psychotherapy is to comprehend and change the maladaptive thoughts, behaviors, and affects that control the lives and relationships of clients suffering from personality disorders. The foundation of treatment is the development of an empathic therapeutic alliance built on cooperation and guided discovery, where the therapist serves as the client's role model. Clients with paranoid, schizoid, schizotypal, borderline, dependent, narcissistic, and obsessive compulsive personality disorders are recommended candidates for interpersonal psychotherapy.

7.6.2. Psychoanalytical Psychotherapy

Psychoanalytical psychotherapy has been the preferred course of treatment for people with histrionic personality disorder (Skodol and Gunderson, 2008). The goal of treatment is to address the underlying causes of the inability to commit to a committed, long-term relationship and the unconscious desire for complete fulfillment from other people.

7.6.3. Milieu or Group Therapy

People with antisocial personality disorder benefit most from this treatment because they react in a more adaptable way to peer support and criticism. Peer feedback is more beneficial in milieu or group therapy settings than it is in individual sessions with therapists. For clients with avoidant personality disorder, group therapy—especially homogeneous supportive groups emphasizing social skill development—may be beneficial in helping them overcome social anxiety and build rapport and interpersonal trust. Groups that promote feminist consciousness can be helpful for dependent clients who are having trouble overcoming stereotypes of social roles.

7.6.4. Cognitive/Behavioral Therapy

Behavioral tactics provide encouragement for constructive modification. Assertiveness and social skills training provide different approaches to handling frustration. Cognitive techniques assist the client in identifying and modifying false internal mental schemas. Clients with avoidant, antisocial, and obsessive compulsive personality disorders may benefit from this kind of therapy.

7.6.5. Dialectical Behavior Therapy

The psychotherapy modality known as dialectical behavior therapy (DBT) was first created by Marsha Linehan, PhD, to address the persistent self-harming and suicidal tendencies of her borderline personality disorder patients (Sadock and Sadock, 2007). The treatment is multifaceted and eclectic, incorporating Eastern mindfulness practices with concepts from cognitive, behavioral, and interpersonal therapies (Dimeff & Linehan, 2001).

Dimeff and Linehan (2001) identify the following five functions of DBT:

- To enhance behavioral capabilities;
- To improve motivation to change;
- To ensure that new capabilities generalize to the natural environment;
- To structure the treatment environment such that client and therapist capabilities are supported and effective behaviors are reinforced;
- To enhance therapist capabilities and motivation to treat clients effectively.

The four primary modes of treatment in DBT include the following:

- **Group Skills Training:** In these groups, clients are taught skills considered relevant to the particular problems experienced by people with borderline personality disorder, such as core mindfulness skills, interpersonal effectiveness skills, emotion modulation skills, and distress tolerance skills (Kiehn & Swales, 2013).
- **Individual Psychotherapy:** Weekly sessions in which dysfunctional behavioral patterns, personal motivation, and skills strengthening are addressed.
- **Telephone Contact:** The therapist is available to the client by telephone, usually on a 24-hour per day basis, but according to limits set by the therapist. Kiehn and Swales (2013) state, "Telephone contact is to give the patient help and support in applying the skills that she is learning to her real life situation between sessions and to help her find ways of avoiding self-injury."
- **Therapist Consultation/Team Meeting:** Therapists meet regularly to review their work with their clients. These meetings are focused specifically on providing support for each other, keeping the therapists motivated, and providing effective treatment to their clients (Dimeff & Linehan, 2001).

DBT has been demonstrated to reduce self-destructive behaviors in clients with borderline personality disorder in controlled studies. DBT has also been demonstrated to reduce treatment attrition and hospitalization rates. Dimeff and Linehan (2001) have reported improvements in global and social adjustment scores, as well as in the reduction of anger. Other disorders such as eating disorders, schizophrenia, substance use disorders, and post-traumatic stress disorder are now being treated with this approach (Sadock & Sadock, 2007).

7.6.6. Psychopharmacology

In some cases, psychopharmacology might be beneficial. While these medications do not directly treat the disorder, they can provide some symptomatic relief. According to Skodol and Gunderson (2008), antipsychotic drugs are useful in treating psychotic decompensations that patients with paranoid, schizotypal, and borderline personality disorders encounter. Many pharmaceutical treatments have been applied to individuals with borderline personality disorder. Monoamine oxidase inhibitors (MAOIs) and SSRIs have been effective in reducing impulsivity and self-destructive behavior in these patients. Nonetheless, due to worries about dietary restrictions being broken and the increased risk of overdosing, MAOIs are not often used. Patients with borderline personality disorder who exhibit dysphoria, mood instability, and impulsivity have found success with the combination of an SSRI and an atypical antipsychotic (Schatzberg, Cole, & DeBattista, 2010). Some patients' illusions, ideas of reference, paranoid thinking, anxiety, and hostility have improved as a result of taking antipsychotics. For the violent episodes seen in clients with antisocial personality disorder, lithium carbonate and propranolol (Inderal) may be helpful (Coccaro & Siever, 2000). Prescribing medication outside of a structured setting requires caution due to the increased risk of substance abuse by these individuals. Anxiolytics can be useful for clients with avoidant personality disorder whenever they attempt to engage in previously avoided behavior. The client may find that just having the medication will provide them with enough comfort to get through this trying time. If panic disorder develops in these clients, antidepressants like paroxetine (Paxil) and sertraline (Zoloft) may be helpful.

A Closer Look

Male Body Dysmorphic Disorder

According to the Anxiety and Depression Association of America, Body Dysmorphic Disorder (BDD) is characterized by an intense preoccupation with perceived flaws in one's appearance, even when these flaws are minor or nonexistent. This mental illness can lead individuals to believe they look unattractive or ugly due to these perceived imperfections. As a result, people with BDD may spend countless hours fixating on various body parts or their overall body shape, unable to stop thinking about these perceived flaws. This relentless focus can severely interfere with daily functioning and the ability to maintain healthy relationships. To correct these perceived flaws, individuals may turn to cosmetic procedures or anabolic steroids, yet these measures often fail to alleviate BDD symptoms.

A person's body image, or their perception and feelings about their body, is influenced by a wide range of factors including friends, family, peers, past experiences, cultural norms, and media messages. Movies, television shows, and advertisements frequently present hyper-idealized standards of beauty, creating unrealistic expectations that can negatively impact mental health, particularly among men. Traditional notions of masculinity often emphasize "dominance" and "power," leading some men to pursue unrealistic physical goals. Social media exacerbates this issue by promoting distorted images of the "ideal" male body through filters and photoshopping, setting unattainable standards.

These dynamics can have profound psychological effects. The pressure to meet these unrealistic standards can cause many men to compare themselves unfavorably to others, resulting in low self-esteem and potentially contributing to the development of BDD. According to the Diagnostic and Statistical Manual of Mental Disorders (DSM-5), BDD is defined by a fixation on perceived flaws in appearance that are not apparent to others. This disorder can cause significant distress and disrupt various aspects of life. The obsessive focus on physical imperfections often leads to compulsive behaviors such as excessive grooming, body checking, and seeking reassurance. Some individuals may also avoid social situations due to their negative self-image. Additionally, those with BDD are more likely to experience other mental health conditions like anxiety disorders, depression, eating disorders, and substance use disorders. Without treatment, BDD can have serious physical and mental health consequences.

BDD can affect individuals of any gender, race, ethnicity, sexual orientation, and socioeconomic status, with specific aspects of a person's identity potentially influencing their experience with the disorder. For instance, research indicates that men with BDD are more likely to be concerned with muscularity and body build, a condition known as muscle dysmorphia. This form of BDD involves an obsessive focus on the idea that one's body is too small or insufficiently muscular, and it is more prevalent among men.

Furthermore, societal stigmas surrounding men seeking help can create additional barriers for those with BDD. The harmful narrative that seeking help is a sign of "weakness" often discourages men from pursuing treatment. Promoting open conversations and education about BDD can help reduce stigma and encourage more men to seek the help they need.

Body dysmorphic disorder can involve a range of signs and symptoms, and it may look different from one person to the next. Some of the common signs of BDD can include:

- An obsession with appearance or physical features;
- Excessive mirror-checking or avoidance of mirrors;
- Compulsive behaviors such as skin-picking or hair-pulling;
- Low self-esteem and feelings of shame, guilt, or worthlessness;
- Strong desire for cosmetic surgery or other treatments;
- Social isolation or a fear of being judged by others.

Individuals with body dysmorphic disorder may deny their condition or be unaware of how far-reaching its effects can be. As BDD progresses, the symptoms you experience may be more severe. For example, someone with BDD may find themselves relying on protein supplements or other performance-enhancing drugs to increase muscle mass. As the disorder worsens, more extreme measures may be taken to alter physical appearance, such as plastic surgery or dermatological treatments. When left untreated, male BDD can lead to severe physical and mental health conditions such as depression, anxiety, suicidal thoughts, and addiction.

Summary

- Obsessive compulsive disorder (OCD) was previously classified as an anxiety disorder due to the sometimes extreme anxiety that people experience. However, it varies from other anxiety disorders in significant ways.
- Obsessions are recurrent, persistent, intrusive, and unwanted thoughts, images, or impulses that cause marked anxiety and interfere with interpersonal, social, or occupational function. The person knows these thoughts are excessive or unreasonable but believes he or she has no control over them.
- Excoriation disorder, skin-picking, also known as dermatillomania, is categorized as a self-soothing behavior' that is, the behavior is an attempt of people to soothe or comfort themselves, not that picking itself is necessarily a positive sensation.
- Trichotillomania, or chronic repetitive hair-pulling, is a self-soothing behavior that can cause distress and functional impairment. Onset in childhood is most common, but it can also persist into adulthood with the development of anxiety and depression.
- Hoarding disorder is a progressive, debilitating, compulsive disorder only recently diagnosed on its own. Hoarding had been a symptom of OCD previously but differs from OCD in significant ways. Diagnosis most commonly occurs between the ages of 20 to 30.
- Onychophagia, or chronic nail-biting, is a self-soothing behavior. The typical onset is childhood, with a decrease in behavior by age 18. However, some nail-biting persists into adulthood. It may lead to psychosocial problems or cause complications involving the nails and oral cavity.
- Body identity integrity disorder (BIID) is the term given to people who feel "overcomplete," or alienated from a part of their body and desire amputation. This condition is also known as amputee identity disorder and apotemnophilia or "amputation love."
- The nurse assesses the client's appearance and behavior. Clients with OCD often seem tense, anxious, worried, and fretful.
- Personality traits may be defined as characteristics with which an individual is born or develops early in life. They influence how he or she perceives and relates to the environment and are quite stable over time.
- Individuals with schizotypal personality disorder are aloof and isolated and behave in a bland and apathetic manner. Magical thinking, ideas of reference, illusions, and depersonalization are part of their everyday world.
- Antisocial personality disorder is a pattern of socially irresponsible, exploitative, and guiltless behavior that reflects a general disregard for the rights of others. These individuals exploit and manipulate others for personal gain and are unconcerned with obeying the law.
- Depression is so common in clients with this disorder that before the inclusion of borderline personality disorder in the DSM, many of these clients were diagnosed with depressive disorder.

- Splitting is a primitive ego defense mechanism that is common in people with borderline personality disorder. It arises from their lack of achievement of object constancy and is manifested by an inability to integrate and accept both positive and negative feelings.
- Nursing diagnoses are formulated from the data gathered during the assessment phase and with background knowledge regarding predisposing factors to the disorder.

References

1. Albano, A. A., & Pimentel, S. S. (2017). Cognitive-behavioral therapy for children and adolescents. In B. J. Sadock, V. A. Sadock, & P. Ruiz (Eds.), *Comprehensive Textbook of Psychiatry* (Vol. 2, 10th ed., pp. 3749–3759). Philadelphia, PA: Wolters Kluwer/Lippincott.
2. American Psychiatric Association. (2013). *Diagnostic and Statistical Manual of Mental Disorders* (5th ed.). Washington, DC: Author. Retrieved from: http://emedicine.medscape.com/article/294307-overview (accessed on 7 September 2024).
3. Black, D. W., & Andreasen, N. C. (2011). *Introductory Textbook of Psychiatry* (5th ed.). Washington, DC: American Psychiatric Publishing.
4. Bosson, J. K., & Prewitt-Freilino, J. L. (2007). Overvalued and ashamed: Considering the roles of self-esteem and self-conscious emotions in covert narcissism. In J. L. Tracy, R. W. Robins, & J. P. Tangney (Eds.), *The Self-Conscious Emotions: Theory and Research*. New York, NY: Guilford Press.
5. Brakoulias, V., Starcevic, V., Belloch, A., Dell'Osso, L., Ferrão, Y. A., Fontenelle, L. F., & Viswasam, K. (2016). International prescribing practices in obsessive compulsive disorder (OCD). *Human Psychopharmacology, 31*(4), 319–324.
6. Candea, D. M., & Szentagotai-Tata, A. (2018). Shame-proneness, guilt-proneness and anxiety symptoms: A meta-analysis. *Journal of Anxiety Disorders, 58*, 78–106.
7. Casale, A. D., Sorice, S., Padovano, A., Simmaco, M., Ferracuti, S., Lamis, D. A., Rapinesi, C., & Pompili, M. (2018). Psychopharmacological treatment of obsessive-compulsive disorder (OCD). *Current Neuropharmacology*. doi:10.2174/1570159X16666180813155017.
8. Cison, H., Kus, A., Popowicz, E., Szyca, M., & Reich, A. (2018). Trichotillomania and trichophagia: Modern diagnostic and therapeutic methods. *Dermatology and Therapy, 8*(3), 389–398.
9. Coccaro, E. F., & Siever, L. J. (2000). The neuropsychopharmacology of personality disorders. In *Psychopharmacology: The Fourth Generation of Progress*. The American College of Neuropsychopharmacology. Retrieved from: www.acnp.org/G4/GN401000152/CH148.html (accessed on 7 September 2024).
10. Cummings, J. L., & Mega, M. S. (2003). *Neuropsychiatry and Behavioral Neuroscience*. New York, NY: Oxford University Press.
11. Dimeff, L., & Linehan, M. M. (2001). Dialectical behavior therapy in a nutshell. *The California Psychologist, 34*, 10–13.
12. Dozier, M. E., Porter, B., & Ayers, C. R. (2016). Age of onset and progression of hoarding symptoms in older adults with hoarding disorder. *Aging & Mental Health, 20*(7), 736–742.
13. Fischer, M., Barkley, R. A., Smallish, L., & Fletcher, K. (2002). Young adult follow-up of hyperactive children: Self-reported psychiatric disorders, comorbidity, and the role of childhood conduct

problems and teen CD. *Journal of Abnormal Child Psychology, 30*(5), 463–475.

14. Gorman, L., & Sultan, D. F. (2008). *Psychosocial Nursing for General Patient Care* (3rd ed.). Philadelphia, PA: F.A. Davis.
15. Grant, J. E., & Chamberlain, S. R. (2018). Symptom severity and its clinical correlates in kleptomania. *Annals of Clinical Psychiatry, 30*(2), 97–101.
16. Gunderson, J. G. (2011). An introduction to borderline personality disorder: Diagnosis, origins, course, and treatment. *National/8 Education Alliance—Borderline Personality Disorder*. Retrieved from: www.borderlinepersonalitydisorder.com/understanding-bpd/a-bpd-brief/ (accessed on 7 September 2024).
17. Halteh, P., Scher, R. K., & Lipner, S. R. (2017). Onychophagia: A nail-biting conundrum for physicians. *Journal of Dermatological Treatment, 28*(2), 166–172.
18. Hill, J. (2003). Early identification of individuals at risk for antisocial personality disorder. *British Journal of Psychiatry, 182*(Suppl. 44), s11–s14.
19. Hong, K., Nezgovorova, V., & Hollander, E. (2018). New perspectives in the treatment of body dysmorphic disorder. *F1000Research, 7*, 361.
20. Isomura, K., Nordsletten, A. E., Rück, C., Ljung, R., Ivarsson, T., Larsson, H., & Mataix-Cols, D. (2016). Pharmacoepidemiology of obsessive-compulsive disorder: A Swedish nationwide cohort study. *European Neuropsychopharmacology, 26*(4), 693–704.
21. Kiehn, B., & Swales, M. (2013). An overview of dialectical behavior therapy in the treatment of borderline personality disorder. *Psychiatry Online*. Retrieved from: http://www.priory.com/dbt.htm (accessed on 7 September 2024).
22. Leite, P. L., & Silva, A. C. (2016). Psychiatric and socioeconomic aspects as possible predictors of compulsive buying behavior. *Trends in Psychiatry and Psychotherapy, 38*(3), 141–146.
23. Lubit, R. H. (2011). Borderline personality disorder. *eMedicine Psychiatry*. Retrieved from: http://emedicine.medscape.com/article/913575-overview (accessed on 7 September 2024).
24. Martinez-Lewi, L. (2008). *Freeing Yourself from the Narcissist in Your Life*. New York, NY: Penguin Group.
25. Millon, T. (2004). *Personality Disorders in Modern Life* (2nd ed.). Hoboken, NJ: John Wiley and Sons.
26. Oldham, J. M., Gabbard, G. O., Goin, M. K., Gunderson, J., Soloff, P., Spiegel, D., Stone, M., & Phillips, K. A. (2006). Practice guideline for the treatment of patients with borderline personality disorder. In *The American Psychiatric Association Practice Guidelines for the Treatment of Psychiatric Disorders, Compendium 2006*. Washington, DC: American Psychiatric Publishing.
27. Ramsland, K. (2013). The childhood psychopath: Bad seed or bad parents? Retrieved from: http://www.trutv.com/library/crime/criminal_mind/psychology/psychopath/2.html (accessed on 7 September 2024).
28. Stein, D. J., & Lochner, C. (2017). Obsessive compulsive and related disorders. In B. J. Sadock, V. A. Sadock, & P. Ruiz (Eds.), *Comprehensive Textbook of Psychiatry* (Vol. 1, 10th ed., pp. 1785–1798). Philadelphia, PA: Wolters Kluwer/Lippincott.
29. Torales, J., Barrios, J., & Villalba, J. (2017). Alternative therapies of excoriation (skin-picking) disorder: A brief update. *Advances in Mind-Body Medicine, 31*(1), 10–13.

30. Williams, M. T., & Jahn, M. E. (2017). Obsessive compulsive disorder in African American children and adolescents: Risks, resiliency, and barriers to treatment. *American Journal of Orthopsychiatry, 87*(3), 291–303.

31. Yue, W., Cheng, W., Liu, Z., Tang, Y., Lu, T., Zhang, D., & Huang, Y. (2016). Genome-wide DNA methylation analysis in obsessive compulsive disorder patients. *Scientific Reports, 6*, 31333.

Chapter

SCHIZOPHRENIA SPECTRUM AND OTHER PSYCHOTIC DISORDERS

8

Contents

Introduction

The Swiss psychiatrist Eugen Bleuler first used the term "schizophrenia" in 1908. The Greek words "skhizo" (split) and "phren" (mind) are the origin of the word. The idea of schizophrenia has been the subject of much discussion over time. Numerous treatment approaches have been put forth, and different definitions of the disorder have developed over time, but none have shown to be consistently successful or adequate. Two general factors seem to be gaining traction among clinicians despite the ongoing controversy. The first is that there is likely more than one cause for schizophrenia and that it is instead the product of a complex interplay between genetic susceptibility, physiological variables, biochemical malfunction, and psychosocial stress. The second factor is that there isn't a single treatment that can cure the disorder, and there probably never will be. Rather, a thorough, multidisciplinary approach is needed for effective treatment, which includes medication and different types of psychosocial care like family therapy, social skills training, living skills training, and rehabilitation and recovery.

Schizophrenia is most likely the mental illness that causes longer hospital stays, more chaos in families, the highest costs to both individuals and governments, and the greatest amount of fear among all the mental illnesses that cause suffering in society. It has likely been studied more than any other mental disorder because it poses such a serious threat to happiness and life, and because its causes remain a mystery. One of the main concerns for patients with schizophrenia is their potential for suicide. A third of individuals with schizophrenia attempt suicide, and one in ten of them end their lives as a result. According to research cited by Addington (2006), between 40% and 55% of people with schizophrenia exhibit evidence of suicidal ideation, and between 20% and 50% attempt suicide.

Orientation and Directional Terms

Term	Definition	Illustration
Psychosocial stress	Psychosocial stress is a form of stress that is experienced due to changes in social situations. When psychosocial stress becomes chronic, the effects can be physically debilitating and lead to heart disease, high blood pressure, and even addictive behavior.	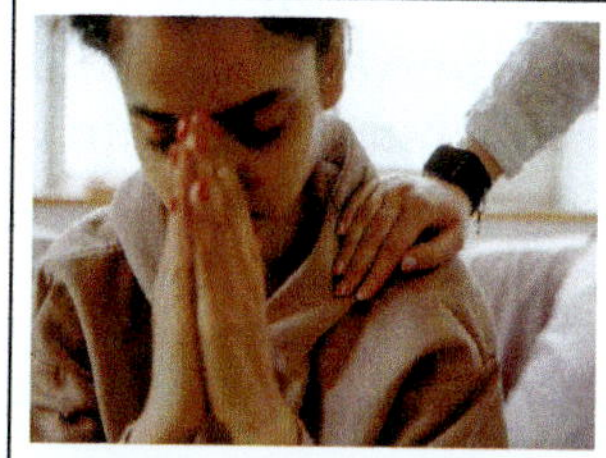
Schizophrenia	Schizophrenia is a serious mental health condition that affects how people think, feel and behave. It may result in a mix of hallucinations, delusions, and disorganized thinking and behavior. Hallucinations involve seeing things or hearing voices that aren't observed by others.	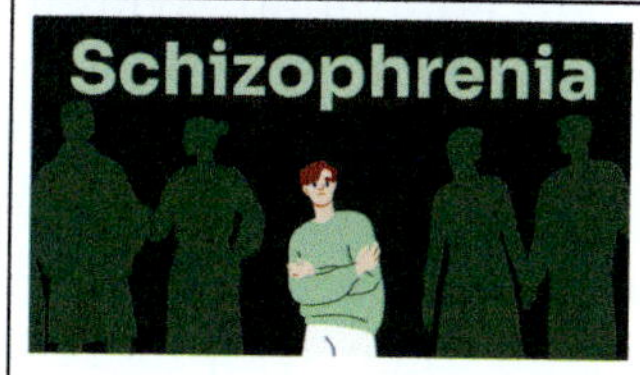
Very early-onset schizophrenia (VEOS)	Very early-onset schizophrenia (VEOS) is a form of schizophrenia that manifests before the age of 13 years and is characterized by the presence of positive, negative, and disorganized symptoms.	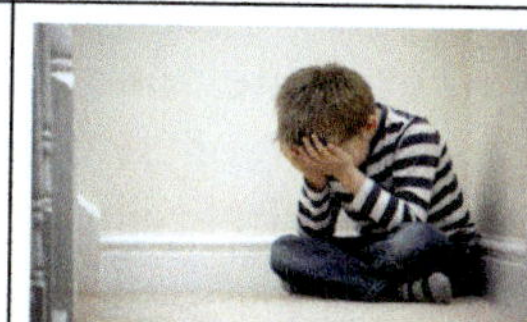
Gamma-aminobutyric acid (GABA)	GABA is the chief inhibitory neurotransmitter in the developmentally mature mammalian central nervous system. Its principal role is reducing neuronal excitability throughout the nervous system. GABA is sold as a dietary supplement in many countries.	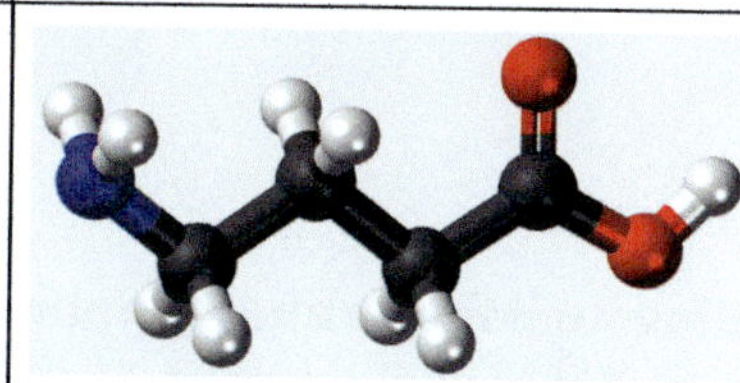
Delusional disorder	Delusional disorder, traditionally synonymous with paranoia, is a mental illness in which a person has delusions, but with no accompanying prominent hallucinations, thought disorder, mood disorder, or significant flattening of affect. Delusions are a specific symptom of psychosis.	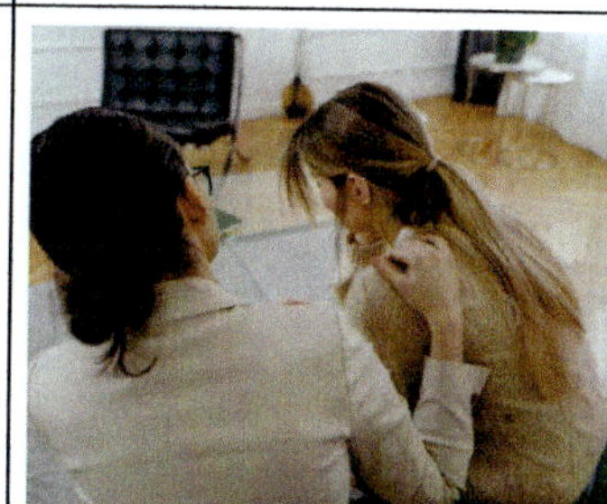

8.1. Nature of the Disorder

Schizophrenia is a psychological disorder that can be extremely debilitating. Disturbances in cognition, perception, and affect are typically associated with a marked decline in social and professional functioning. In the general population, the lifetime prevalence of schizophrenia is approximately 1% (Puri and Treasaden, 2011). Although they can happen in middle or late adulthood, symptoms typically manifest in late adolescence or early adulthood. Early-onset schizophrenia (EOS) is suspected when symptoms appear before the age of 17. Very early-onset schizophrenia (VEOS) is the diagnosis made when symptoms appear before the age of 13, which is extremely uncommon (Mattai, Hill, & Lenroot, 2010). According to certain research, men experience symptoms earlier than women. The four phases of the pattern of development of schizophrenia are the prodromal phase, the residual phase, the active psychotic phase (schizophrenia), and the premorbid phase.

8.1.1. Phase I: The Premorbid Phase

According to Mindzenberg, Yoon, and Carter (2008), social maladjustment, social withdrawal, irritability, and antagonistic thoughts and behavior are common indicators of the premorbid personality. Measures of premorbid personality and behavior that have been identified include extreme shyness and withdrawal, poor peer relationships, subpar academic performance, and antisocial behavior. Sadock and Sadock (2007) stated:

- In the common, though not always the case, premorbid history of schizophrenia, patients exhibited quiet, passive, introverted schizoid or schizotypal personalities' they also typically had few childhood friends. Adolescents with preschizophrenia might not date, have any close friends, or participate in team sports. They might prioritize [solitary activities] over social ones.

8.1.2. Phase II: The Prodromal Phase

An illness's early warning signs and symptoms are referred to as the prodrome, and they occur before the acute, fully developed illness's typical manifestations. When premorbid functioning changes, the prodromal phase of schizophrenia commences and lasts until the onset of overt psychotic symptoms. The prodromal phase can last for a few weeks or months, but most research suggests that it lasts for two to five years on average. According to Lehman and colleagues (2006), the prodromal phase is characterized by a significant reduction in functioning and nonspecific symptoms like fatigue, poor concentration, anxiety, irritability, depression, sleep disturbance, and behavioral deficits like social disengagement and declining role functioning. Positive symptoms that indicate the impending onset of psychosis include ideas of reference, suspiciousness, and perceptual abnormalities. These symptoms emerge late in the prodromal phase.

Identifying the behaviors linked to the prodromal phase offers a chance for early intervention that may improve long-term results. Therapy interventions that provide assistance with identified issues, cognitive therapies to minimize functional impairment, family interventions to enhance coping, and school involvement to lessen the likelihood of failure are all recommended by current treatment guidelines. The usefulness of pharmacological therapy during the prodromal phase is a topic of some debate. According to Minzenberg, Yoon, and Carter (2008), "the use of [antipsychotic] medications to treat symptoms that are below the threshold of psychosis has to date been poorly studied," it is possible to delay or even prevent the onset of psychosis by providing interventions, including pharmacologic treatments.

8.1.3. Phase III: Schizophrenia

In the active phase of the disorder, psychotic symptoms are prominent. Following are the Diagnostic and Statistical Manual of Mental Disorders, Fifth Edition (DSM-5) diagnostic criteria for schizophrenia:

- Two (or more) of the following, each present for a significant portion of time during a 1-month period (or less if successfully treated). At least one of these must be (1), (2), or (3):
  - Delusions;
  - Hallucinations;
  - Disorganized speech (e.g., frequent derailment or incoherence);
  - Grossly disorganized or catatonic behavior;
  - Negative symptoms (i.e., diminished emotional expression or avolition).
- When the disturbance first appears, the person's functioning in one or more major areas—like work, relationships with others, or self-care—is significantly lower than it was before the disturbance started. Alternatively, if the disturbance starts in childhood or adolescence, the person does not reach the expected level of academic, occupational, or interpersonal functioning.
- The disturbance is continuously present for at least six months. This 6-month period must include periods of prodromal or residual symptoms, as well as at least one month's worth of symptoms (or less if treatment is successful) that satisfy Criterion A, or active-phase symptoms. The symptoms of the disturbance can appear during these prodromal or residual periods as a single negative symptom or as two or more attenuated symptoms listed in Criterion A (e.g., strange beliefs, unusual perceptual experiences).
- Because either (1) no significant manic or depressive episodes have occurred concurrently with the active-phase symptoms, or (2) if mood episodes have occurred during active-phase symptoms, they have only been present for a small portion of the total duration of the active and residual periods of the illness, schizoaffective disorder and depressive or bipolar disorder with psychotic features have been ruled out.
- The disturbance is not attributable to the physiological effects of a substance (e.g., a drug of abuse, a medication) or another medical condition.
- The additional diagnosis of schizophrenia is only made if prominent delusions or hallucinations are present for at least one month (or less if successfully treated) in addition to the other necessary symptoms of schizophrenia in the presence of a history of autism spectrum disorder or childhood-onset communication disorders.

8.1.4. Phase IV: Residual Phase

There are phases of remission and exacerbation in schizophrenia. Usually, an active phase of the illness (symptoms listed in Phase III) is followed by a residual phase. The acute stage's symptoms are either nonexistent or less noticeable during the residual phase. Recurring negative symptoms are possible, and role functioning impairment and flat affect are frequent. In the intervals between active psychotic episodes, residual impairment frequently worsens.

8.1.5. Prognosis

While it is difficult to predict exactly what will happen in a schizophrenia case, it is uncommon for full premorbid functioning to return. Nonetheless, a number of variables have been linked to a better result. These include the following: minimal residual symptoms, absence of structural brain abnormalities, normal neurological functioning, good premorbid functioning, later age at onset, female gender, abrupt onset of symptoms with obvious precipitating factor (as opposed to gradual insidious onset of symptoms), associated mood disturbance, fast resolution of active-phase symptoms, minimal residual symptoms, and no family history of schizophrenia.

8.2. Predisposing Factors

Schizophrenia still has an unknown cause. It is highly likely that no single factor can be linked to the etiology' rather, a variety of factors, including biological, psychological, and environmental ones, combine to cause the disease.

8.2.1. Biological Factors

Review of the biological implications of psychiatric illness.

8.2.1.1. Genetics

An increasing amount of evidence points to a genetic susceptibility to schizophrenia. Research indicates that the likelihood of relatives of individuals with schizophrenia developing the illness is significantly higher than that of the general population. While most population studies show that the lifetime risk of schizophrenia is approximately 1%, siblings of an identified client are at 10% risk, and children of a parent with schizophrenia are at 5% to 6% risk of developing the disorder. It's unclear how schizophrenia is inherited. There is currently no conclusive biological marker available. Research is still being conducted to find out which genes play a significant role in schizophrenia susceptibility and whether one or more genes are involved. While some people may only have a weak genetic basis for the illness, others may have a strong genetic link. This theory supports the idea of multiple causalities even more.

When it comes to dizygotic (fraternal) twins, the rate of schizophrenia is four times higher than that of identical twins, and it is roughly 50 times higher than that of the general population. The illness develops in identical twins raised apart at the same rate as in twins raised together. Some researchers think that environmental factors interact with genetic ones in schizophrenia because only one out of a pair of monozygotic twins develops the disorder in about half of cases. Adopted children of schizophrenic mothers were compared with adopted children whose mothers did not have a mental illness in studies done by Danish and American researchers. Compared to comparison control groups, children born to mothers diagnosed with schizophrenia had a higher risk of developing the illness (Minzenberg et al., 2008). Research also suggests that children raised by parents with schizophrenia but not by parents without the illness do not appear to experience schizophrenia more frequently than general controls. These results add to the body of evidence supporting the genetic origins of schizophrenia.

8.2.1.2. Biochemical Factors

The most established and extensively studied biological theory explaining schizophrenia identifies aberrant brain biochemistry as a pathogenic factor. Some theorists as far back as the mid-19th century proposed the idea of a "chemical disturbance" as the cause of insanity.

The Dopamine Hypothesis

This theory postulates that an excess of dopamine-dependent neuronal activity in the brain could be the cause of schizophrenia or symptoms similar to schizophrenia. This overactivity could be caused by an excess of dopamine receptors, an increase in the substance's production or release at nerve terminals, or a combination of these mechanisms. There is pharmacological evidence to support this theory. Psychotomimetic symptoms are brought on by amphetamines, which raise dopamine levels. The antipsychotics (e.g., haloperidol or chlorpromazine) inhibit dopamine receptors in the brain to lower dopamine levels. This lessens schizophrenia symptoms, including amphetamine-induced ones (Figure 8.1).

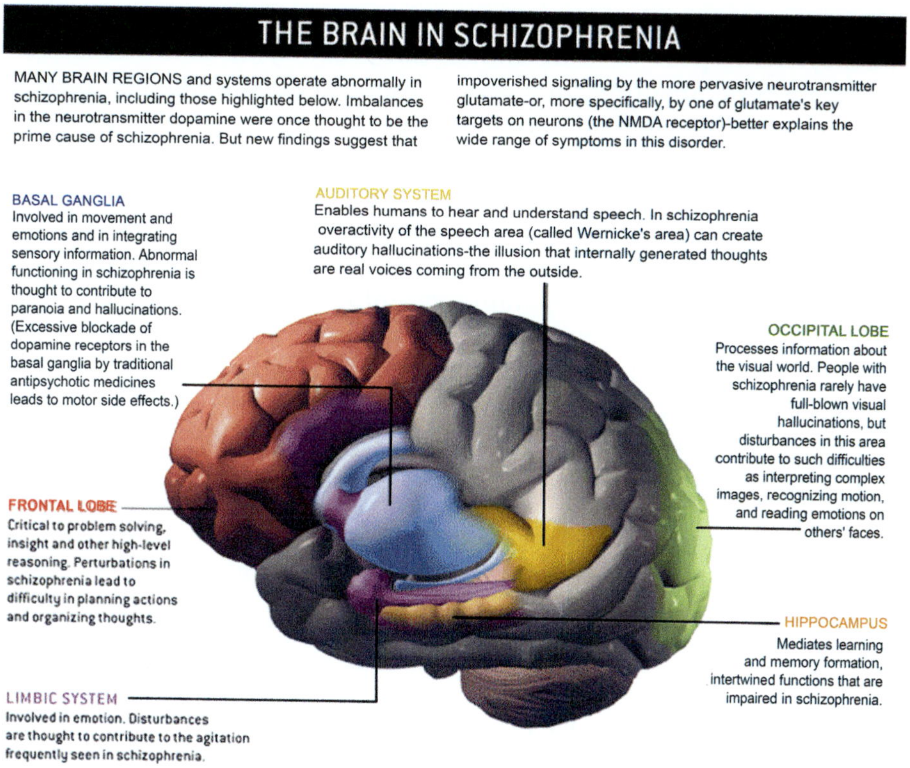

Figure 8.1. *Neurobiology of schizophrenia.*

Source: By Jurgitta - Own work, CC BY-SA 4.0, https://commons.wikimedia.org/w/index.php?curid=45787706.

The average number of dopamine receptors in the brains of people who had schizophrenia was found to be significantly higher in about two-thirds of the brains examined in postmortem investigation. It is possible that not all people with schizophrenia will have a significant increase in dopamine. When taking antipsychotic medications, patients with acute symptoms—such as delusions and hallucinations—respond more effectively than those with chronic symptoms. , indifference, lack of inspiration, and demotivation). According to current theories regarding the dopamine hypothesis, acute schizophrenia symptoms could be linked to an increase in dopamine receptors in the brain, which would make them responsive to antipsychotic medications that block these receptors. Antipsychotic medications are unlikely to be as helpful in treating the chronic symptoms of schizophrenia, and it is likely that the number of dopamine receptors has no bearing on the symptoms of the condition.

Other Biochemical Hypotheses

Numerous additional biochemicals have been connected to the susceptibility to schizophrenia. The neuroregulators prostaglandins and endorphins as well as the neurotransmitters norepinephrine, serotonin, acetylcholine, and gamma-aminobutyric acid (GABA) have been implicated in abnormalities. Glutamate, a neurotransmitter, has been linked to the genesis of schizophrenia in recent studies. Glycine and glutamate are two neurotransmitters that activate the N-methyl-D-aspartate (NMDA) receptor. Psychopharmacological research has demonstrated that the glutamate antagonist drug class, which includes phencyclidine [PCP] and ketamine, can cause symptoms similar to schizophrenia in people who do not have the disorder. In a recent study, ketamine-induced psychotic symptoms resembling schizophrenia were managed with a glycine transporter-1 inhibitor medication trial. It has been demonstrated that this drug lessens the effects of ketamine's NMDA receptor antagonistic effects. Enhancing glutamate function by stimulating the glycine site of the NMDA receptor with glycine, D-serine, or medications that block glycine reuptake may be therapeutically beneficial for schizophrenia, according to the researchers. The majority of currently prescribed conventional antipsychotic drugs target the brain's dopamine receptors. Serotonergic receptors are strongly favored by more recent novel antipsychotics. The glutamate model of schizophrenia raises the prospect of novel therapeutic targets, such as metabotropic glutamate receptor agonists, glycine transport inhibitors, and NMDA agonists.

8.2.1.3. Physiological Factors

In the medical literature, several physical factors that may have etiological significance have been identified. Uncertainty surrounds their precise mechanisms in the context of schizophrenia.

Viral Infection

Epidemiological data show a high incidence of schizophrenia following prenatal influenza exposure, according to Sadock and Sadock (2007). They said: *Physical anomalies at birth, pregnancy and birth complications, seasonality of birth consistent with viral infection, geographic clusters of adult cases, and seasonality of hospitalizations are additional data supporting a viral hypothesis.* Another study discovered a link between childhood-onset viral infections of the central nervous system and adult-onset schizophrenia.

Anatomical Abnormalities

Individuals diagnosed with schizophrenia have been found to have structural brain abnormalities using neuroimaging technologies. The most frequent finding is ventricular enlargement, though cerebellar atrophy and sulci enlargement have also been noted. "Ventricular enlargement is associated with poor premorbid functioning, negative symptoms, poor response to treatment, and cognitive impairment," according to Black and Andreasen (2011). An increased capacity to image in multiple planes is offered by magnetic resonance imaging (MRI). MRI studies have suggested that patients with schizophrenia may have smaller brain and intracranial volumes. A smaller frontal lobe has also been reported in studies, though this has not been as reliably confirmed. In the brains of individuals with schizophrenia, MRI has been used to investigate potential abnormalities in particular subregions, including the temporal lobes, basal ganglia, hippocampus, and amygdala.

Histological Changes

Microscopic studies of schizophrenia-related brain alterations have also been conducted. It has been proposed that there is a "disordering" or disarray of the pyramidal cells near the hippocampus. The normal alignment of the cells in the brains of patients without the disorder has been compared to this state of disarray. According to certain theories, this change in hippocampus cells takes place in the second trimester of pregnancy and could be caused by an influenza virus that the mother contracts during this time. To ascertain whether schizophrenia development and this birth defect are related, more research is needed.

Physical Conditions

According to certain research, there may be a connection between schizophrenia and the following conditions: Huntington's disease, birth trauma, adult head trauma, alcoholism, cerebral tumors (especially those affecting the limbic system), cerebrovascular accidents, systemic lupus erythematosus, myxedema, parkinsonism, and Wilson's disease.

8.2.2. Psychological Factors

Early theories of schizophrenia emphasized the importance of family relationships in the illness's development, most likely due to the clear lack of evidence supporting a biological basis. These antiquated theories, which linked dysfunctional family structures and bad parent-child relationships to schizophrenia, are no longer credible. Scholars currently concentrate their research on schizophrenia as a neurological condition. However, as noted by Sadock and Sadock (2007), clinicians ought to take into account the biological as well as psychosocial aspects that influence schizophrenia. Individual patients are affected by the disorder, and each has a distinct psychological profile. Though many psychodynamic theories regarding the pathophysiology of schizophrenia appear antiquated, astute clinical observations can assist modern clinicians in comprehending the potential psychological effects of the illness on a patient.

8.2.3. Environmental Influences

8.2.3.1. Sociocultural Factors

Numerous research projects have tried to establish a connection between schizophrenia and socioeconomic status. In fact, epidemiological data have demonstrated that a higher proportion of people from lower socioeconomic classes than from higher socioeconomic groups suffer from symptoms related to schizophrenia. The circumstances of living in poverty, such as cramped living quarters, poor nutrition, lack of prenatal care, a lack of resources for handling difficult circumstances, and a hopeless feeling about changing one's way of life, are some explanations for this phenomenon. An alternative perspective is the downward drift hypothesis, which postulates that people with schizophrenia "drift down" to a lower socioeconomic level (or fail to rise out of a lower socioeconomic group) due to their inability to maintain gainful employment as a result of the disorder's characteristic symptoms. Advocates of this perspective believe that schizophrenia is a result of social conditions rather than a cause.

8.2.3.2. Stressful Life Events

Research has been done to try and ascertain whether stressful life events can trigger psychotic episodes. There isn't any proof from science that stress leads to schizophrenia. Nonetheless, there's a good chance that stress plays a role in the intensity and progression of the sickness. Severe stress has been shown to have the ability to trigger psychotic episodes. In fact, stress can exacerbate symptoms in those with a genetic susceptibility to schizophrenia. Stressful life events may also be linked to higher relapse rates and an aggravation of schizophrenia symptoms.

8.2.4. The Transactional Model

Uncertainty surrounds the cause of schizophrenia. No one theory or hypothesis has been put forth that provides a conclusive explanation for the illness. As it happens, the idea of multiple causation in the development of schizophrenia appears to be supported by an increasing body of evidence with each new study that is undertaken. The prevailing theory at the moment seems to be that schizophrenia is a biologically based illness whose onset is impacted by environmental factors (internal or external). (Addington, 2006' American Psychiatric Association, 2013).

Figure 8.2 presents how the Transactional Model of Stress/Adaptation explains the dynamics of schizophrenia.

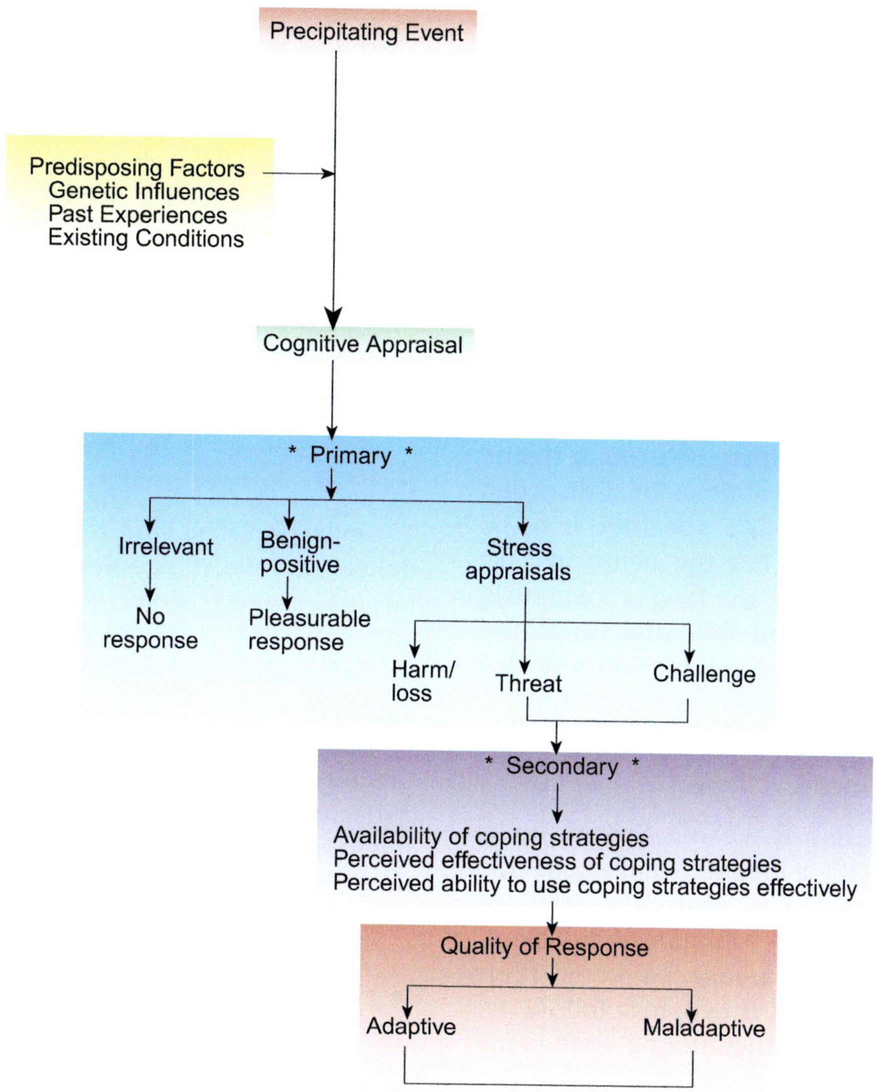

Figure 8.2. *The dynamics of schizophrenia using the Transactional Model of Stress/Adaptation.*

Source: https://repository.poltekkes-kaltim.ac.id/625/1/Psychiatric%20Mental%20Health%20Nursing%20Concepts%20of%20Care%20in%20Evidence-Based%20Practice%20by%20Mary%20C.%20Townsend%20DSN%20%20PMHCNS-BC%20(z-lib.org).pdf.

8.3. Types of Schizophrenia and Other Psychotic Disorders

A range of psychotic disorders are recognized by the DSM-5, which is arranged to show a gradient of psychopathology ranging from mild to severe. The intensity, quantity, and duration of psychotic symptoms and signs define the severity. There is a possibility that some of the disorders also have catatonic features specified. This specifier may be used to describe the following disorders: substance-induced psychotic disorder, schizoaffective disorder, schizophrenia, brief psychotic disorder, and schizophreniform disorder. Major depressive disorder, bipolar disorders I and II, and neurodevelopmental disorders can all benefit from its application. Schizotypal personality disorder is the first disorder on the spectrum according to the DSM-5.

8.3.1. Delusional Disorder

The presence of delusions that the person has had for at least a month is what defines delusional disorder. Hallucinations are not severe, if they are present at all, and behavior is not odd. The predominate delusional theme determines the subtype of delusional disorder. According to the DSM-5, a specifier may be added to indicate whether the delusions are deemed abnormal (i.e., if the idea is "obviously unrealistic, incomprehensible, and unrelated to everyday life experiences." Subtypes of delusional disorder include the following:

8.3.1.1. Erotomanic Type

This kind of delusion is when a person thinks they are in love with someone, usually someone who is more important to them. Celebrities are frequently the focus of erotomaniac delusions. While some people choose to keep their delusions to themselves, others may follow, get in touch with, or make other attempts to pursue the target of their delusions.

8.3.1.2. Grandiose Type

Grandiose delusions cause people to have unreasonable beliefs about their own abilities, abilities, knowledge, or power. They might think they have a unique bond with a well-known person, or they might even take on the persona of a well-known person, thinking the real one is a fraud. The assumption of the identity of a deity or religious leader can result from grandiose delusions of a religious nature.

8.3.1.3. Jealous Type

The belief that one's sexual partner is unfaithful lies at the heart of jealous delusions. Even though the belief is illogical and unfounded, the person who is delusional looks for proof to support it. The suspected infidelity is brought up to the sexual partner, who may even be physically assaulted in the process. The target of the attack could also be the sexual partner's presumed "lover". It's not uncommon to try to limit the sexual partner's autonomy in an attempt to put an end to the perceived infidelity.

8.3.1.4. Persecutory Type

The most prevalent kind of delusions, persecutory delusions, involve people thinking they are the targets of malice or persecution. Being followed and spied on, drugged or poisoned, cheated or defrauded, and being plotted against are common themes. A small rejection (real or imagined) may cause the person to become fixated on it and exaggerate it to the point where it becomes the center of a delusional system. If legal authorities receive repeated complaints, they may become dissatisfied and resort to violence against the target of their delusion.

8.3.1.5. Somatic Type

Somatic delusions cause a person to think they have a general medical condition.

8.3.1.6. Mixed Type

When the disorder is mixed, delusions are prominent, but no single theme is predominant.

8.3.2. Brief Psychotic Disorder

The abrupt onset of psychotic symptoms, which may or may not be preceded by a severe psychosocial stressor, is the hallmark of this disorder. There is a complete return to the premorbid level of functioning after these symptoms subside after at least one day but less than a month. The person is filled with intense emotional turmoil, overwhelming confusion, or perplexity. Delusions, hallucinations, disorientation, incoherent speech, and strange behavior are examples of symptoms of impaired reality testing. This disorder seems to be more likely to affect people who have a history of personality disorders, most commonly borderline, schizotypal, paranoid, histrionic, and narcissistic disorders. This disorder may also be linked to catatonic features.

8.3.3. Substance/Medication-Induced Psychotic Disorder

The main causes of the delusions and hallucinations linked to this illness are determined to be drug or toxin exposure, substance intoxication or withdrawal, or both. When the symptoms exceed and worsen beyond what is typically seen with intoxication or withdrawal syndrome, this diagnosis is made. The presence of substance intoxication or withdrawal, or exposure to a medication or toxin, is linked to the onset of symptoms, as demonstrated by the medical history, physical examination, and laboratory results. Table 8.1 lists substances that are thought to cause psychotic disorders. This disorder may also be linked to catatonic features.

8.3.4. Psychotic Disorder Due to Another Medical Condition

The main characteristics of this illness are strong delusions and hallucinations that are clearly related to another medical condition. If the symptoms appear while the patient is experiencing delirium, no diagnosis is made. Table 8.2 lists several medical conditions that can result in psychotic symptoms.

Table 8.1. *Substances That May Cause Psychotic Disorders*

Drugs of Abuse	Alcohol
	Amphetamines and related substances
	Cannabis
	Cocaine
	Hallucinogens
	Inhalants
	Opioids
	Phencyclidine and related substances
	Sedatives, hypnotics, and anxiolytics
Medications	Anesthetics and analgesics
	Anticholinergic agents
	Anticonvulsants
	Antidepressant medication
	Antihistamines
	Antihypertensive agents
	Cardiovascular medications
	Antimicrobial medications
	Antiparkinsonian agents
	Chemotherapeutic agents
	Corticosteroids
	Disulfiram
	Gastrointestinal medications
	Muscle relaxants
	Nonsteroidal anti-inflammatory agents
Toxins	Anticholinesterase
	Organophosphate insecticides
	Nerve gases
	Carbon monoxide
	Carbon dioxide
	Volatile substances (e.g., fuel or paint)

Source: APA (2013)' Black & Andreasen (2011)' Eisendrath & Lichtmacher (2012)' Fohrman & Stein (2006)' Freudenreich (2010).

8.3.5. Catatonic Disorder Due to Another Medical Condition

The symptoms listed can be used to diagnose catatonic disorder. This diagnosis is established when the symptomatology is directly attributable to the physiological aftereffects of another medical condition, as demonstrated by the patient's medical history, physical examination, or laboratory results. Medical conditions of the following kinds have been linked to catatonic disorder: metabolic disorders (e.g. , vitamin B12 deficiency, hepatic encephalopathy, hypo- and hyperthyroidism, hypo- and hyperadrenalism, and neurological disorders (e.g. epilepsy, encephalitis, head trauma, tumors, and cerebrovascular disease).

Table 8.2. *General Medical Conditions That May Cause Psychotic Symptoms*

Neurological Conditions	Neoplasms Cerebrovascular disease Huntington's disease Epilepsy Auditory nerve injury Deafness Migraine headache CNS infections
Endocrine Conditions	Hyperthyroidism Hypothyroidism Hyperparathyroidism Hypoparathyroidism Hypoadrenocorticism
Metabolic Conditions	Hypoxia Hypercarbia Hypoglycemia
Autoimmune Disorders	Systemic lupus erythematosus
Others	Fluid or electrolyte imbalances Hepatic or renal diseases

Source: APA (2013)' Black & Andreasen (2011)' Freudenreich (2010)' Sadock & Sadock (2007).

8.3.6. Schizophreniform Disorder

The main distinction between schizophreniform disorder and schizophrenia is that the former has prodromal, active, and residual phases lasting at least one month but less than six months. A diagnosis is considered "provisional" if it is given while the patient is still experiencing symptoms but has not been for longer than six months. If the symptoms last longer than six months, the diagnosis is revised to schizophrenia. A person with schizophrenia-form illness is considered to have a good prognosis if their affect is not flattened or blunted, if psychotic symptoms appear quickly after the unusual behavior is observed, or if their premorbid social and occupational functioning was satisfactory.

8.3.7. Schizoaffective Disorder

Schizophrenic behaviors characterize this disorder, which has a significant component of symptomatology linked to mood disorders (mania or depression). In addition to psychomotor retardation, suicidal thoughts, and a depressed appearance, the client may also exhibit exuberance, grandiosity, and hyperactivity. The presence of hallucinations and/or delusions that last for at least two weeks without a significant mood episode is the determining factor in the diagnosis of schizoaffective disorder. Significant symptoms of a mood disorder must, however, be present most of the time. Schizoaffective disorder has a worse prognosis than mood disorders alone, but it is generally better than other schizophrenic disorders. (Addington, 2006' American Psychiatric Association, 2013)

8.4. Application of the Nursing Process

8.4.1. Schizophrenia—Background Assessment Data

Schizophrenia represents the active phase of the disorder, and symptoms of the diagnosis may manifest in stages. Signs and symptoms related to the active phase. The nurse compiles a database in the first stage of the nursing process, from which nursing diagnoses are made and a care plan is created. This is the most crucial step in the nursing process because without a proper assessment, it is impossible to accurately identify the problem, determine the goals of care, and establish the outcome criteria.

The process of evaluating a client who has schizophrenia may be intricate and involve gathering data from various sources. Rarely are clients who are experiencing a severe episode of their illness able to add much to their history. Information can be gathered from other people who have been in a position to report on the client's behavioral development, from family members, if that is feasible, or from previous records, if they are available. For the nurse to properly assess a client with schizophrenia, they must be knowledgeable about behaviors typical of the illness. Positive and negative symptoms are frequently used to characterize schizophrenia symptoms. While negative symptoms indicate a reduction or loss of normal functions, positive symptoms typically indicate an alteration or distortion of normal mental functions. Most patients display a combination of the two categories of symptoms.

Positive symptoms are linked to reasonably good treatment responses and normal brain structures on computed tomography (CT) scans. "Not only are [negative symptoms] difficult to treat and respond less well to antipsychotics than positive symptoms, but they are also the most destructive because they render the patient inert and unmotivated," according to Ho, Black, and Andreasen (2003). The behavioral abnormalities linked to schizophrenia. Positive or negative, they are classified and taken into account in eight domains of functioning: thought form, thought content, perception, affect, sense of self, volition, relationship to the outside world and interpersonal functioning, and psychomotor behavior. There are also other impairments that fall outside of these eight categories.

8.4.1.1. Positive Symptoms

Content of Thought

False personal beliefs that are out of line with one's IQ or cultural background are known as delusions. Even when there is clear evidence that the belief is illogical or incorrect, the person nevertheless holds onto it. Delusions are classified based on the content of each one. Some of the more common ones are listed here.

- **Delusion of Persecution:** The individual feels threatened and believes that others intend harm or persecution toward him or her in some way (e.g., "The FBI has 'bugged' my room and intends to kill me." "I can't take a shower in this bathroom' the nurses have put a camera in there so that they can watch everything I do").
- **Delusion of Grandeur:** The individual has an exaggerated feeling of importance, power, knowledge, or identity (e.g., "I am Jesus Christ").
- **Delusion of Reference:** All events within the environment are referred by the psychotic person to him- or herself (e.g., "Someone is trying to get a message to me through the articles in this magazine [or newspaper or TV program]' I must break the code so that I can receive the message"). Ideas of reference are less rigid than delusions of reference. An example of an idea of reference is irrationally assuming that, when in the presence of others, one is the object of their discussion or ridicule.
- **Delusion of Control or Influence:** The individual believes certain objects or persons have control over his or her behavior (e.g., "The dentist put a filling in my tooth' I now receive transmissions through the filling that control what I think and do").
- **Somatic Delusion:** The individual has a false idea about the functioning of his or her body (e.g., "I'm 70 years old and I will be the oldest person ever to give birth. The doctor says I'm not pregnant, but I know I am.").

- **Nihilistic Delusion:** The individual has a false idea that the self, a part of the self, others, or the world is nonexistent (e.g., "The world no longer exists." "I have no heart.").

Excessive display of or fixation with religious concepts and practices is called religiosity. Reliability is frequently challenging to measure since people differ widely in their degree of spiritual commitment and religious beliefs. The person suffering from schizophrenia might try to give his or her behavior a logical purpose and structure by incorporating religious concepts. Thus, religious obsession in this way could be regarded as a symptom of the disease. It is important to remember that clients who find solace in their religious convictions shouldn't be dissuaded from using this kind of assistance. A person who believes the voice they hear is from God and who constantly consults the Bible for clarification is considered religious.

People who suffer from paranoia are extremely wary of other people, their actions, and their perceived intentions (e.g. "I refuse to consume this food. I am aware that it is poisoned. "). When someone engages in magical thinking, they feel as though they have control over particular circumstances or individuals (e.g. the mother who thought her son would be taken away from her if she reprimanded him in any way). Children frequently think in magical ways (e.g. "The sky is depressing' it is raining.". I wished fervently that it would snow last night, and it did").

Form of Thought

- Thinking is characterized by speech in which ideas shift from one unrelated subject to another. With associative looseness, the individual is unaware that the topics are unconnected. When the condition is severe, speech may be incoherent (e.g., "We wanted to take the bus, but the airport took all the traffic. Driving is the ticket when you want to get somewhere. No one needs a ticket to heaven. We have it all in our pockets.").
- The psychotic person invents new words, or neologisms, that are meaningless to others but have symbolic meaning to the psychotic person (e.g., "She wanted to give me a ride in her new uniphorum.").
- Concreteness, or literal interpretations of the environment, represents a regression to an earlier level of cognitive development. Abstract thinking is very difficult. For example, the client with schizophrenia would have great difficulty describing the abstract meaning of sayings such as "I'm climbing the walls" or "It's raining cats and dogs."
- Choice of words is governed by sounds. Clang associations often take the form of rhyming. For instance, "It is very cold. I am cold and bold. The gold has been sold."
- A word salad is a group of words that are put together randomly, without any logical connection (e.g., "Most forward action grows life double plays circle uniform.").
- With circumstantiality, the individual delays in reaching the point of a communication because of unnecessary and tedious details. The point or goal is usually met but only with numerous interruptions by the interviewer to keep the person on track of the topic being discussed.

- Tangentiality differs from circumstantiality in that the person never really gets to the point of the communication. Unrelated topics are introduced, and the focus of the original discussion is lost.
- Mutism is an individual's inability or refusal to speak.
- The individual who exhibits perseveration persistently repeats the same word or idea in response to different questions.

8.4.1.2. Perception

Any one of the five senses may be involved in hallucinations, which are defined as false sensory perceptions that are not connected to actual external stimuli. A few types of hallucinations include the following:

- **Auditory:** Auditory hallucinations are false perceptions of sound. Most commonly they are of voices, but the individual may report clicks, rushing noises, music, and other noises. Command hallucinations may place the individual or others in a potentially dangerous situation. "Voices" that issue commands for violence to self or others may or may not be heeded by the psychotic person. Auditory hallucinations are the most common type in psychiatric disorders.
- **Visual:** These are false visual perceptions. They may consist of formed images, such as of people, or of unformed images, such as flashes of light.
- **Tactile:** Tactile hallucinations are false perceptions of the sense of touch, often of something on or under the skin. One specific tactile hallucination is formication, the sensation that something is crawling on or under the skin.
- **Gustatory:** This type is a false perception of taste. Most commonly, gustatory hallucinations are described as unpleasant tastes.
- **Olfactory:** Olfactory hallucinations are false perceptions of the sense of smell.

Illusions are misperceptions or misinterpretations of real external stimuli.

8.4.1.3. Sense of Self

A person's sense of self encapsulates their sense of distinctiveness and individuality. The person with schizophrenia lacks this sense of individuality and is greatly confused about who they are due to incredibly weak ego boundaries.

- Echolalia is the term for when a person with schizophrenia repeats words they hear. This is an effort to empathize with the speaker. (For example, John, it's time for lunch, says the nurse. "It's time for lunch, it's time for lunch," or occasionally "Lunch, lunch, lunch, lunch," is how the client may reply.
- The client who exhibits echopraxia may purposelessly imitate movements made by others.
- Identification, which occurs on an unconscious level, and imitation, which occurs on a conscious level, are ego defense mechanisms used by individuals with schizophrenia and reflect their confusion regarding self-identity. Because they have difficulty knowing where their ego boundaries end and another person's begins, their behavior often

takes on the form of that which they see in the other person.

- The unstable self-identity of an individual with schizophrenia may lead to feelings of unreality (e.g., feeling that one's extremities have changed in size' or a sense of seeing oneself from a distance).

8.4.1.4. Negative Symptoms

Affect

Affect describes the behavior associated with an individual's feeling state or emotional tone.

- Affect is inappropriate when the individual's emotional tone is incongruent with the circumstances (e.g., a young woman who laughs when told of the death of her mother).
- Affect is described as bland when the emotional tone is very weak. The individual with flat affect appears to be void of emotional tone (or overt expression of feelings).
- The client with schizophrenia often demonstrates an indifference to or disinterest in the environment. The bland or flat affect is a manifestation of the emotional apathy.

Volition

Impaired volition has to do with the inability to initiate goal-directed activity. In the individual with schizophrenia, this may take the form of inadequate interest, motivation, or ability to choose a logical course of action in a given situation.

- Ambivalence in the client with schizophrenia refers to the coexistence of opposite emotions toward the same object, person, or situation. These opposing emotions may interfere with the person's ability to make even a very simple decision (e.g., whether to have coffee or tea with lunch). Underlying the ambivalence is the difficulty the client with schizophrenia has in fulfilling a satisfying human relationship. This difficulty is based on the need fear dilemma—the simultaneous need for and fear of intimacy.
- Personal grooming and selfcare activities may be neglected. The client with schizophrenia may appear disheveled and untidy and may need to be reminded of the need for personal hygiene.

Interpersonal Functioning and Relationship to the External World

Impairment in social functioning may be reflected in social isolation, emotional detachment, and lack of regard for social convention.

- Some clients with acute schizophrenia cling to others and intrude on the personal space of others, exhibiting behaviors that are not socially and culturally acceptable.
- Individuals with schizophrenia sometimes focus inward on themselves to the exclusion of the external environment.

Psychomotor Behavior

- Anergia is a deficiency of energy. The individual with schizophrenia may lack sufficient energy to carry out activities of daily living or to interact with others.

- Waxy flexibility describes a condition in which the client with schizophrenia allows body parts to be placed in bizarre or uncomfortable positions. Once placed in position, the arm, leg, or head remains in that position for long periods, regardless of how uncomfortable it is for the client. For example, the nurse may position the client's arm in an outward position to take a blood pressure measurement. When the cuff is removed, the client may maintain the arm in the position in which it was placed to take the reading.
- This symptom is manifested by the voluntary assumption of inappropriate or bizarre postures.
- Pacing back and forth and body rocking (a slow, rhythmic, backward-and-forward swaying of the trunk from the hips, usually while sitting) are common psychomotor behaviors of the client with schizophrenia.

Associated Features

- Anhedonia is the inability to experience pleasure. This is a particularly distressing symptom that compels some clients to attempt suicide.
- Regression is the retreat to an earlier level of development. Regression, a primary defense mechanism of schizophrenia, is a dysfunctional attempt to reduce anxiety. It provides the basis for many of the behaviors associated with schizophrenia (Addington, 2006' American Psychiatric Association, 2013).

8.4.2. Diagnosis/Outcome Identification

The nurse fills out the client database with the data gathered from the assessment, which is then used to choose the most appropriate nursing diagnoses. Care plans for clients with psychotic disorders can be formulated using the list of client behaviors in Table 8.3 and the corresponding NANDA International (NANDA-I) nursing diagnoses.

8.4.2.1. Outcome Criteria

The following criteria may be used for measurement of outcomes in the care of the client with schizophrenia.

The Client:

- Demonstrates an ability to relate satisfactorily with others;
- Recognizes distortions of reality;
- Has not harmed self or others;
- Perceives self realistically;
- Demonstrates the ability to perceive the environment correctly;
- Maintains anxiety at a manageable level;
- Relinquishes the need for delusions and hallucinations;
- Demonstrates the ability to trust others;
- Uses appropriate verbal communication in interactions with others;
- Performs self-care activities independently.

Table 8.3. *Assigning Nursing Diagnoses to Behaviors Commonly Associated With Psychotic Disorders*

BEHAVIORS	NURSING DIAGNOSES
Impaired communication (inappropriate responses), disordered thought sequencing, rapid mood swings, poor concentration, disorientation, stops talking in midsentence, tilts head to side as if to be listening	Disturbed sensory perception*
Delusional thinking; inability to concentrate; impaired volition; inability to problem solve, abstract, or conceptualize; extreme suspiciousness of others; inaccurate interpretation of the environment	Disturbed thought processes*
Withdrawal, sad dull affect, need-fear dilemma, preoccupation with own thoughts, expression of feelings of rejection or of aloneness imposed by others, uncommunicative, seeks to be alone	Social isolation
Risk factors: Aggressive body language (e.g., clenching fists and jaw, pacing, threatening stance), verbal aggression, catatonic excitement, command hallucinations, rage reactions, history of violence, overt and aggressive acts, goal-directed destruction of objects in the environment, self-destructive behavior, or active aggressive suicidal acts	Risk for violence: Self-directed or other-directed
Loose association of ideas, neologisms, word salad, clang associations, echolalia, verbalizations that reflect concrete thinking, poor eye contact, difficulty expressing thoughts verbally, inappropriate verbalization	Impaired verbal communication
Difficulty carrying out tasks associated with hygiene, dressing, grooming, eating, and toileting	Self-care deficit
Neglectful care of client in regard to basic human needs or illness treatment, extreme denial or prolonged overconcern regarding client's illness, depression, hostility and aggression	Disabled family coping
Inability to take responsibility for meeting basic health practices, history of lack of health-seeking behavior, lack of expressed interest in improving health behaviors, demonstrated lack of knowledge regarding basic health practices	Ineffective health maintenance
Unsafe, unclean, disorderly home environment; household members express difficulty in maintaining their home in a safe and comfortable condition	Impaired home maintenance

Source: https://repository.poltekkes-kaltim.ac.id/625/1/Psychiatric%20Mental%20Health%20Nursing%20Concepts%20of%20Care%20in%20Evidence-Based%20Practice%20by%20Mary%20C.%20Townsend%20DSN%20%20PMHCNS-BC%20(z-lib.org).pdf.

8.5. Treatment Modalities for Schizophrenia and other Psychotic Disorders

Psychological Treatments

Individual Psychotherapy

The type of individual psychotherapy that psychiatrists use when prescribing medication usually entails a synthesis of different psychotherapeutic techniques and interventions, even though intense psychodynamic and insight-oriented psychotherapy is generally discouraged. Problem-solving, reality testing, psychological counseling, and supportive and cognitive-behavioral methods based on a compassionate therapeutic alliance with the patient are a few of these. Such individual psychotherapy aims to prevent relapse, improve social and occupational functioning, and increase medication compliance.

The best method of individual psychotherapy for schizophrenia is reality-oriented therapy. In all cases, efforts to reduce anxiety and boost trust must be the main focus. Developing a relationship can be especially challenging for individuals with schizophrenia, as they often experience extreme loneliness and resist intimacy and trust. Attempts at intimacy are likely to be met with suspicion, anxiety, aggression, or regression from him or her. When an intervention is conducted with integrity, straightforwardness, and consideration for the client's privacy and human dignity, it can be successful. Proclamations of friendship and excessive warmth are likely to be viewed with skepticism and confusion. Through examination of the client's behavior in relationships, reality orientation is preserved once a therapeutic interpersonal relationship has been established. Education is given to the client to assist them in recognizing potential dangers and knowing how to respond appropriately. There are attempts to improve emotional expression, interpersonal communication, and frustration tolerance. For patients with schizophrenia, individual psychotherapy is viewed as a long-term process requiring the healthcare provider to be patient and to be able to accept the possibility that significant change may not happen. In certain instances, it takes years for clients to regain some degree of independent functioning after treatment.

Group Therapy

It has been demonstrated that group therapy for people with schizophrenia is beneficial, especially for outpatients and when paired with medication treatment. For individuals with schizophrenia, group therapy typically focuses on relationships, problems, and plans from everyday life. Certain researchers question the usefulness of insight therapy and dynamic interpretation for typical schizophrenia patients. However, group therapy helps patients with schizophrenia feel less alone in society, feel more cohesive, and perform better on reality tests. Inpatient settings yield lower productivity from group therapy. When social disarray and symptomatology are at their worst, inpatient treatment is typically necessary. The client would benefit most from as little stimulation as possible at this time. Group therapy can be counterproductive early in treatment because it can be intense and very stimulating. For schizophrenia, group therapy has proven most beneficial when the condition is treated long-term. For these clients, the social interaction, feeling of unity, identification, and reality testing that occur in a group environment have proven to be extremely therapeutic processes. Organizations that provide a nurturing atmosphere seem to benefit schizophrenia patients more than those that take a more aggressive stance (Addington, 2006' American Psychiatric Association, 2013).

Behavior Therapy

There is evidence that behavior modification can decrease the frequency of odd, upsetting, and deviant behaviors while increasing the frequency of appropriate behaviors. Features that have led to the most positive results include:

- Clearly defining goals and how they will be measured.
- Attaching positive, negative, and aversive reinforcements to adaptive and maladaptive behavior.
- Using simple, concrete instructions and prompts to elicit the desired behavior.

For patients who are unable to modify their unwanted behaviors, behavior therapy can be an effective therapeutic method. In the context of treatment, the medical professional can assist the patient with schizophrenia in lowering the frequency of maladaptive or deviant behaviors by using praise and other forms of positive reinforcement. One drawback of this kind of therapy is that some people with schizophrenia are unable to apply what they have learned in the treatment environment to their everyday lives.

Social Skills Training

One of the most popular psychosocial interventions in the treatment of schizophrenia is social skills training. The fundamental idea of social skills training is that sophisticated interpersonal abilities entail the seamless fusion of several less complicated behaviors, such as nonverbal ones (e.g., eye contact, and facial expression)' paralinguistic elements (e.g. , affect and volume of the voice)' verbal content (i.e. , the suitability of the remarks made)' and interactive harmony (e.g. response time, duration of conversation). These particular abilities can be methodically imparted, and via the shaping process (i.e., encouraging incremental approaches to the desired behavior), intricate behavioral repertoires can be learned. One of schizophrenia's hallmarks is social dysfunction. One of the defining diagnostic criteria for schizophrenia is impairment in interpersonal relations (DSM-5). These clients' social skill development is currently receiving a lot of attention.

Role-playing is a key component of the social skills training curriculum. Several succinct situations are chosen. These ought to be graduated in terms of difficulty and representative of the kinds of scenarios that clients encounter on a daily basis. The medical professional could act as an example of certain behaviors. For instance, "Notice how I look at your face and nod my head up and down while you talk." After this demonstration, the client role-plays". Feedback on the client's presentation is given right away. It takes innumerable tries for the response to finally become effortless and fluid. Development is tailored to the needs and constraints of the client. Small behavioral units are the main focus, and the training goes very slowly. Extremely dangerous situations are avoided in favor of functional abilities that are applicable to day-to-day activities.

8.5.1. Social Treatments

8.5.1.1. Milieu Therapy

Certain medical professionals think milieu therapy may be a suitable course of treatment for a patient suffering from schizophrenia. Studies indicate that when combined with milieu therapy, psychotropic medication is more successful at all care levels. Meanwhile, milieu therapy is more successful when combined with these medications. The majority of milieu therapy programs place a strong emphasis on social and group interaction' peer pressure mediates norms and expectations and normalizes adaptation. The patient's role becomes hazy when they are perceived as responsible individuals.

Milieu therapy emphasizes interdisciplinary participation, goal-oriented, clear communication, as well as a patient's rights to goals, freedom of movement, and an informal relationship with staff. Patients with schizophrenia who receive only milieu therapy need to stay in the hospital longer than those who receive both medication and psychosocial therapy. The use of milieu therapy in the treatment of schizophrenia is restricted by additional financial factors, such as the requirement for a high staff-to-client ratio and the lengthier admission period. Nonetheless, the milieu environment can be used effectively in outpatient programs, including day and partial hospitalization.

8.5.1.2. Family Therapy

Some medical professionals treat schizophrenia as a family illness rather than just the patient's. The mental health status of family members is significantly impacted when a family member has the illness, even in cases where the family seems to be coping well. The loss of a once-promising child or relationship is a terrible event that causes great pain and grief for the family when a family member suffers from a serious mental illness. The recognition of the growing role that families play in the aftercare of relatives with schizophrenia has sparked interest in family intervention programs that aim to maintain the client in the community, support the family system, and prevent or delay relapse. These psychoeducational programs emphasize concrete problem solving and particular helpful behaviors for stress management, treating the family as a resource rather than a source of stress. These programs acknowledge the biological underpinnings of schizophrenia as well as the detrimental effects of stress on the functioning of the client. Psychoeducational programs lessen the chance of the client's relapse and the potential emergence of mental illness in previously unaffected relatives by educating the family about the illness and offering coping strategies.

Mueser et al (2002) stated that although models of family intervention with schizophrenia differ in their characteristics and methods, effective treatment programs share many common features:

- All programs are long-term (usually 9 months to 2 years or more).
- They all provide the client and family with information about the illness and its management.
- They focus on improving adherence to prescribed medications.
- They strive to decrease stress in the family and improve family functioning.

Asen (2002) suggested the following interventions with families of individuals with schizophrenia:

- Forming a close alliance with the caregivers;
- Lowering the emotional intrafamily climate by reducing stress and burden on relatives;
- Increasing the ability of relatives to anticipate and solve problems;
- Reducing the expressions of anger and guilt by family members;
- Maintaining reasonable expectations for how the ill family member should perform;
- Encouraging relatives to set appropriate limits while maintaining some degree of separateness;
- Promoting desirable changes in the relatives' behaviors and belief systems.

A shorter program of family education about schizophrenia and a longer program of family contact are the usual components of family therapy. The former aims to lessen overt conflict manifestations and enhances family communication and problem-solving skills. This kind of therapy has had a very noticeable response. Research has unequivocally demonstrated that integrating the family system into the care plan can lead to a better result for the patient with schizophrenia.

8.5.2. Organic Treatment

8.5.2.1. Psychopharmacology

In 1952, chlorpromazine, also known as thorazine, was first made available in the US. It was then used in surgical anesthesia in combination with barbiturates. The drug's psychic qualities became apparent with continued use, and by 1954 it was being sold in the US as an antipsychotic. The production and distribution of additional antipsychotic medications ensued in quick succession. Major tranquilizers, also known as neuroleptics, are other names for antipsychotic drugs. They work well in maintenance therapy to stop the worsening of schizophrenia symptoms as well as in the treatment of both acute and chronic manifestations of the disease. 72% of people who have had a psychotic episode relapse within a year if they do not receive drug treatment. With ongoing medication administration, this relapse rate can be lowered to roughly 23%.

Table 8.4. *Antipsychotic Agents*

CATEGORY	GENERIC (TRADE NAME)	PREGNANCY CATEGORIES/ HALF-LIFE (hr)	DAILY DOSAGE RANGE (mg)
Typical Antipsychotic Agents (First Generation; Conventional)	Chlorpromazine	C/ 24	40–400
	Fluphenazine	C/ HCl: 18 hr Decanoate: 6.8–9.6 days	2.5–10
	Haloperidol (Haldol)	C/ ~18 (oral); ~3 wk (IM decanoate)	1–100
	Loxapine	C/ 8	20–250
	Perphenazine	C/ 9–12	12–64
	Pimozide (Orap)	C/ ~55	1–10
	Prochlorperazine	C/ 3–5 (oral) 6.9 (IV)	15–150
	Thioridazine	C/ 24	150–800
	Thiothixene (Navane)	C/ 34	6–30
	Trifluoperazine	C/ 18	4–40
Atypical Antipsychotic Agents (Second Generation; Novel)	Aripiprazole (Abilify)	C/ 75–146	10–30
	Asenapine (Saphris)	C/ 24	10–20
	Clozapine (Clozaril)	B/ 8 (single dose); 12 (at steady state)	300–900
	Iloperidone (Fanapt)	C/ 18–33	12–24
	Lurasidone (Latuda)	B/ 18	40–80
	Olanzapine (Zyprexa)	C/ 21–54	5–20
	Paliperidone (Invega)	C/ 23	6–12
	Quetiapine (Seroquel)	C/ ~6	300–400
	Risperidone (Risperdal)	C/ 3–20	4–8
	Ziprasidone (Geodon)	C/ ~7 (oral); 2–5 (IM)	40–160

Source: https://repository.poltekkes-kaltim.ac.id/625/1/Psychiatric%20Mental%20Health%20Nursing%20Concepts%20of%20Care%20in%20Evidence-Based%20Practice%20by%20Mary%20C.%20Townsend%20DSN%20%20PMHCNS-BC%20(z-lib.org).pdf.

Schizophrenia prognoses are frequently presented using a paradigm of thirds. A third of the population experiences notable and long-lasting improvement. They might never go through another psychotic episode after the first one. A third may show some improvement, but they will still have residual disability and sporadic relapses. Their illness may have caused a decline in their occupational level, or they may be socially isolated. Lastly, a third become severely and permanently incapacitated. They frequently don't get better with medicine and suffer from severe illness for a long time. Women respond better to antipsychotic medication treatment' men experience worse outcomes.

Adjunctive psychosocial therapy improves the effectiveness of antipsychotic medications, as was previously mentioned. Clients tend to cooperate better with psychosocial therapies because the medication reduces the psychotic manifestations of the illness. Nevertheless, it takes a few weeks for antipsychotics to effectively treat positive symptoms' this fact frequently results in the medication being stopped. The necessity of waiting, frequently for several weeks, to find out if the medication will work is something that needs to be explained to clients and their families.

These medications are classified as either "typical" (first-generation, conventional antipsychotics) or "atypical" (the newer, novel antipsychotics). Examples of commonly used antipsychotic agents are presented in Table 8.4. A detailed description of these medications follows (Lehman et al., 2006).

Indications

Antipsychotic drugs are used to treat psychotic disorders such as schizophrenia. A few specific medications (olanzapine, aripiprazole, chlorpromazine, quetiapine, risperidone, asenapine, ziprasidone) are used to treat bipolar mania. Some are used to treat intractable hiccoughs (chlorpromazine), to treat antiemetics (chlorpromazine, perphenazine, prochlorperazine), to control tics and vocal utterances in Tourette's disorder (haloperidol, pimozide).

Action

The way that typical antipsychotics function is by preventing postsynaptic dopamine receptors in the medulla, brainstem, limbic system, and basal ganglia from functioning. They also exhibit different levels of affinity for histaminic, cholinergic, and alpha1-adrenergic receptors. The inhibition of dopamine-mediated synaptic impulse transmission is another potential explanation for antipsychotic effects. Atypical antipsychotics have a stronger antagonistic effect on serotonin (5-hydroxytryptamine) type 2A (5HT2A) receptors than conventional antipsychotics do on dopamine receptors. Adrenergic, histaminic, and cholinergic receptors are also antagonistic to them.

Contraindications/Precautions

Clients with a history of hypersensitivity should not take typical antipsychotics (cross-sensitivity between phenothiazines may exist). They should not be administered to comatose patients, exhibit clear central nervous system (CNS) depression, have blood dyscrasias, have Parkinson's disease or narrow-angle glaucoma, have liver, renal, or cardiac insufficiency, have poorly controlled seizure disorders, or are elderly and have psychosis associated with neurocognitive disorder (NCD). Since haloperidol, pimozide, and thioridazine have been demonstrated to lengthen the QT interval, they should not be administered to a patient who is also taking other medications that cause this side effect. Patients who are elderly, very sick, or incapacitated, as well as those with diabetes, respiratory insufficiency, prostatic hypertrophy, or intestinal obstruction, should be treated with caution when taking these medications. The seizures threshold may be lowered by antipsychotics. When taking antipsychotic medication, people should limit their exposure to extreme temperatures. There is no proven safety during pregnancy or lactation.

In cases of hypersensitivity, comatose or severely depressed patients, elderly patients with psychosis related to non-communicable disease, and lactation, atypical antipsychotics should not be administered. Patients with a history of QT prolongation or cardiac arrhythmias, recent myocardial infarction (MI), uncompensated heart failure, or concurrent use with other medications that prolong the QT interval should not take ziprasidone, risperidone, paliperidone, asenapine, or iloperidone. Patients who have uncontrolled epilepsy, myeloproliferative disorders, or a history of clozapine-induced agranulocytosis or severe granulocytopenia should not take clozapine. Strong inhibitors of cytochrome P450 isozyme 3A4 (CYP3A4), such as lurasidone, should not be used together for example ketoconazole) and potent CYP3A4 inducers (e.g., rifampin). When giving these medications to elderly or disabled patients, those with heart, liver, or kidney insufficiency, people with a history of seizures, people with diabetes or those at risk for developing the disease, people exposed to extreme temperatures, people experiencing hypotension due to dehydration, hypovolemia, or antihypertensive medication treatment, pregnant women, or children, care should be taken (safety not established).

Interactions

Conventional antipsychotics exhibit additive effects on the central nervous system (CNS) when combined with antihypertensive agents, additive effects on the brain when combined with CNS depressants, and additive effects on the anticholinergic system when combined with anticholinergic medications. Oral anticoagulants may become less effective when taken with phenothiazines. Severe hypotension may occur if phenothiazines or haloperidol are used concurrently with dopamine or adrenaline. When haloperidol, thioridazine, or pimozide are taken in addition to other medications that prolong the QT interval, additive effects of QT prolongation happen. It is not recommended to take pimozide with CYP3A inhibitors or thioridazine with inhibitors of cytochrome P450 isozyme 2D6 (CYP2D6). When haloperidol and carbamazepine are taken together, the therapeutic effects of the former are enhanced and the latter is diminished.

A typical antipsychotics combined with antihypertensive medications cause additive hypotensive effects, and when combined with CNS depressants, they cause additive CNS effects. When taken with other medications that also have anticholinergic qualities, risperidone or paliperidone can have additive anticholinergic effects. When zipramide, risperidone, paliperidone, asenapine, and iloperidone are taken with other medications that prolong the QT interval, additive effects of QT prolongation happen. When ziprasidone, olanzapine, quetiapine, risperidone, or paliperidone are used concurrently, the effects of levodopa and dopamine agonists are lessened. CYP3A4 inhibitors cause increased effects from ziprasidone, clozapine, quetiapine, aripiprazole, lurasidone, and iloperidone. CYP3A4 inducers cause lurasidone's effects to be lessened. CYP2D6 inhibitors increase the effects of iloperidone. Asenapine, aripiprazole, clozapine, olanzapine, risperidone, paliperidone, asenapine, and CYP450 isozyme 1A2 (CYP1A2) inducers have reduced effects while CYP1A2 inhibitors have increased effects. The therapeutic effects of asenapine are reduced and those of paroxetine are increased when both medications are used at the same time. Along with other medications that also cause this side effect, risperidone, paliperidone, iloperidone, and others can result in additive orthostatic hypotension.

Side Effects

These drugs block a variety of receptors for

which they have varying degrees of affinity, which is related to their effects. Positive symptoms of schizophrenia are thought to be controlled by blocking dopamine receptors. In addition, prolactin elevation (gynecomastia' galactorrhea) and extrapyramidal symptoms (EPS) are caused by dopamine blockage. Anticholinergic side effects (dry mouth, blurred vision, constipation, urine retention, tachycardia) are brought on by cholinergic blockade. Alpha1-adrenergic receptor blockage results in reflex tachycardia, tremors, orthostatic hypotension, and lightheadedness. Weight gain and drowsiness are linked to histamine blockade.

Table 8.5. *Comparison of Side Effects Among Antipsychotic Agents*

CLASS	GENERIC (TRADE) NAME	EPS†	SEDATION	ANTI-CHOLINERGIC	ORTHOSTATIC HYPOTENSION	WEIGHT GAIN
Typical Antipsychotic Agents	Chlorpromazine	3	4	3	4	*
	Fluphenazine	5	2	2	2	
	Haloperidol (Haldol)	5	2	2	2	
	Loxapine	3	2	2	2	*
	Perphenazine	4	2	2	2	*
	Pimozide (Orap)	4	2	3	2	*
	Prochlorperazine	3	2	2	2	*
	Thioridazine	2	4	4	4	*
	Thiothixene (Navane)	4	2	2	2	*
	Trifluoperazine	4	2	2	2	*
Atypicals	Aripiprazole (Abilify)	1	2	1	3	2
	Asenapine (Saphris)	1	3	1	3	4
	Clozapine (Clozaril)	1	5	5	4	5
	Iloperidone (Fanapt)	1	3	2	3	3
	Lurasidone (Latuda)	1	3	1	3	3
	Olanzapine (Zyprexa)	1	3	2	2	5
	Paliperidone (Invega)	1	2	1	3	2
	Quetiapine (Seroquel)	1	3	1	3	4
	Risperidone (Risperdal)	1	2	1	3	4
	Ziprasidone (Geodon)	1	3	1	2	2

Key: 1 = Very low' 2 = Low' 3 = Moderate' 4 = High' 5 = Very high *Weight gain occurs, but incidence is unknown. †EPS = Extrapyramidal symptoms.

Source: Adapted from Black & Andreasen (2011)' Drug Facts and Comparisons (2014)' and Schatzberg, Cole, & DeBattista (2010).

Monitoring for the following antipsychotic medication side effects should be part of the care plan. An asterisk (*) indicates the nursing implications associated with each side effect. Table 8.5 presents a profile of side effects comparing different antipsychotic medications.

- Anticholinergic Effects
- Dry Mouth:
  - Provide the client with sugarless candy or gum, ice, and frequent sips of water.
  - Ensure that the client practices strict oral hygiene.
- Blurred Vision:
  - Explain that this symptom will most likely subside after a few weeks.
  - Advise the client not to drive a car until their vision clears.
  - Clear small items from the pathway to prevent falls.

- Constipation:
  - Order foods high in fiber' encourage an increase in physical activity and fluid intake if not contraindicated.
  - Urinary retention
  - Instruct client to report any difficulty urinating' monitor intake and output.
  - Nausea' gastrointestinal (GI) upset (may occur with all classifications)
  - Tablets or capsules may be administered with food to minimize GI upset (Lehman et al., 2006).
- **Concentrates:** may be diluted and administered with fruit juice or other liquid' they should be mixed immediately before administration.
- **Skin Rash:** (may occur with all classifications)
  - Report the appearance of any rash on the skin to the physician.
  - Avoid spilling any of the liquid concentrate on the skin' contact dermatitis can occur with some medications.
- Sedation:
  - Discuss with a physician the possibility of administering the drug at bedtime.
  - Discuss with the physician a possible decrease in dosage or an order for a less sedating drug.
  - Instruct client not to drive or operate dangerous equipment while experiencing sedation.
- Orthostatic Hypotension:
  - Instruct the client to rise slowly from a lying or sitting position.
  - Monitor blood pressure (lying and standing) each shift' document and report significant changes.
- **Photosensitivity:** (may occur with all classifications) *Ensure that the client wears a sunblock lotion, protective clothing, and sunglasses while spending time outdoors.
- **Hormonal Effects:** (may occur with all classifications, but are more common with typical antipsychotics)
- **Decreased Libido, Retrograde Ejaculation:** (the discharge of seminal fluid into the bladder rather than through the urethra), gynecomastia (men)
  - Provide an explanation of the effects and reassurance of reversibility. If necessary, discuss with the physician the possibility of ordering alternate medication.
- **Amenorrhea:** (absence of menstruation) (women)
  - Offer reassurance of reversibility' instruct the client to continue the use of contraception, because amenorrhea does not indicate cessation of ovulation.
- **Weight Gain:** (may occur with all classifications' has been problematic with the atypical antipsychotics)

- Weigh client every other day' order calorie-controlled diet' provide opportunity for physical exercise' provide diet and exercise instruction.

- **Electrocardiogram:** (ECG) changes. A prolongation of the QT interval is one of the possible ECG changes associated with most antipsychotics. This is especially true for the medications clozapine, asenapine, haloperidol, pimozide, thioridazine, ziprasidone, and paliperidone. When prescribing these drugs to people who have a history of arrhythmias, caution is advised. When prescribing, it is important to consider conditions like diuretic therapy or diarrhea that can result in hypokalemia and/or hypomagnesemia. Regular ECGs should be carried out both before and occasionally during therapy. Other cardiac events like ischemic changes, arrhythmias, congestive heart failure, myocarditis, and cardiomyopathy have also been linked to clozapine.
  - Monitor vital signs every shift.
  - Observe for symptoms of dizziness, palpitations, syncope, weakness, dyspnea, and peripheral edema.

- **Reduction of Seizure Threshold:** (more common with the typical than the atypical antipsychotics, except clozapine)
  - Closely observe clients with history of seizures. Note: This is particularly important with clients taking clozapine (Clozaril), with which seizures have been frequently associated. Dose appears to be an important predictor, with a greater likelihood of seizures occurring at higher doses. Extreme caution is advised in prescribing clozapine for clients with a history of seizures.

- **Agranulocytosis:** (more common with the typical than the atypical antipsychotics, except clozapine)
  - Agranulocytosis usually occurs within the first 3 months of treatment. Observe for symptoms of sore throat, fever, and malaise. A complete blood count should be monitored if these symptoms appear.
  - EXCEPTION: Clozapine (Clozaril) carries a significant risk of agranulocytosis. The blood condition known as agranulocytosis can be fatal and cause a patient's white blood cell (WBC) count to plummet to dangerously low levels. Before starting clozapine therapy, a baseline WBC count and an absolute neutrophil count (ANC) must be obtained. These tests must also be performed every week for the first six months of the medication. Medication is only given out in doses of one week at a time. Should the counts hold true within the permissible ranges (i.e. blood counts may be checked every two weeks for the duration of the 6-month period (WBC at least 3,500/mm3 and the ANC at least 2,000/mm3). Following this, a two-week supply of medication may be given. After

the six-month biweekly period, if the counts stay within the acceptable range, they can then be checked every four weeks. Weekly WBC counts are maintained for an extra four weeks after the medication is stopped (Table 8.6).

Table 8.6. *Antiparkinsonian Agents Used to Treat Extrapyramidal Side Effects of Antipsychotic Drugs*

Indication	Used to treat parkinsonism of various causes and drug-induced extrapyramidal reactions.		
Action	Restores the natural balance of acetylcholine and dopamine in the CNS. The imbalance is a deficiency in dopamine that results in excessive cholinergic activity.		
Contraindications/ Precautions	Antiparkinsonian agents are contraindicated in individuals with hypersensitivity. Anticholinergics should be avoided by individuals with angle-closure glaucoma; pyloric, duodenal, or bladder neck obstructions; prostatic hypertrophy; or myasthenia gravis. Caution should be used in administering these drugs to clients with hepatic, renal or cardiac insufficiency; elderly and debilitated clients; those with a tendency toward urinary retention; or those exposed to high environmental temperatures.		
Common side effects	Anticholinergic effects (dry mouth, blurred vision, constipation, paralytic ileus, urinary retention, tachycardia, elevated temperature, decreased sweating), nausea/GI upset, sedation, dizziness, orthostatic hypotension, exacerbation of psychoses.		
CHEMICAL CLASS	GENERIC (TRADE NAME)	PREGNANCY CATEGORIES/ HALF-LIFE (hr)	DAILY DOSAGE RANGE (mg)
Anticholinergics	Benztropine (Cogentin) Biperiden (Akineton) Trihexyphenidyl	C/UKN C/18.4–24.3 C/5.6–10.2	1–8 2–6 1–15
Antihistamines	Diphenhydramine (Benadryl)	C/4–15	25–200
Dopaminergic Agonists	Amantadine	C/10–25	200–300

Source: https://repository.poltekkes-kaltim.ac.id/625/1/Psychiatric%20Mental%20Health%20Nursing%20Concepts%20of%20Care%20in%20Evidence-Based%20Practice%20by%20Mary%20C.%20Townsend%20DSN%20%20PMHCNS-BC%20(z-lib.org).pdf.

- **Hypersalivation:** (most common with clozapine)
  - A significant number of clients receiving clozapine (Clozaril) therapy experience extreme salivation. Offer support to the client because this may be an embarrassing situation. It may even be a safety issue (e.g., risk of aspiration) if the problem is very severe. Management has included the use of sugarfree gum to increase the swallowing rate, as well as the prescription of medications such as an anticholinergic (e.g., scopolamine patch) or alpha2- adrenoceptor agonist (e.g., clonidine).
- Extrapyramidal Symptoms:
  - Observe for symptoms and report' administer antiparkinsonian drugs, as ordered.
- **Pseudoparkinsonism:** (tremor, shuffling gait, drooling, rigidity)
  - Symptoms may appear 1 to 5 days following initiation of antipsychotic medication' occurs most often in women, the elderly, and dehydrated clients.
- **Akinesia:** (muscular weakness)
  - Same as for pseudoparkinsonism.

- **Akathisia:** (continuous restlessness and fidgeting)
  - This occurs most frequently in women' symptoms may occur 50 to 60 days following initiation of therapy.
- **Dystonia:** (involuntary muscular movements [spasms] of face, arms, legs, and neck)
  - This occurs most often in men and in people younger than 25 years of age.
- **Oculogyric Crisis :**(uncontrolled rolling back of the eyes)
  - This may appear as part of the syndrome described as dystonia. It may be mistaken for seizure activity. Dystonia and oculogyric crisis should be treated as an emergency situation. The physician should be contacted, and intravenous benztropine mesylate (Cogentin) is commonly administered. Stay with the client and offer reassurance and support during this frightening time.
- **Tardive Dyskinesia:** (bizarre facial and tongue movements, stiff neck, and difficulty swallowing' may occur with all classifications, but is more common with typical antipsychotics)
  - All clients receiving long-term (months or years) antipsychotic therapy are at risk.
  - The symptoms are potentially irreversible.
  - The drug should be withdrawn at the first sign, which is usually vermiform movements of the tongue' prompt action may prevent irreversibility.
  - The Abnormal Involuntary Movement Scale (AIMS) is a rating scale that was developed in the 1970s by the National Institute of Mental Health to measure involuntary movements associated with tardive dyskinesia. The AIMS aids in early
  - Symptoms include severe parkinsonian muscle rigidity, very high fever, tachycardia, tachypnea, fluctuations in blood pressure, diaphoresis, and rapid deterioration of mental status to stupor and coma.
  - Discontinue antipsychotic medication immediately.
  - Monitor vital signs, degree of muscle rigidity, intake and output, level of consciousness.
  - The physician may order bromocriptine (Parlodel) or dantrolene (Dantrium) to counteract the effects of neuroleptic malignant syndrome.
- **Diabetes and Hyperglycemia:** (more prevalent with atypical antipsychotics). Atypical antipsychotic patients may be more susceptible to treatment-emergent hyperglycemia-related adverse events, according to studies (e.g. clozepine, asenapine, olanzapine, quetiapine, ziprasidone, paliperidone, iloperidone, lurasidone, aripiprazole, and risperidone). The U.S. Food and Drug Administration (FDA) recommends

that clients with diabetes starting on atypical antipsychotic drugs be monitored regularly for worsening of glucose control.

- Patients who have diabetes risk factors should have fasting blood glucose tests done before starting treatment and then on a regular basis after that. Polydipsia, polyuria, polyphagia, and weakness are signs of hyperglycemia that should be kept an eye out for in all of the patients taking these drugs. If these symptoms develop while the patient is receiving treatment, a fasting blood glucose test should be performed.

- Increased risk of mortality in elderly patients with psychosis related to neurocognitive disorder (NCD). Studies have indicated that elderly patients with NCD-related psychosis who are treated with antipsychotic drugs are at increased risk of death, compared with placebo. Causes of death are most commonly related to infections or cardiovascular problems. All antipsychotic drugs now carry blackbox warnings to this effect. They are not approved for treatment of elderly patients with NCD-related psychosis (Lehman et al., 2006).

A Closer Look

Dealing with Psychosis

Psychosis is a collection of symptoms associated with the loss of touch with reality. People with psychosis experience disturbances in their thoughts and perceptions. They experience difficulty differentiating between what is real and what is not during a psychotic episode. Psychosis typically begins in young adulthood and is often a symptom of another mental health condition such as severe depression, anxiety, bipolar disorder, or schizophrenia.

Psychosis is a complex and multifaceted mental health condition characterized by a disconnection from reality, manifesting primarily through hallucinations, delusions, disorganized thinking, and impaired insight. Hallucinations, often auditory, involve hearing voices or sounds that are not present, while visual, tactile, olfactory, or gustatory hallucinations are less common but still significant. Delusions, which are strongly held false beliefs, can be paranoid, grandiose, or involve thoughts of persecution. Disorganized thinking is evident in incoherent speech and thought patterns, making communication challenging. Psychosis can occur in various psychiatric disorders, including schizophrenia, schizoaffective disorder, bipolar disorder, and severe depression, as well as in substance-induced psychotic disorders and due to medical conditions such as brain injuries or infections.

The etiology of psychosis is multifactorial, involving genetic predispositions, neurobiological abnormalities, and environmental influences. Genetic factors play a significant role, with family studies indicating a higher risk among first-degree relatives of individuals with psychotic disorders. Neurobiologically, imbalances in neurotransmitters such as dopamine and glutamate are implicated in the pathophysiology of psychosis. Structural brain abnormalities, including changes in the volume of the hippocampus, amygdala, and prefrontal cortex, are often observed in individuals experiencing psychosis. Environmental factors such as prenatal exposure to infections, malnutrition, and psychosocial stressors during critical developmental periods further contribute to the risk of developing psychosis.

The onset of psychosis typically occurs in late adolescence or early adulthood, although it can appear at any age. Early signs, known as prodromal symptoms, may include social withdrawal, unusual thoughts or perceptions, and a decline in functioning. Early intervention during this prodromal phase is crucial, as it can significantly improve long-term outcomes and reduce the severity of the disorder. Comprehensive assessment and diagnosis involve detailed clinical interviews, the use of standardized diagnostic criteria such as the DSM-5, and ruling out other potential causes through medical and neurological evaluations.

Treatment for psychosis is multifaceted, aiming to manage symptoms, prevent relapses, and improve overall functioning. Antipsychotic medications are the cornerstone of treatment, effectively reducing the severity of hallucinations and delusions. These medications are classified into typical (first-generation) and atypical (second-generation) antipsychotics, with the latter being preferred due to a more favorable side effect profile. Psychosocial interventions, including cognitive-behavioral therapy (CBT), social skills training, and family therapy, play a crucial role in addressing the cognitive and social impairments associated with psychosis. Early intervention programs that provide comprehensive, coordinated care have been shown to improve outcomes significantly.

The impact of psychosis on individuals and their families is profound, affecting personal relationships, educational and occupational attainment, and overall quality of life. Stigma and misconceptions surrounding psychosis further exacerbate these challenges, often leading to social isolation and reluctance to seek help. Public education and awareness campaigns are essential in reducing stigma and promoting understanding and acceptance. Additionally, ongoing research into the underlying mechanisms of psychosis and the development of novel treatment approaches holds promise for more effective and personalized interventions.

Living with psychosis requires a holistic approach to care, encompassing medical treatment, psychosocial support, and efforts to enhance social integration and quality of life. Advocacy for better mental health services, increased funding for research, and policies supporting early intervention and continuous care are critical in addressing the needs of those affected by psychosis. Overall, understanding and managing psychosis necessitates a comprehensive, compassionate, and multidisciplinary approach to improve the lives of individuals experiencing this challenging condition.

Summary

- Schizophrenia causes psychosis and is associated with considerable disability and may affect all areas of life including personal, family, social, educational, and occupational functioning.
- A person with schizotypal personality disorder has irrational, obsessive thought patterns and fears that interfere with their ability to form and maintain relationships. They are not disconnected from reality like someone with schizophrenia, but they can develop significant social problems and are often perceived as behaving oddly or inappropriately.
- The prodrome of an illness refers to certain signs and symptoms that precede the characteristic manifestations of the acute, fully developed illness. The prodromal phase of schizophrenia begins with a change from premorbid functioning and extends until the onset of frank psychotic symptoms.
- The body of evidence for genetic vulnerability to schizophrenia is growing. Studies show that relatives of individuals with schizophrenia have a much higher probability of developing the disease than does the general population.
- Pharmacological support for this hypothesis exists. Amphetamines, which increase levels of dopamine, induce psychotomimetic symptoms. The antipsychotics (e.g., chlorpromazine or haloperidol) lower brain levels of dopamine by blocking dopamine receptors, thus reducing the schizophrenic symptoms, including those induced by amphetamines.
- Delusional disorder is characterized by the presence of delusions that have been experienced by the individual for at least 1 month. If present at all, hallucinations are not prominent, and behavior is not bizarre.
- The prominent hallucinations and delusions associated with this disorder are found to be directly attributable to substance intoxication or withdrawal or to exposure to a medication or toxin.
- Catatonic disorder is identified by the symptoms described. This diagnosis is made when the symptomatology is evidenced from medical history, physical examination, or laboratory findings to be directly attributable to the physiological consequences of another medical condition.

References

1. Addington, D. E. (2006). Reducing suicide risk in patients with schizophrenia. *Medscape Psychiatry & Mental Health*. Retrieved from: https://www.medscape.com/editorial/cmetogo/5793.
2. American Psychiatric Association (APA). (2013). *Diagnostic and Statistical Manual of Mental Disorders* (5th ed.). Washington, DC: American Psychiatric Publishing.
3. Asen, E. (2002). Outcome research in family therapy: Family intervention for psychosis. *Advances in Psychiatric Treatment, 8*, 230–238.
4. Assertive Community Treatment Association (ACTA). (2013). ACT model. Retrieved from: http://www.actassociation.org/actModel (accessed on 7 September 2024).

5. Black, D. W., & Andreasen, N. C. (2011). *Introductory Textbook of Psychiatry* (5th ed.). Washington, DC: American Psychiatric Publishing.
6. Citrome, L. (2011). Neurochemical models of schizophrenia: Transcending dopamine. *Supplement to Current Psychiatry, 10*(9), S10–S14.
7. D'Souza, D. C., Singh, N., Elander, J., Carbuto, M., Pittman, B., Udo de Haes, J., Sjogren, M., Peeters, P., Ranganathan, M., & Schipper, J. (2012). Glycine transporter inhibitor attenuates the psychotomimetic effects of ketamine in healthy males: Preliminary evidence. *Neuropsychopharmacology, 37*, 1036–1046.
8. Dixon, L. B., Lehman, A. F., & Levine, J. (2010). Conventional antipsychotic medications for schizophrenia. Retrieved from: http://www.mental-health-matters.com (accessed on 7 September 2024).
9. Drug facts and comparisons. (2014). St. Louis, MO: Wolters Kluwer.
10. Eisendrath, S. J., & Lichtmacher, J. E. (2012). Psychiatric disorders. In S. J. McPhee, M. A. Papadakis, & M. W. Rabow (Eds.), *Current Medical Diagnosis and Treatment 2012* (pp. 1010–1064). New York, NY: McGraw-Hill.
11. Fohrman, D. A., & Stein, M. T. (2006). Psychosis: Six steps rule out medical causes in kids. *The Journal of Family Practice Online, 5*(2). Retrieved from: http://www.jfponline.com/pages.asp?aid=3887 (accessed on 7 September 2024).
12. Freudenreich, O. (2010). Differential diagnosis of psychotic symptoms: Medical "mimics." *Psychiatric Times, 27*(12), 52–61.
13. Hashimoto, K. (2006). Glycine transporter inhibitors as therapeutic agents for schizophrenia. *Recent Patents on CNS Drug Discovery, 1*, 43–53.
14. Ho, B. C., Black, D. W., & Andreasen, N. C. (2003). Schizophrenia and other psychotic disorders. In R. E. Hales & S. C. Yudofsky (Eds.), *Textbook of Clinical Psychiatry* (4th ed., pp. 379–438). Washington, DC: American Psychiatric Publishing.
15. Institute of Medicine. (2003). *Health Professions Education: A Bridge to Quality*. Washington, DC: Author.
16. Jonsson, S. A., Luts, A., Guldberg-Kjaer, N., & Brun, A. (1997). Hippocampal pyramidal cell disarray correlates negatively to cell number: Implications for the pathogenesis of schizophrenia. *European Archives of Psychiatry and Clinical Neuroscience, 247*(3), 120–127.
17. Lehman, A. F., Lieberman, J. A., Dixon, L. B., McGlashan, T. H., Miller, A. L., Perkins, D. O., & Kreyenbuhl, J. (2006). Practice guideline for the treatment of patients with schizophrenia, 2nd edition. *American Psychiatric Association Practice Guidelines for the Treatment of Psychiatric Disorders, Compendium 2006*. Washington, DC: American Psychiatric Publishing.
18. Levenson, J. L. (2009). Medical aspects of catatonia. *Primary Psychiatry, 16*(3), 23–26.
19. Lysaker, P. H., Roe, D., & Buck, K. D. (2010). Recovery and wellness amidst schizophrenia: Definitions, evidence, and the implications for clinical practice. *Journal of the American Psychiatric Nurses Association, 16*(1), 36–42.
20. Mattai, A. K., Hill, J. L., & Lenroot, R. K. (2010). Treatment of early-onset schizophrenia. *Current Opinion in Psychiatry, 23*(4), 304–310.

21. Minzenberg, M. J., Yoon, J. H., & Carter, C. S. (2008). Schizophrenia. In R. E. Hales, S. C. Yudofsky, & G. O. Gabbard (Eds.), *Textbook of Psychiatry* (5th ed., pp. 407–456). Washington, DC: American Psychiatric Publishing.

22. Mueser, K. T., Bond, G. R., & Drake, R. E. (2002). Community-based treatment of schizophrenia and other severe mental disorders: Treatment outcomes. *Medscape Psychiatry & Mental Health eJournal*. Retrieved from: http://www.medscape.com/viewarticle/430529 (accessed on 7 September 2024).

23. NANDA International (NANDA-I). (2012). *Nursing Diagnoses: Definitions & Classification 2012–2014*. Philadelphia, PA: NANDA-I.

24. National Alliance on Mental Illness (NAMI). (2013). PACT: Program of assertive community treatment. Retrieved from: http://www.nami.org (accessed on 7 September 2024).

25. Puri, B. K., & Treasaden, I. H. (2011). *Textbook of Psychiatry* (3rd ed.). Philadelphia, PA: Churchill Livingstone Elsevier.

26. Puri, B. K., Laking, P. J., & Treasaden, I. H. (1996). *Textbook of Psychiatry*. Churchill Livingstone.

27. Rantakallio, P., Jones, P., Moring, J., & Von Wendt, L. (1997). Association between central nervous system infections during childhood and adult-onset schizophrenia and other psychoses: A 28-year follow-up. *International Journal of Epidemiology, 26*, 837–843.

28. Sadock, B. J., & Sadock, V. A. (2007). *Synopsis of Psychiatry: Behavioral Sciences/Clinical Psychiatry* (10th ed.). Philadelphia, PA: Lippincott Williams & Wilkins.

29. Safier, E. (1997). Our families, the context of our lives. *Menninger Perspective, 28*(1), 4–9.

30. Schatzberg, A. F., Cole, J. O., & DeBattista, C. (2010). *Manual of Clinical Psychopharmacology* (7th ed.). Washington, DC: American Psychiatric Publishing.

31. Stahl, S. M. (2008). *Stahl's Essential Psychopharmacology: Neuroscientific Basis and Practical Applications* (3rd ed.). New York, NY: Cambridge University Press.

32. The Joint Commission. (2010). *The Comprehensive Accreditation Manual for Hospitals: The Official Handbook*. Oakbrook Terrace, IL: Joint Commission Resources.

33. Weiden, P. J. (2010). Is recovery attainable in schizophrenia? *Medscape Psychiatry & Mental Health*. Retrieved from: http://www.medscape.com/viewarticle/729750 (accessed on 7 September 2024).

Chapter 9

MOOD DISORDERS

Contents

Introduction

Mood disorders are a broad category of emotional disturbances that have a substantial impact on day-to-day functioning and overall quality of life. Depression is one of the most common and incapacitating of these. Millions of people worldwide suffer from depression, which is characterized by a protracted sense of sadness, a loss of interest in once-enjoyed activities, and a variety of cognitive and physical symptoms. Depression is a complicated illness that can be brought on by a number of things, such as a genetic predisposition, biochemical imbalances, and environmental stressors. It is not just a fleeting feeling of melancholy or a reaction to life's hardships. The most prevalent type, major depressive disorder (MDD), can cause serious impairment in social, professional, and personal spheres. Depressed mood, exhaustion, altered sleep and eating patterns, trouble concentrating, guilt or worthlessness feelings, and, in extreme situations, suicidal thoughts are some of the symptoms of Major Depressive Disorder (MDD). A comprehensive clinical evaluation that includes the patient's history, a symptom assessment, and occasionally the use of standardized screening instruments is required to diagnose depression. Healthcare professionals need to make the distinction between bipola and depression among other mood disorders.

Pharmacological therapy, lifestyle changes, and psychotherapy are commonly used in the treatment of depression. Counseling techniques such as cognitive-behavioral therapy (CBT) can assist people in changing negative thought patterns and creating coping mechanisms. Underlying biochemical imbalances can be corrected by antidepressant medications, such as selective serotonin reuptake inhibitors (SSRIs). A thorough treatment plan should also include social support, a balanced diet, and regular physical activity. Even though there are effective treatments available, people are frequently discouraged from seeking help due to stigma and ignorance. Destigmatization initiatives and public education are crucial in motivating those impacted to get the care they require. Depression is a severe mood illness that has a significant impact on people's lives as well as society. For individuals impacted, better outcomes and an improved quality of life can result from an understanding of its complexity and the promotion of effective interventions.

Orientation and Directional Terms

Term	Definition	Illustration
Mood disorder	Mood disorder is a type of mental health condition where there is a disconnect between actual life circumstances and the person's state of mind or feeling. A mood disorder can negatively affect your ability to function normally.	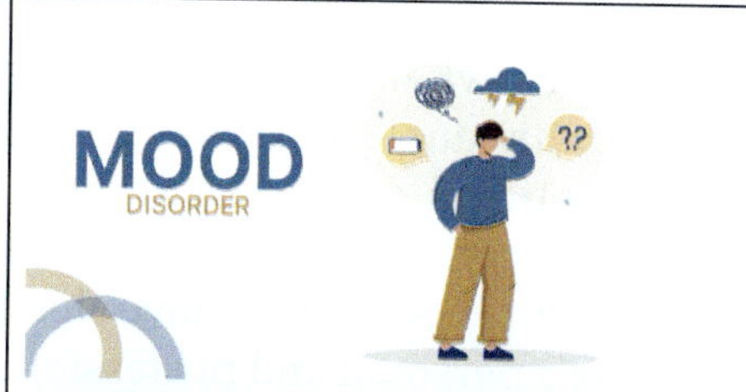
Depression	Depression is a common but serious mood disorder. It causes severe symptoms that affect how a person feels, thinks, and handles daily activities, such as sleeping, eating, or working.	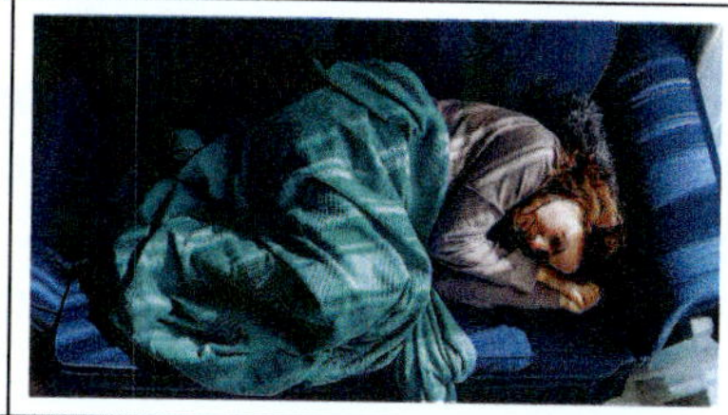
Substance Abuse and Mental Health Services Administration	Substance Abuse and Mental Health Services Administration is a branch of the U.S. Department of Health and Human Services. SAMHSA is charged with improving the quality and availability of treatment and rehabilitative services in order to reduce illness, death, disability, and the cost to society resulting from substance abuse and mental illnesses.	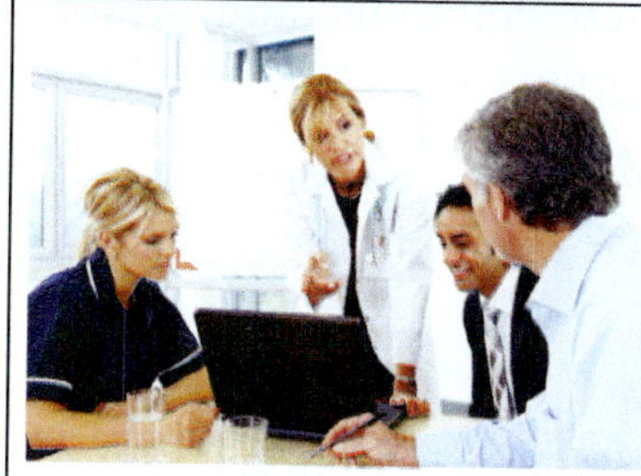
Nerve gases	Nerve gases, are a class of organic chemicals that disrupt the mechanisms by which nerves transfer messages to organs. The disruption is caused by the blocking of acetylcholinesterase (AChE), an enzyme that catalyzes the breakdown of acetylcholine, a neurotransmitter.	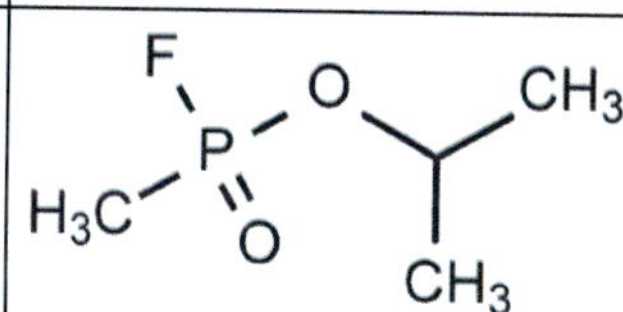
Cerebrovascular accidents	Cerebrovascular accidents are caused by blood clots and broken blood vessels in the brain. Symptoms include dizziness, numbness, weakness on one side of the body, and problems with talking, writing, or understanding language.	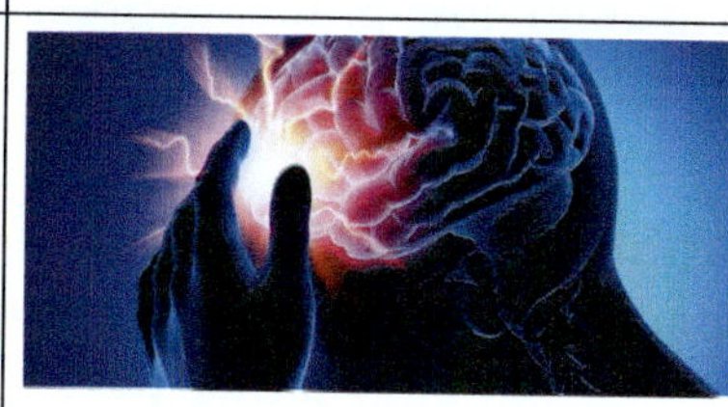

9.1. Overview of Mood Disorders

A mental health condition known as mood disorder occurs when there is a discrepancy between an individual's true life circumstances and their emotional or mental state. Having a mood disorder can make it difficult for you to carry out daily tasks. It may have detrimental effects on one's personal and professional life in equal measure. Mood disorders can affect adults, teenagers, and children. But the symptoms that adults experience aren't always the same in kids and teenagers. Children's mood disorders are more difficult to diagnose. This is due to the fact that children may not always be able to articulate their emotions, and symptoms may not always appear the same in adults.

Therapy, medicines, support and self-care can help treat mood disorders.

9.1.1. Types of Mood Disorders

These are the most common types of mood disorders:

- **Major Depression:** Having less interest in normal activities, feeling sad or hopeless, and other symptoms for at least 2 weeks may mean depression.
- **Dysthymia:** This is an ongoing (chronic), low-grade, depressed, or irritable mood that lasts for at least 2 years.
- **Bipolar Disorder:** With this condition, a person has times of depression alternating with times of mania or a higher mood.
- **Mood Disorder Linked to Another Health Condition:** Many health conditions (including cancer, injuries, infections, and chronic illnesses) can trigger symptoms of depression.
- **Substance-Induced Mood Disorder:** Symptoms of depression may be caused by drug abuse, alcohol use disorder, exposure to toxins, or side effects of medicines.

9.1.2. Causes Mood Disorders

Mood disorders are caused by numerous factors. They most likely result from a chemical imbalance in the brain. Events in life, like traumatic life transitions, can also contribute to depression. Moreover, mood disorders frequently run in families.

9.1.3. Risk for Mood Disorders

Everyone has moments of sadness or depression. However, mood disorders are more severe and persistent. They are also more difficult to control than typical depressive symptoms. Having a parent with a mood disorder increases the likelihood that children, teens, or adults will experience a mood disorder themselves. However, stress and life events can reveal or exacerbate depressive or melancholic feelings. This complicates the management of the emotions. Depression can occasionally be triggered by life's problems. Certain life events can be challenging, like losing a loved one, getting divorced, getting fired from your job, experiencing a death in the family, and having money problems. It might be difficult to handle the pressure. Depressive or melancholic feelings may be triggered by these life events and stress. Or they may make it more difficult to control a mood disorder. Compared to men, women are almost twice as likely to experience depression. Siblings and offspring are more likely to receive the same diagnosis if an individual in the family has it.

9.1.4. Symptoms of Mood Disorders

Depending on age and the type of mood disorder, a person may have different symptoms when they become depressed. The following are the most common symptoms of a mood disorder:

- Ongoing sad, anxious, or "empty" mood;
- Feeling hopeless or helpless;
- Having low self-esteem;
- Feeling inadequate or worthless;
- Excessive guilt;
- Not interested in normal activities or activities that were once enjoyed, including sex;
- Relationship problems;
- Trouble sleeping or sleeping too much;
- Changes in appetite or weight;
- Decreased energy;
- Trouble focusing;
- Less able to make decisions;
- Frequent physical complaints (for example, headache, stomachache, or tiredness) that don't get better with treatment;
- Running away or threats of running away from home;
- Very sensitive to failure or rejection;
- Irritability, hostility, or aggression;
- Repeated thoughts of death or suicide, planning for death, or wishing to die.

These emotions are stronger in mood disorders than they might be in a regular person. Concerning is also raised if these emotions persist in the long run. Alternatively, if they get in the way of someone's interest in their job, community, friends, or family. Anyone experiencing suicidal thoughts should seek medical attention as soon as possible. If your primary care physician isn't available right away, visit a respectable mental health facility in your neighborhood. Don't wait to do it. Mood disorder symptoms can mimic those of other illnesses or mental health issues. For a diagnosis, always consult a healthcare professional.

9.1.5. Mood Disorders Treated

Mood disorders can often be treated with success. Treatment may include:

- **Antidepressant and Mood-Stabilizing Medicines:** These medicines work very well in treating mood disorders, especially when combined with psychotherapy.
- **Psychotherapy (most often Cognitive-Behavioral or Interpersonal Therapy):** This kind of therapy is focused on changing the person's distorted view of themselves and their environment. It also helps to improve relationship skills. And it can help the person identify stressors in the environment and learn how to avoid or manage them.

- **Family Therapy:** A mood disorder can affect all aspects of a family (emotional, physical, occupational, and financial). Professional support can help both the person with the diagnosis and family members.
- **Other Therapies:** These may include transcranial stimulation and electroconvulsive therapy for refractory depression (treatment-resistant depression).

Families play a vital supportive role in any treatment process. A person with a mood disorder may experience periods of stability followed by recurrence of symptoms. Continuous, long-term care can help the patient maintain their health and manage their symptoms. Mood disorders can be effectively diagnosed and treated to allow for stable, productive, and healthy lives.

9.2. Epidemiology

A major contributing factor to disability in the US is major depression. A total of 14.3 million people, or 6% of those who were 18 years of age or older, reported having at least one major depressive episode in 2008. The Substance Abuse and Mental Health Services Administration [SAMHSA], 2009 reported that 4.2%, or 9.5 million individuals, experienced a major depressive episode with severe impairment in the previous year. Over the course of their lives, approximately 13% of men and 21% of women will experience clinical depression. Several researchers have referred to depression as "the common cold of psychiatric disorders" and this generation as the "age of melancholia" as a result of this prevalence. "

9.2.1. Age and Gender

According to research, women are nearly twice as likely as men to experience depressive disorder. Beginning at around age 10 and continuing through midlife, women experience depression at a higher rate than men (Kornstein, 2006). Between the ages of 44 and 65, there is less of a gender difference' however, after 65, women are once more likely than men to experience depression. This phenomenon could potentially be associated with variations in social roles, economic and social prospects between genders, and age-related changes. Gender socialization, or the creation of gender stereotypes, encourages stereotypically feminine traits like emotionality, passivity, and helplessness—all of which are linked to depression. Conversely, some research suggests that traits that are traditionally associated with men are linked to lower levels of depression and higher levels of self-esteem.

9.2.2. Social Class

Research findings have demonstrated a negative correlation between one's social class and their report of depressive symptoms. Still, the relationship between mental illness and socioeconomic status lacks a clear causal structure. According to Hudson (2005), depression and personality disorders have been found to be outcomes of low socioeconomic status most frequently. Does this mean that people with preexisting, biologically based mental illnesses drift into poor socioeconomic circumstances, or does it mean that people with poor socioeconomic conditions are predisposed to mental disability?

9.2.3. Race and Culture

Research has not consistently demonstrated a connection between affective disorder and race. Reviewing racial comparisons can present challenges, one of which is the socioeconomic status of the race under investigation. Non-white client sample populations are frequently compared to white populations from middle and upper social classes, with a preponderance of lower-class members. Additional research points to a second troubling aspect of the racial comparison study. When treating patients from racial or cultural backgrounds distinct from their own, clinicians frequently overdiagnoses schizophrenia and underdiagnose mood disorders (Sadock and Sadock, 2007). Language barriers between patients and doctors who are not familiar with the cultural nuances of non-White patients' language and behavior may be the cause of this incorrect diagnosis.

Recent results from the National Study of American Life, a survey of black American mental health, show that while depression is more common in white people than in black people, it is also more severe, persistent, and incapacitating in black people, and they are less likely to receive treatment (Williams et al., 2007). Not even among blacks with severe or very severe symptoms were 48% of African Americans and 21% of Blacks from the Caribbean receiving any kind of treatment. The findings, according to the authors, underscore the significance of identifying high-risk subgroups within racial populations and the necessity of directing affordable interventions towards them.

9.2.4. Marital Status

Many research have revealed that married people have better psychological outcomes than single people or people who do not have a close relationship with another person. According to LaPierre (2004), there might be a limit to the validity of marital status alone, and the impact of marital status on depression might depend on an individual's age. In her research, she discovered that while depression was not significantly predicted by being single in any of the other age groups (18–25, 26–36, and 50+), it was in the 37–49 year old age group. She provided the following explanation for her findings: The 37–49 year old age group is likely to experience a decline in mental health and an increase in depressive symptomatology as they come to terms with the fact that marriage and the accompanying children are becoming increasingly unlikely. This is especially true for women in this age group who feel they may have to give up the traditional role of motherhood if they do not find a partner with whom to have children when their childbearing years come to an end. The 50+ age group saw a subsequent decrease in depressive symptomatology.

Age may mitigate the impact of marital status on depression, according to other research. George (1992) discovered that only in the oldest age group (65+) did marriage (as opposed to being separated or divorced) have a protective effect against major depression. Her findings also indicated that never getting married (as opposed to. Separated or divorced) was linked to a higher risk of major depression in the age groups of 65 and older and 40 to 64.

9.2.5. Seasonality

Seasonal patterns and mood disorders have been the subject of several studies. Two seasons that are commonly involved are spring (March, April, and May) and fall (September, October, and November), according to these studies. According to Davidson (2005), there is a considerable peak in the spring and a smaller one in October for suicide rates, which is similar to this pattern. A number of etiologies associated with this trend have been postulated (Hakko, 2000). Some of these include the following:

- A meteorological factor associating drastic temperature and barometric pressure changes with human mental instability;
- Sociodemographic variables, such as the seasonal increase in social intercourse (e.g., increased social activity with the commencement of an academic year);
- Biochemical variables due to seasonal variations in various peripheral and central aspects of

serotonergic function involved in depression and suicide.

9.3. Types of Depressive Disorders

9.3.1. Major Depressive Disorder

A depressed mood or a lack of interest in or enjoyment from routine activities are characteristics of major depressive disorder (MDD). There must be evidence of reduced social and occupational functioning that has persisted for at least two weeks, no prior history of manic behavior, and symptoms that are not related to drug use or a general medical illness. Furthermore, whether an episode is a recurrent episode (the person has a history of previous episodes) or a single episode (the person's first encounter) determines the diagnosis of MDD. Along with determining whether there is evidence of psychotic or catatonic features, the diagnosis will also determine whether the symptoms are mild, moderate, or severe, and whether a seasonal pattern can be identified. When symptoms appear four weeks after childbirth, they are referred to as postpartum onset.

9.3.2. Dysthymic Disorder

The traits associated with dysthymic disorder are comparable to those of major depressive disorder, albeit a little milder. People who experience this type of mood disturbance characterize themselves as depressed or feeling "down in the dumps" (American Psychiatric Association [APA], 2000). No signs of psychotic symptoms are present. A chronically depressed mood (or possibly an irritable mood in children or adolescents) for the majority of the day, most days, for at least two years—one year for children and adolescents—is the essential feature. The diagnosis is classified as either late onset (occurring at age 21 or older) or early onset (occurring before age 21).

9.3.3. Premenstrual Dysphoric Disorder

While premenstrual dysphoric disorder is not recognized as an official diagnostic category in the DSM-IV-TR (APA, 2000), it does offer a set of research criteria to encourage additional investigation into the condition. The primary characteristics are a markedly depressed mood, excessive anxiety, mood swings, and a decreased interest in activities in the week before menstruation, which subsides soon after (APA, 2000).

9.3.4. Other Depressive Disorders

9.3.4.1. Mood Disorder (Depression) Due to a General Medical Condition

Prominent and ongoing depression, which is thought to be the direct physiological effect of a general medical condition, is the hallmark of this disorder (APA, 2000). Clinically significant distress or impairment in social, occupational, or other important domains of functioning are caused by the depression. The discussion of the etiological implications for depression includes various types of physiological influences.

9.3.4.2. Substance-Induced Mood Disorder (Depression)

The physiological effects of a substance (such as an abuse drug, medication, or exposure to toxins) are thought to be the direct cause of the depressed mood associated with substance-induced mood disorders, which can lead to clinically significant distress or impairment in social, occupational, or other important areas of functioning. Intoxication from drugs like alcohol, cocaine, amphetamines, hallucinogens, inhalants, opioids, phencyclidine, sedatives, hypnotics, and anxiolytics is linked to mood disorders. Withdrawal symptoms from drugs like cocaine, alcohol, amphetamines, sedatives, hypnotics, and anxiolytics can appear. Mood symptoms can also be brought on by heavy metals and poisons, such as paint, gasoline, nerve gases, carbon monoxide, and carbon dioxide (APA, 2000). Mood symptoms have been reported to be induced by several medications. Anaesthetics, analgesics, cardiac medications, oral contraceptives, anticholinergics, anticonvulsants, antihypertensives, antiparkinsonian agents, antiulcer agents, psychotropic medications, muscle relaxants, steroids, and sulfonamides are among the classifications. The topic of includes a few particular instances.

9.4. Etiological Implications

Depression's exact cause is unknown. There isn't a single theory or hypothesis that provides a conclusive explanation for the illness. A person's susceptibility to depression can be influenced by a combination of genetic, biochemical, and psychosocial factors, as evidence for multiple causations keeps growing. Here are some theoretical postulates that are put forth.

9.4.1. Biological Theories

9.4.1.1. Genetics

Considerable research has been done on the significance of genetic factors in affective illness. Numerous studies have indicated a genetic connection, but no clear-cut method of genetic transmission has been established as of yet.

Twin Studies

Twin research points to a significant hereditary component in the etiology of emotional disorders. According to Joska and Stein (2008), research on monozygotic twins suggests that recurrent major depression has a roughly 37% heritability. Genes determine approximately 37% of the risk of major depression in people who share all or nearly all of their genetic makeup. A significant amount of the residual risk is likely due to the influence of an individual's environment and the interaction between genes and that environment.

Family Studies

According to the majority of family studies, first-degree biological relatives of individuals with the disorder have major depression 1.5–3 times more frequently than the general population (APA, 2000). It's true that there is strong evidence linking positive family history to a higher risk of depressive illness in people. Random environmental factors are unlikely to be the cause of the illness concentration observed in families.

Adoption Studies

Research on adopted children of biological parents with affective disorders provides more evidence that heritability plays a role in the etiology of depression. According to these studies, even when raised by adoptive parents who are not affected by the disorder, biological children of parents with mood disorders are more likely to experience a mood disorder themselves (Dubovsky, Davies, and Dubovsky, 2003).

9.4.1.2. Biochemical Influences

Biogenic Amines

The neurotransmitters norepinepherine, serotonin, and dopamine may be deficient at functionally significant receptor sites in the brain, which has been linked to depression. Reserpine, which depletes amines in the brain, has historically been linked to the onset of depression syndrome, which gave rise to the biogenic amine hypothesis of mood disorders (Slattery, Hudson, and Nutt, 2004). It has been determined that the catecholamine norepinephrine plays a crucial role in the body's mobilization in response to stressful events. Many psychobiological processes, including mood, anxiety, arousal, vigilance, irritability, thinking, cognition, appetite, aggression, and circadian rhythm, are crucially regulated by serotonin-containing neurons (Dubovsky et al., 2003).

It has been demonstrated that tryptophan, the amino acid precursor of serotonin, can sometimes act as an antidepressant on its own and can also improve the effectiveness of antidepressant drugs. Dopamine levels in the brain's mesolimbic system are assumed to have a significant impact on people's moods and behaviors. A diminished supply of these biogenic amines inhibits the transmission of impulses from one neuronal fiber to another, causing a failure of the cells to fire or become charged.

Acetylcholine is another neurotransmitter that has been added to the biogenic amine theory more recently. A possible explanation for the observed effects of cholinergic agents on mood, electroencephalogram, sleep, and neuroendocrine function is an imbalance between acetylcholine and biogenic amines, which has been proposed as the cause of depression and mania. According to Dubovsky et al. (2003), cholinergic transmission is assumed to be insufficient in mania and excessive in depression. It's unclear exactly what part any neurotransmitter plays in the genesis of depression. Undoubtedly, as the corpus of research expands, a deeper understanding of biogenic amines will lead to improved diagnostic and therapeutic tools for affective disorders.

9.4.1.3. Neuroendocrine Disturbances

The etiology or persistence of depression may be influenced by neuroendocrine disorders. This idea has emerged in light of the noticeable mood disruptions linked to the administration of specific hormones or the existence of endocrine diseases that develop on their own.

Hypothalamic-Pituitary-Adrenocortical Axis

The typical system of hormonal inhibition malfunctions in depressed clients, leading to an excess of cortisol being secreted. The dexamethasone suppression test, which is occasionally used to assess whether a patient has depression that can be treated somatically, is based on this elevated serum cortisol level.

Hypothalamic-Pituitary-Thyroid Axis

Thyroid-stimulating hormone (TSH) is released from the anterior pituitary gland in response to thyrotropin-releasing factor (TRF) from the hypothalamus. TSH then causes the thyroid gland to become active. About 25% of people with depression exhibit a diminished TSH response to TRF administration. In the future, this lab test may be used to identify patients who are highly susceptible to affective disorders.

9.4.1.4. Physiological Influences

Secondary depression refers to depressive symptoms that arise from a non-mood disorder or as a side effect of specific medications. Medication side effects, neurological disorders, hormonal or electrolyte imbalances, nutritional deficiencies, and other physiological or psychological conditions can all contribute to secondary depression.

Medication Side Effects

A variety of drugs can cause a depressive syndrome, either by themselves or in conjunction with other prescription drugs. Among these medications, those that directly affect the central nervous system are the most prevalent. Examples of these include the anxiolytics, antipsychotics, and sedative-hypnotics. Certain antihypertensive medications, such as propranolol and reserpine, have been known to produce depressive symptoms. A recent Canadian study found a statistically significant association between the acne medication isotretinoin (Accutane) and depression (Azoulay et al., 2008). Depressed mood may also occur with any of the following medications, although the list is by no means all-inclusive (Sadock & Sadock, 2007):

- **Steroids:** prednisone and cortisone;
- **Hormones:** estrogen and progesterone;
- **Sedatives:** barbiturates and benzodiazepines;
- **Antibacterial and Antifungal Drugs:** ampicillin, cycloserine, tetracycline, and sulfonamides;
- **Antineoplastics:** vincristine and zidovudine;
- **Analgesics and Anti-Inflammatory Drugs:** opiates, ibuprofen, and phenylbutazone;
- **Antiulcer:** cimetidine.

Neurological Disorders

A person who has had a cardiovascular accident (CVA) could feel depressed for reasons unrelated to how bad the CVA was. These are real mood disorders, and treatment with antidepressant medications may be necessary. Depression is a common side effect of brain tumors, especially those located in the temporal lobe. Huntington's, Parkinson's, and Alzheimer's disease-related clinical manifestations may include agitated depression. In a person with multiple sclerosis, agitation and restlessness could also be signs of an underlying depression.

Electrolyte Disturbances

Depression symptoms can be brought on by deficiencies in magnesium and sodium as well as excessive amounts of calcium or sodium bicarbonate. Additionally, the depression syndrome is linked to potassium. Both cases of potassium depletion and excess potassium in the body have been linked to symptoms.

Hormonal Disturbances

Depression is associated with dysfunction of the adrenal cortex and is commonly observed in both Addison's disease and Cushing's syndrome. Other endocrine conditions that may result in symptoms of depression include hypoparathyroidism, hyperparathyroidism, hypothyroidism, and hyperthyroidism.

An imbalance of the hormones estrogen and progesterone has been implicated in the predisposition to premenstrual dysphoric disorder. It is postulated that excess estrogen or a high estrogen-to-progesterone ratio during the luteal phase of the menstrual cycle is responsible for the symptoms associated with premenstrual syndrome, although the exact etiology is unknown (Sadock & Sadock, 2007).

Nutritional Deficiencies

Depression symptoms may be brought on by deficiencies in vitamin B1 (thiamine), vitamin B6 (pyridoxine), vitamin B12, niacin, vitamin C, iron, folic acid, zinc, calcium, and potassium (Schimelpfening, 2009). The etiology of premenstrual dysphoric disorder has also been linked to several nutritional changes. According to Frakiewicz and Shiovitz (2001), these include insufficiencies in linolenic acid, calcium, magnesium, manganese, vitamin E, and the B vitamins. Variations in glucose tolerance, aberrant fatty acid metabolism, and alcohol and caffeine sensitivity may also contribute to the symptoms of this disorder. There is insufficient evidence to substantiate the existence of any particular dietary modification in the aetiology of these symptoms.

Other Physiological Conditions

Additional conditions that have been linked to secondary depression include infections like encephalitis, hepatitis, mononucleosis, pneumonia, and syphilis' metabolic disorders like diabetes mellitus and porphyria' collagen disorders like polyarteritis nodosa and systemic lupus erythematosus (SLE)' and cardiovascular disease like cardiomyopathy, congestive heart failure, myocardial infarction, and cerebrovascular accident (stroke).

9.4.2. Psychosocial Theories

9.4.2.1. Psychoanalytical Theory

Freud (1957) presented his classic paper "Mourning and Melancholia" in 1917. He defined the distinguishing features of melancholia as:

> An excruciatingly agonizing sense of hopelessness, a loss of interest in the outside world, the inability to love, inhibition of all activities, and a reduction in self-esteem to the point where self-loathing and self-reproaches become uttered, ultimately leading to a misunderstanding of punishment. He noted that melancholy follows the loss of a loved one, either physically or emotionally through rejection, or the loss of any other abstraction that holds significance for the person. According to Sadock and Sadock (2007), Freud suggested that in melancholia, the angry depressed patient directs their anger inward due to their identification with the misplaced object. Freud thought that ambivalence in romantic relationships was a trait of the melancholic. Therefore, he conjectured that the hostile aspect of the ambivalence felt for the lost object is turned inward against the ego once the loss has been absorbed into the self (ego).

9.4.2.2. Learning Theory

The "learned helplessness" model originates from Seligman's (1973) canine experiments. The animals were subjected to electrical stimulation that they were unable to resist. When they were later given the chance to avoid the traumatic event, they reacted helplessly and didn't try to flee. People who have failed many times in their lives—real or imagined—experience a similar sense of helplessness. The person gives up on trying to succeed in the future. According to Seligman's theory, people who experience learned helplessness are more likely to experience depression because they feel like they have no control over their circumstances. They experience depression as a result of feeling powerless and realizing that their efforts are in vain. Because emotional development later on depends heavily on having a sense of control over one's surroundings, this can be particularly harmful very early in life.

9.4.2.3. Object Loss Theory

According to the theory of object loss, experiencing separation or abandonment from a significant other within the first six months of life can lead to depressive illness. The mother is viewed as the "object" during this time because she serves as the child's primary source of security. This lack of attachment, which can be emotional or physical, causes hopelessness and despair, which fuels recurring patterns of depression in the wake of loss throughout one's life. René Spitz, a psychiatrist, coined the term "anaclitic depression" in 1946 to describe the depression that some infants experienced during the first year of life when they were separated from their mothers for an extended period of time (Cartwright, 2004). Excessive crying, anorexia, withdrawal, psychomotor retardation, stupor, and a generalized impairment in the normal process of growth and development were among the behaviors associated with the condition. According to certain researchers, individuals who have experienced loss in their early childhood are more susceptible to depression in adulthood.

9.4.2.4. Cognitive Theory

Beck and colleagues (1979) proposed a theory suggesting that the primary disturbance in depression is cognitive rather than affective. The underlying cause of the depressive effect is seen as cognitive distortions that result in negative, defeated attitudes. Beck identifies three cognitive distortions that he believes serve as the basis for depression:

- Negative expectations of the environment;
- Negative expectations of the self;
- Negative expectations of the future.

A defect in cognitive development causes these cognitive distortions, which make the person feel unworthy, inadequate, and rejected by others. There is a bleak and depressing outlook for the future. According to cognitive theorists, depressive thoughts are the result of negative thinking. This is in contrast to other theorists who contend that depression causes one to think negatively. The goal of cognitive therapy is to assist the patient in modifying their mood through thought changes. The person is trained to manage negative thought distortions that cause low self-esteem, procrastination, sluggishness, and pessimism.

9.5. Developmental Implications

9.5.1. Childhood

Only in recent years has a consensus developed among investigators that major depressive disorder as an entity in children and adolescents can be identified using criteria similar to those used for adults (APA, 2000' Dubovsky et al., 2003). It is not uncommon, however, for the symptoms of depression to be manifested differently in childhood, and the picture changes with age (Joska & Stein, 2008' Harvard Medical School, 2002' Tempfer, 2006):

- **Up to Age 3:** Signs may include feeding problems, tantrums, lack of playfulness and emotional expressiveness, failure to thrive, or delays in speech and gross motor development.
- **From Ages 3 to 5:** Common symptoms may include accident proneness, phobias, aggressiveness, and excessive self-reproach for minor infractions.
- **From Ages 6 to 8:** There may be vague physical complaints and aggressive behavior. They may cling to their parents and avoid new people and challenges. They may lag behind their classmates in social skills and academic competence.
- **At Ages 9 to 12:** Common symptoms include morbid thoughts and excessive worrying. They may reason that they are depressed because they have disappointed their parents in some way. There may be a lack of interest in playing with friends.

Hyperactivity, delinquency, academic difficulties, psychosomatic complaints, eating and sleeping disorders, social isolation, delusional thinking, and suicidal thoughts or deeds are some additional signs of childhood depression. A child may experience depression for a variety of reasons. There is a hereditary component to depression in many children, and the illness is triggered by stressful events. A move, academic failure, physical illness, parental separation or divorce, the physical or emotional detachment of the primary caregiver, the death of a loved one (person or pet), and so on are common precipitating factors. Either way, loss is the common denominator. The goal of therapy for depressed children is to reduce symptoms and improve the child's ability to cope and adjust, in the hopes that future psychological issues may be avoided. Untreated childhood depression has been linked to problems in adolescence and adulthood, according to certain studies. The majority of children receive outpatient care.

A depressed child is typically admitted to the hospital only in the following situations: when the child is actively considering suicide, when the home environment makes it difficult for them to follow a treatment plan, or when they need to be removed from the house due to psychosocial deprivation.

Parental and family therapy are commonly used to help the younger depressed child. Recovery is facilitated by emotional support and guidance to family members. Children older than age 8 years usually participate in family therapy. In some situations, individual treatment may be appropriate for older children. Medications, such as antidepressants, can be important in the treatment of children, especially for the more serious and recurrent forms of depression. The selective serotonin reuptake inhibitors (SSRIs) have been used with success, particularly in combination with psychosocial therapies. However, because there has been some concern that the use of antidepressant medications may cause suicidal behavior in young people, the U.S. Food and Drug Administration (FDA) has applied a "black box" label warning (described in the next section) to all antidepressant medications. The National Institute of Mental Health (2009) states:

Those who are prescribed an [antidepressant] medication should receive ongoing medical monitoring. Children already taking an [antidepressant] should remain on the medication if it has been helpful, but should be carefully monitored by a doctor for side effects. Parents should promptly seek medical advice and evaluation if their child or adolescent experiences suicidal thinking or behavior, nervousness, agitation, irritability, mood instability, or sleeplessness that either emerges or worsens during treatment with [antidepressant] medications.

9.5.2. Adolescence

Adolescent depression may be even more difficult to diagnose than younger childhood depression. Depression-related feelings of melancholy, loneliness, anxiety, and hopelessness may be mistaken for typical emotional strains of growing up. As a result, many young people who have symptoms that are thought to be "normal adjustments" associated with adolescence do not receive the necessary assistance. Teenage depression is a major contributing factor to suicide, which ranks third among all causes of death for those between the ages of 15 and 24 (National Center for Health Statistics [NCHS], 2009).

Inappropriately expressed anger, aggression, fleeing, delinquency, social disengagement, sexual acting out, substance abuse, restlessness, and apathy are typical signs of depression in adolescents. Psychosomatic complaints, eating and sleeping disorders, and low self-esteem are also prevalent. The best clue for a mood disorder is a visible manifestation of behavioral change that lasts for several weeks. But what distinguishes mood disorder from the usual stormy behavior of adolescence? Examples include the once-extroverted and outgoing teenager who has turned inward and antisocial' the good student who used to get good grades but is now failing and missing classes' and the once-self-assured teenager who is now acting inappropriately defensive and irritable toward others.

The same causes that were covered under the section on childhood depression also apply to adolescents experiencing depression. However, depression is a common adolescent symptom of the stress and conflicts related to independence that come with normal maturation. Depression can also be the result of a breakup with a boyfriend or girlfriend, or the death of a parent, other relative, or friend. The most common direct cause of teenage suicide is believed to be the perception of parental or closest peer abandonment. Adolescent depression is typically treated as an outpatient procedure. Hospitalization might be necessary in situations involving severe depression or the threat of suicide, when family dynamics make treatment in the home impractical, when the adolescent's physical condition makes it impossible for them to take care of their biological needs on their own, or when they have expressed a desire to hurt themselves or other family members.

Antidepressant therapy may be used in conjunction with supportive psychosocial intervention to treat mood disorders in adolescents. As was previously mentioned, the FDA has cautioned the public in a public health advisory about the higher risk of suicidal thoughts and actions in children and adolescents receiving antidepressant medication. All antidepressant drugs come with a black box warning label that outlines this risk and stresses the importance of closely monitoring patients who begin taking these drugs. It is not forbidden to use antidepressants in children and adolescents under the new warning language. Instead, it alerts prescribers to the possibility of suicidality and urges them to weigh that risk against clinical necessity.

The only drug currently approved to treat depression in children and adolescents is fluoxetine, better known by its brand name, Prozac. While venlafaxine, a serotonin-norepinephrine reuptake inhibitor (SNRI) antidepressant, and other SSRI drugs like sertraline, citalopram, and paroxetine have been prescribed to children by doctors for "off-label use," or uses other than those for which the FDA has approved them, these drugs have not been approved for the treatment of depression in children or adolescents. The FDA advised against treating major depressive disorder in children and adolescents with paroxetine in June 2003.

9.5.3. Senescence

The most prevalent psychiatric illness among the elderly, who comprise 12.8% of the US population overall, is depression (Administration on Aging, 2010). Given the disproportionate value our society places on youth, vigor, and continuous productivity, this is not surprising. As people age, these cultural attitudes intensify and become more prevalent, feeding feelings of hopelessness, powerlessness, and low self-worth. Furthermore, significant stressors like financial difficulties, physical illness, changes in bodily functioning, and a growing awareness of impending death may pose a serious threat to the aging person's adaptive coping strategies. The issue is frequently made worse by the multiple losses people go through during this stage of life, including those of a spouse, friends, child, home, and independence. When people suffer so many losses in their lives that they are unable to finish one grieving process before another one starts, it's known as bereavement overload. Older people who have experienced a lot of loss are more likely to suffer from depression.

The elderly account for roughly 16% of suicides in the US, despite making up less than 13% of the population (NCHS, 2009). White men 85 years of age and older commit suicide at a rate more than four times higher than the national average. Depression symptoms in older adults are not all that dissimilar from those in younger adults. However, other illnesses linked to aging frequently cause confusion with depressive syndromes. Depression symptoms are frequently misdiagnosed as senile dementia, even though depression may be the cause of memory loss, disorientation, or apathy which are signs of dementia. Many older adults who are not depressed share the early awakening and decreased appetite that are typical of depression. The fact that many medical conditions, including endocrinological, neurological, nutritional, and metabolic disorders, frequently present with the traditional symptoms of depression exacerbates the situation. Numerous drugs that are frequently taken by the elderly, like analgesics, corticosteroids, and antihypertensives, can also have depressant effects.

Depression does accompany many of the illnesses that afflict older people, such as Parkinson's disease, cancer, arthritis, and the early stages of Alzheimer's disease. Treating depression in these situations can reduce unnecessary suffering and help afflicted individuals cope with their medical problems.

The most effective treatment of depression in the elderly individual is thought to be a combination of psychosocial and biological approaches. Antidepressant medications are administered with consideration for age-related physiological changes in absorption, distribution, elimination, and brain receptor sensitivity. Because of these changes, plasma concentrations of these medications can reach very high levels despite moderate oral doses.

One of the safest and most successful treatments for major depression in the elderly is still electroconvulsive therapy (ECT). With age, the response to ECT seems to slow down, and the treatment benefits are transient. For older people who pose an immediate risk of suicide or who cannot take antidepressant medication, it might be the preferred course of treatment. Interpersonal, behavioral, cognitive, group, and family psychotherapies are additional therapeutic modalities. An elderly person who is depressed may experience relief from their suffering and a renewed sense of productivity with appropriate treatment.

9.5.4. Postpartum Depression

A postpartum depressive episode can range in intensity from the "blues," to moderate depression, to psychotic depression, or melancholia. Between 50% and 85% of women who give birth report having the "blues" after delivery (Mehta and Sheth, 2006). 10% to 20% of people experience moderate depression. Severe depression, also known as psychotic depression, affects only 1-2 out of every 1,000 postpartum women. The "maternity blues" manifest in the early puerperium as feelings of tearfulness, despondency, anxiety, and subjectively impaired concentration. Mehta and Sheth (2006) state that the symptoms typically start 48 hours after delivery, peak in 3–5 days, and last for about 2 weeks. Moderate postpartum depression symptoms include mood swings, with more bad days than good, with a tendency to get worse in the evening, and physical and emotional exhaustion, irritability, appetite loss, sleep disturbances, and sexual dysfunction. The new mother also lets it be known how worried she is about not being able to provide for her child. It takes a few weeks to several months for these symptoms to go away, and they start a little later than the "maternity blues" symptoms.

An abnormal attitude toward bodily functions, agitation, indecision, lack of concentration, guilt, and depressed mood are the hallmarks of postpartum melancholia, also known as depressive psychosis. There can be a morbid fear that the baby will be harmed, or there might be rejection or lack of interest in the child. The dangers of infanticide and suicide should not be disregarded. Although they can appear later, these symptoms typically appear in the initial days after delivery (Mehta and Sheth, 2006). Postpartum depression-its etiology is still unknown. Early postpartum hormone fluctuations, tryptophan metabolism, or modifications in membrane transport may all be linked to "maternity blues.". A woman with moderate to severe symptoms is likely susceptible to depression due to hereditary factors, upbringing, early experiences, personality, or social circumstances, in addition to experiencing these same somatic changes. Some women who suffer from this disorder lament their husbands' lack of support and marital discontent. Postpartum depression is most likely the result of a confluence of hormonal, metabolic, and psychosocial factors. Depending on how severe the condition is, postpartum depression is treated differently. Antidepressant medication, supportive psychotherapy, group therapy, and possibly family therapy are all possible treatments for psychotic depression. Supportive psychotherapy and ongoing help with home management can help relieve moderate depression symptoms until they go away. The only treatment for "maternity blues" is usually a word of comfort from the doctor or nurse that these emotions are normal and will pass quickly. Additional consolation and support from significant others is also crucial.

9.6. Application of the Nursing Process

9.6.1. Background Assessment Data

Depression symptoms can be categorized along a spectrum based on how severe the condition is. Everyone experiences depression from time to time. These are the fleeting signs that go along with life's regular setbacks. Breaking up with a boyfriend or girlfriend or failing an exam are two examples of disappointments. The momentary depressive symptoms go away rather quickly as the person works toward other objectives. When the loss of a valuable item sets off the grieving process, mild depressive episodes transpire. This can happen when you lose a home, a significant other, a pet, or a loved one. After going through the grieving process, the loss is acknowledged, symptoms go away, and after a few weeks, daily activities can be resumed. If this doesn't happen, the symptoms worsen and the grieving process is prolonged or exaggerated.

When mourning is prolonged or exaggerated, moderate depression develops. Anger is directed inward toward oneself as the person becomes stuck in the anger phase of the grieving process. The person exaggerates all of the typical grieving emotions to the point of being unable to function without help. One instance of mild depression is dysthymic disorder. A worsening of the symptoms linked to a moderate level of depression is known as severe depression. Serious depression can also manifest as a disconnection from reality in the affected person. Suicidal thoughts are frequently entertained at this level, which is linked to an absolute lack of enjoyment in all activities. An instance of severe depression is a major depressive disorder. Four domains of human functioning—affective, behavioral, cognitive, and physiological—can be altered by depressive symptoms. The degree of severity of symptomatology influences the changes within these spheres.

9.6.1.1. Transient Depression

Symptoms at this level of the continuum are not necessarily dysfunctional. Alterations include the following:

- **Affective**: Sadness, dejection, feeling downhearted, having the "blues"'
- **Behavioral:** Some crying is possible;
- **Cognitive:** Some difficulty getting mind off of one's disappointment;
- **Physiological:** Feeling tired and listless.

9.6.1.2. Mild Depression

Symptoms at the mild level of depression are identified by those associated with normal grieving. Alterations at the mild level include the following:

- **Affective:** Denial of feelings, anger, anxiety, guilt, helplessness, hopelessness, sadness, despondency
- **Behavioral:** Tearfulness, regression, restlessness, agitation, withdrawal
- **Cognitive:** Preoccupation with the loss, self-blame, ambivalence, blaming others
- **Physiological:** Anorexia or overeating, insomnia or hypersomnia, headache, backache, chest pain, or other symptoms associated with the loss of a significant other.

9.6.1.3. Moderate Depression

A more problematic disturbance is dysthymic disorder, which is an example of moderate depression. (Figure 9.1).Symptoms associated with this disorder include the following:

- **Affective:** Feelings of sadness, dejection, helplessness, powerlessness, hopelessness' gloomy and pessimistic outlook' low self-esteem' difficulty experiencing pleasure in activities.

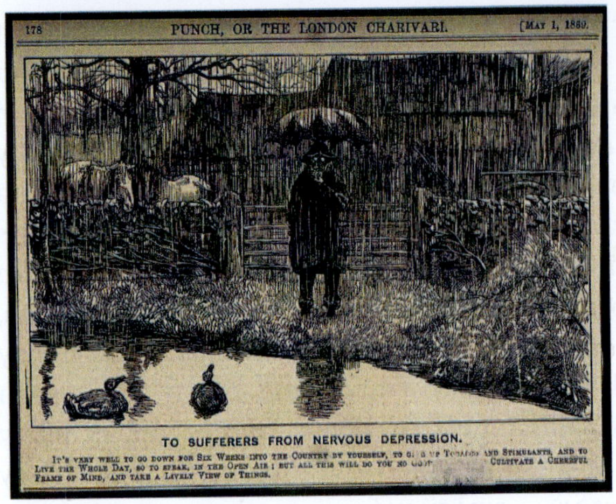

Figure 9.1. *A continuum of depression.*

Source: By https://wellcomeimages.org/indexplus/obf_images/25/74/c53e54147ac535b0b7bba3d96ef8.jpgGallery: https://wellcomeimages.org/indexplus/image/V0011388.htmlWellcome Collection gallery (2018-03-21): https://wellcomecollection.org/works/cwpqt4df CC-BY-4.0, Public Domain, https://commons.wikimedia.org/w/index.php?curid=36463277.

- **Behavioral:** Reduced kinetic energy (i.e. psychomotor retardation)' hunched posture' sluggish speech' limited verbalizations, potentially comprising of self-centered thoughts about past mistakes or regrets' social disengagement with an emphasis on oneself' potential for increased substance use' potential for self-destructive behavior' and diminished interest in personal grooming and hygiene.
- **Cognitive:** Thinking processes that are delayed' trouble focusing and maintaining focus' recurrent, obsessive thoughts that are usually depressing' verbalizations and actions indicative of suicidal thoughts.

- **Physiological:** Anorexia, overeating, hypersomnia, insomnia, headaches, backaches, chest pain, abdominal pain, low energy, exhaustion, and listlessness' feeling best in the morning and getting worse throughout the day' amenorrhea' decreased libido' and so on. This might be connected to the fluctuations in neurotransmitter levels throughout the day that impact mood and activity level.

9.6.1.4. Severe Depression

The symptoms of moderate depression are characterized by an intensification in cases of severe depression. Bipolar depression and major depressive disorder are two instances of severe depression.

Symptoms at the severe level of depression include the following:

- **Affective:** Sensations of complete hopelessness, worthlessness, and despair' a flat, emotionless facial expression' a general sense of emptiness and nothingness' apathy' loneliness' melancholy' and the incapacity to experience pleasure.
- **Behavioral:** Psychomotor behavior can take many forms, such as rapid, agitated, purposeless movements' slumped posture' sitting curled up' slow, rigid walking' virtually nonexistent communication (when verbalizations do occur, they may reflect delusional thinking)' lack of personal hygiene and grooming' and social isolation, which is common with virtually no inclination toward interaction with others. Psychomotor retardation can be so severe that physical movement can literally come to a standstill.
- **Cognitive:** Frequent delusional thinking' confusion, indecision, and difficulty focusing' hallucinations that represent incorrect interpretations of the surroundings' excessive self-blame, self-deprecation, and suicidal thoughts' delusions of persecution and somatic delusions being typical.

Because of the low energy level and retarded thought processes, the individual may be unable to follow through on suicidal ideas. However, the desire is strong at this level.

- **Physiological:** General slowdown of the entire body, reflected in sluggish digestion, constipation, and urinary retention' amenorrhea' impotence' diminished libido' anorexia' weight loss' difficulty falling asleep and awakening very early in the morning' feeling worse early in the morning and somewhat better as the day progresses. As with moderate depression, this may reflect the diurnal variation in the level of neurotransmitters that affect mood and activity.

9.6.2. Diagnosis/Outcome Identification

The nurse fills out the client database with the data gathered from the assessment, which is then used to choose the most appropriate nursing diagnoses. When planning care for a depressed client, Table 9.1 lists common client behaviors along with the NANDA nursing diagnoses that go along with them.

9.6.2.1. Outcome Criteria

The following criteria may be used for measurement of outcomes in the care of the depressed client which includes:

- The Client:
  - Has experienced no physical harm to self.
  - Discusses the loss with staff and family members.
  - No longer idealizes or obsesses about the lost object.
  - Sets realistic goals for self.
  - Is no longer afraid to attempt new activities.
  - Is able to identify aspects of self-control over life situation.
  - Expresses personal satisfaction and support from spiritual practices.
  - Interacts willingly and appropriately with others.
  - Is able to maintain reality orientation.
  - Is able to concentrate, reason, and solve problems.
  - Eats a well-balanced diet with snacks, to prevent weight loss and maintain nutritional status.
  - Sleeps 6 to 8 hours per night and reports feeling well rested.
  - Bathes, washes and combs hair, and dresses in clean clothing without assistance.

Table 9.1. *Assigning Nursing Diagnoses to Behaviors Commonly Associated With Depression*

BEHAVIORS	NURSING DIAGNOSES
Depressed mood; feelings of hopelessness and worthlessness; anger turned inward on the self; misinterpretations of reality; suicidal ideation, plan, and available means	Risk for suicide
Depression, preoccupation with thoughts of loss, self-blame, grief avoidance, inappropriate expression of anger, decreased functioning in life roles	Complicated grieving
Expressions of helplessness, uselessness, guilt, and shame; hypersensitivity to slight or criticism; negative, pessimistic outlook; lack of eye contact; self-negating verbalizations	Low self-esteem
Apathy, verbal expressions of having no control, dependence on others to fulfill needs	Powerlessness
Expresses anger toward God, expresses lack of meaning in life, sudden changes in spiritual practices, refuses interactions with significant others or with spiritual leaders	Spiritual distress
Withdrawn, uncommunicative, seeks to be alone, dysfunctional interaction with others, discomfort in social situations	Social isolation/Impaired social interaction
Inappropriate thinking, confusion, difficulty concentrating, impaired problem-solving ability, inaccurate interpretation of environment, memory deficit	Disturbed thought processes*
Weight loss, poor muscle tone, pale conjunctiva and mucous membranes, poor skin turgor, weakness	Imbalanced nutrition: Less than body requirements
Difficulty falling asleep, difficulty staying asleep, lack of energy, difficulty concentrating, verbal reports of not feeling well rested	Insomnia
Uncombed hair, disheveled clothing, offensive body odor	Self-care deficit (hygiene, grooming)

Source: https://ia800602.us.archive.org/18/items/EssentialsOfPsychiatricMentalHealthNursing-Townsend/PsychBook.pdf.

9.7. Treatment Modalities for Depression

Individual Psychotherapy

Disrupted attachments play a role in the development of depression, and research has shown how important close and satisfying attachments are in preventing depression. The client's present interpersonal relationships are the main focus of interpersonal psychotherapy in light of this idea. The stages and treatments of interpersonal psychotherapy for the depressed patient are as follows.

- **Phase I:** The client is evaluated in the first phase to ascertain the severity of the illness. The patient is then fully informed about the type of depression, its frequency, pattern, and clinical course, as well as available treatment options. Interpersonal psychotherapy has been demonstrated to be more successful when combined with antidepressant medication in cases of severe depression. Throughout therapy, the client is encouraged to carry on working and engaging in routine activities. A mutually beneficial therapy agreement is worked out.
- **Phase II:** The goal of treatment during this stage is to assist the client in resolving complex grief reactions. This could entail helping to forge new connections, replacing the broken relationship temporarily, and resolving any ambivalence about the broken one. The resolution of interpersonal deficits that may impede the client's capacity to form or maintain interpersonal relationships, challenging role transitions at different developmental life cycles, and conflicts between the client and a significant other could all be additional treatment areas of focus.
- **Phase III:** The therapeutic alliance is broken during interpersonal psychotherapy's last stage. Interpersonal psychotherapy has proven effective in assisting depressed individuals in regaining improved social functioning by placing a strong emphasis on reassurance, emotional state clarification, interpersonal communication improvement, perception testing, and performance in interpersonal settings.

9.7.1. Group Therapy

An essential component of the multimodal treatment plan for the depressed patient is group therapy. After a period of acute illness has passed, support groups can offer a safe space for people to talk about personal issues that contribute to, sustain, or result from having a serious affective disorder. Peer support offers a sense of security while uncomfortable or awkward topics are discussed and handled. Certain groups serve specialized functions, such as monitoring medication-related problems or providing a platform for the dissemination of information about affective disorders and their treatments.

Members of support groups are able to better understand their condition and are actively encouraged to connect with others who share similar issues. When a person realizes that they are not the only ones going through an affective illness, a sense of hope is expressed. Another source of support for the depressed client is self-help groups. Typically run by peers, these groups are not intended to replace or compete with formal therapy. Their additional assistance often improves adherence to the prescribed treatment plan. Examples of self-help groups are the Depression and Bipolar Support Alliance (DBSA), Depressives Anonymous, Manic and Depressive Support Group, Recovery Inc., and New Images for Widows. Although self-help groups are not psychotherapy groups, they do provide important adjunctive support experiences, which often have therapeutic benefit for participants.

9.7.2. Family Therapy

Resolving the symptoms and restoring or initiating adaptive family functioning are the ultimate goals when working with the families of clients suffering from mood disorders. Similar to group therapy, a combination of pharmacotherapeutic and psychotherapeutic treatments seems to be the most successful strategy. Sadock and Sadock, (2007) state:

> If the disorder puts the patient's marriage or family dynamics in jeopardy, or if the family environment contributes to or perpetuates the mood disorder, family therapy may be necessary. Family therapy looks at how the mood-disordered family member contributes to the overall psychological health of the group as well as how the patient's symptoms are maintained by the family as a whole.

9.7.3. Cognitive Therapy

The goal of cognitive therapy is to help the patient learn how to manage cognitive distortions, which are thought to play a role in the emergence and persistence of mood disorders. According to the cognitive model, a trio of negative distortions pertaining to expectations of oneself, the environment, and the future characterize depression. The self is unjustly devalued, the surroundings and the things that take place in them are seen as unsatisfying, and there is little hope for the future. Rapid symptom relief, helping the client recognize dysfunctional thought and behavior patterns, and directing the client toward information and reasoning that successfully challenges the validity of the dysfunctional thinking are the main objectives of cognitive therapy. Therapy focuses on changing "automatic thoughts" that occur spontaneously and contribute to the distorted affect. Examples of automatic thoughts in depression include:

- **Personalizing:** "I'm the only one who failed."
- **All or Nothing:** "I'm a complete failure."
- **Mind Reading:** "He thinks I'm foolish."
- **Discounting Positives:** "The other questions were so easy. Any dummy could have gotten them right."

The customer is asked to provide evidence both in favor of and against the automatic thought. The client is then taken through the reasoning behind the inferences. An additional method is to assess what would probably occur if the client's automatic beliefs were accurate. The consequences' ramifications are then talked about. If one technique doesn't seem to work, clients shouldn't give up. No single method is effective for every client. He or she should be reassured that a variety of techniques are available, and that the client and therapist are free to investigate these options. Treatment outcomes for depression with cognitive therapy have been encouraging. According to Rupke, Blecke, and Renfrow (2006), there are instances in which cognitive therapy can be just as effective as antidepressant medication, if not more so. This is supported by the findings of multiple studies conducted on depressed clients.

9.7.4. Electroconvulsive Therapy

The use of electrical current to induce a grand mal (generalized) seizure is known as electroconvulsive therapy, or ECT. When used to treat severe depression and clients who are acutely suicidal, ECT is particularly effective. It also works well for clients who also have psychotic symptoms, psychomotor retardation, and neurovegetative changes, which include irregularities in energy, appetite, and sleep patterns. It is frequently only taken into consideration as a form of therapy after an antidepressant medication trial has failed.

9.7.4.1. Mechanism of Action

It is unclear how precisely ECT produces a therapeutic response. There are other theories, but the biochemical theory is the one that has received the greatest support. Numerous studies have shown that electrical stimulation causes a number of neurotransmitters' circulating levels to rise noticeably (Wahlund and von Rosen, 2003). These neurotransmitters include dopamine, norepinephrine, and serotonin' antidepressant medications also influence these biogenic amines. According to additional data, ECT may also raise glutamate and gamma-aminobutyric acid levels (Grover, Mattoo, & Gupta, 2005). Research on the mechanism behind ECT's effectiveness is still being conducted, and the findings are still up for debate.

9.7.4.2. Side Effects

Transient confusion and memory loss are the most frequent side effects of ECT. Opponents of the therapy contend that these alterations signify permanent harm to the brain. They are transient and reversible, according to supporters. Marangell, Silver, and Yudofsky (2003) state that there is currently no trustworthy evidence linking contemporary ECT to permanent memory loss. Some researchers have hypothesized that some patients may experience variable degrees of memory loss up to six or seven months after receiving ECT (Hall and Bensing, 2009' Popolos, 2009). The debate over whether to use bilateral or unilateral ECT is still going strong. Unilateral electrode placement reduces the degree of memory disruption, according to studies. But in order to equal bilateral ECT's effectiveness in treating depression, unilateral ECT frequently needs more sessions (Geddes, 2003).

9.7.4.3. Risks Associated With ECT

Mortality

According to studies, there are roughly two deaths from ECT for every 100,000 treatments (Marangell et al., 2003' Sadock and Sadock, 2007). Cardiovascular problems, such as acute myocardial infarction or cerebrovascular accident, are the primary cause of death with ECT, despite its rarity. These complications typically affect people whose heart health has already been compromised. In order to lower the morbidity and death rates linked to ECT, it is essential to assess and treat cardiovascular disease before beginning treatment.

Permanent Memory Loss

According to Marangell and colleagues (2003), the initial confusion and cognitive impairments brought on by ECT treatment are typically transient, lasting no more than half an hour. Some patients report that their memory is not as good as it was prior to receiving ECT, while many report no memory problems at all, with the exception of the period immediately following the treatments. As of yet, trustworthy data have not demonstrated that current ECT causes irreversible memory loss. Prospective brain magnetic resonance imaging and computed tomography studies reveal no evidence of structural alterations brought on by ECT. The findings of a long-term study of the clinical and cognitive outcomes in patients with major depression receiving ECT at seven facilities in the New York City metropolitan area were recently published by Sackeim et al. (2007). Subjects were assessed both six months and soon after the ECT course. Data showed a clear correlation between the type of electrode placement and electrical waveform used and cognitive deficits at the 6-month mark. When compared to unilateral electrode placement, bilateral electrode placement caused more severe and long-lasting retrograde amnesia (as determined at the 6-month follow-up). The quantity of ECT treatments received was directly correlated with the degree of amnesia. Additionally, the researchers discovered that short-pulse wave (intermittent) current stimulation produced smaller short- and long-term deficits than sine wave (continuous) current stimulation.

Brain Damage

Even among those who maintain that ECT is a helpful and effective treatment for depression, there is still concern about brain damage from the procedure. ECT critics are steadfast in their conviction that the treatment always causes some degree of immediate brain damage (Frank, 2002). However, the majority of the evidence comes from animal studies where the participants received excessive electrical dosages and the seizures remained unaltered by oxygenation and muscle paralysis (Abrams, 2002). There is no proof that ECT causes any long-term changes in the structure or function of the brain, despite the fact that this is an area that needs more research (Sadock and Sadock, 2007).

9.7.4.4. Medications Used With ECT

There are several drugs connected to ECT. A pretreatment drug is injected intramuscularly about half an hour prior to the treatment, such as atropine sulfate or glycopyrrolate (Robinul). To reduce secretions and reverse the effects of vagal stimulation brought on by the ECT, a doctor may prescribe any one of these drugs. An intravenous short-acting anesthetic, such as methohexital sodium (Brevital) or thiopental sodium (Pentothal), is given by the anesthesiologist in the treatment room. To lessen the risk of fractured or dislocated bones, a muscle relaxant, typically succinylcholine chloride (Anectine), is injected intravenously to stop severe muscle contractions during the seizure. The client is oxygenated with pure oxygen during and after the treatment, with the exception of the brief electrical stimulation interval, until spontaneous respirations return, as succinylcholine also paralyzes respiratory muscles. (Prator, 2006)

9.7.5. Transcranial Magnetic Stimulation

For the treatment of depression, one of the more recent technologies is transcranial magnetic stimulation (TMS). The vast majority of research has been on the impact of TMS on major depression, but it is also being investigated in the treatment of mania, schizophrenia, obsessive compulsive disorder, post-traumatic stress disorder, and other disorders (Pridmore et al., 2001). Using extremely brief magnetic energy pulses, TMS stimulates brain nerve cells in a manner akin to the electrical activity seen with electrical shock therapy (ECT). But unlike ECT, TMS's electrical waves don't cause widespread seizure activity (Rosenbaum and Judy, 2004). The waves are directed toward the parts of the brain responsible for controlling mood via a coil applied to the scalp. While some medical professionals are skeptical, others think TMS has a lot of potential for treating depression. TMS therapy has infrequently been known to cause seizures (Rosenbaum & Judy, 2004). Researchers compared the effectiveness of TMS and ECT in treating severe depression in a recent study conducted at King's College in London (Eranti et al., 2007). They came to the conclusion that ECT was significantly more successful in treating depression in the short term, and they recommended more thorough clinical testing of TMS.

9.7.6. Light Therapy

A seasonal pattern is seen in 15%–25% of individuals with recurrent depressive disorder, where symptoms worsen in the winter and get better in the spring and summer (Thase, 2007). Major Depressive Disorder with Seasonal Pattern is the DSM-IV-TR's classification for this illness. The term Seasonal Affective Disorder (SAD) is a common one. According to Karasu et al. (2006), bright-light therapy has been recommended as a first-line treatment for the winter "blues" and as an adjunct in chronic major depressive disorder or dysthymia with seasonal exacerbations.

The pineal gland's production of the hormone melatonin is thought to be connected to SAD. The biological cycles for activation and sleep are regulated in part by melatonin. It produces itself during the dark cycle and stops during the day. Melatonin production rises during the months with longer dark hours, and this appears to set off the symptoms of SAD in those who are vulnerable.

It has been demonstrated that exposure to light, or light therapy, is a successful treatment for SAD. A 10,000-lux light box that blocks ultraviolet light with a plastic screen covers white fluorescent light tubes is used to administer the light therapy. The person opens his or her eyes and sits in front of the box, but not in direct line with the light. Sessions in therapy typically start out at 10 to 15 minutes and go up to 30 to 45 minutes over time. While some people experience improvement quickly—within a few days—others may not feel better for several weeks. Headache, eyestrain, nausea, irritability, photophobia (sensitivity of the eyes to light), insomnia (when light therapy is used late in the day), and (rarely) hypomania are side effects that seem to be related to dosage (Terman and Terman, 2005). Studies on the treatment of SAD have demonstrated similar efficacy between light therapy and antidepressants. In one recent study, the effectiveness of 20 mg of fluoxetine taken daily against light therapy for SAD was compared (Lam et al., 2006). The authors came to the following conclusion: "There were no other significant differences in outcome between light therapy and antidepressant medication, but light treatment showed earlier response onset and lower rate of some adverse events relative to fluoxetine."

9.7.7. Psychopharmacology

9.7.7.1. Historical Aspects

The genesis of antidepressant medication was coincidental. Iproniazid, a monoamine oxidase inhibitor (MAOI), was used to treat tuberculosis patients in the early 1950s. Despite the medication's ineffectiveness in treating tuberculosis, patients showed a persistent improvement in their mood while taking it (Schatzberg, Cole, and DeBattista, 2007). Because of their perceived low risk-benefit ratio, MAOIs lost some of their initial appeal and were largely ignored for almost 20 years.

The introduction of tricyclic antidepressants (TCAs) was comparable. Iripramine was studied as a potential treatment for schizophrenia in the late 1950s' while it didn't reduce psychotic symptoms, it did seem to improve mood. Tricyclic antidepressants, or TCAs, have been used extensively to treat depression for nearly 50 years. They have undergone hundreds of controlled trials since the discovery of their antidepressant qualities, and their effectiveness in treating depressive illness is now well established. Due to the initial two groups of antidepressants' success, the pharmaceutical industry began looking for compounds that would be just as effective as the MAOIs and TCAs, but with less side effects.

9.7.7.2. Indications

Antidepressant medications are used to treat a variety of conditions, including mental retardation, organic disease, alcoholism, schizophrenia, major depression with melancholia or psychotic symptoms, depressive phase of bipolar disorder, and depression with accompanying anxiety. These medications improve mood and lessen additional symptoms linked to moderate-to-severe depression. Premenstrual dysphoric disorder, bulimia nervosa, and anxiety disorders are also treated with specific agents.

9.7.7.3. Action

In the end, these medications aim to raise the body's levels of dopamine, serotonin, and/or norepinephrine. This is achieved in the brain by preventing these neurotransmitters (TCAs, heterocyclics, SSRIs, and SNRIs) from being reabsorbed by the neurons. It also happens when monoamine oxidase (MAOIs), an enzyme that is known to deactivate dopamine, serotonin, and norepinephrine, is inhibited at different locations throughout the nervous system.

9.7.7.4. Contraindications/Precautions

Hypersensitive people should not take antidepressant medications. When someone has angle-closure glaucoma or is in the acute phase of recovery after a myocardial infarction, TCAs should not be used. Concurrent use of MAOIs and TCAs, heterocyclics, SSRIs, and SNRIs is contraindicated. When giving these medications to elderly or disabled patients as well as those with renal, cardiac, or hepatic insufficiency, caution should be exercised. Usually, the dosage needs to be lowered. Additionally, caution is needed when dealing with clients who are psychotic, have benign prostatic hypertrophy, or have a history of seizures (which may lower the seizure threshold).

9.7.7.5. Interactions

Tricyclic Antidepressants

- Increased effects of tricyclic antidepressants may occur with bupropion, cimetidine, haloperidol, SSRIs, and valproic acid.
- Decreased effects of tricyclic antidepressants may occur with carbamazepine, barbiturates, and rifamycins (Table 9.2).

Table 9.2. *Selected Antidepressants (OTC Drugs or Dietary Supplements) Available in Poland*

Brand Name	Marketing Authorization Holder	Pharmaceutical Form	Active Ingredients (per Dose)	Dosage	Declared Effects by MAH
MIRALO	USP Zdrowie, Warszawa	Capsules	100 mg *Withania somnifera* (ashwagandha) extract (7 mg withanolides), 28 mg saffron stigma extract (0.84 mg crocin and 0.56 mg safranal), 100 mg lemon balm extract (2 mg rosemary acid)	1 capsule a day	Improves mood, helps maintain a state of relaxation, contributes to emotional balance.
JASNUM MOOD	USP Zdrowie, Warszawa	Capsules	30 mg saffron stigma extract, vitamin B6 (1.4 mg), vitamin B12 (100 µg)	1 capsule a day	Alleviates hormonal disorders during menopause that cause mood swings.
DEPRIBON	Bonimed, Żywiec	Capsules	150 mg of St. John's wort extract, 50 mg of Ginseng root extract	1 capsule a day	Improves mood.
INTRACTUM HYPERICI	Phyto Pharm, Klęka	Liquid	Ethanol extract of *Hypericum perforatum*L., *herba* (fresh St. John's wort) *Hyperici herbae recentis intractum* (1:1). Extraction solvent: ethanol 96% (*v/v*)	4 times a day, 5 mL of the preparation in a small amount of liquid. The recommended treatment time is 4 weeks.	Traditional herbal medicine used to relieve temporary states of nervous exhaustion. It also relieves depression.
DEPRESANUM	Novascon, Warszawa	Coated tablets	Inositol 100 mg, L-tryptophan 100 mg, saffron flower extract 15 mg, vitamin B6 0.210 mg, folic acid 100 µg	1 tablet 2 times a day during a meal	Helps maintain a positive mood, reduces fatigue and tiredness, improves nervous system function.
SZAFRACEUM	Lekam, Warszawa	Tablets	Saffron extract 30 mg, inositol 100 mg, L-tryptophan 50 mg, ginseng root extract 50 mg, vitamin B6 1.3 mg, vitamin B2 1.3 mg, vitamin B12 2.5 µg, folic acid 200 µg	1 tablet a day	Helps maintain a positive mood, supports the maintenance of emotional balance.

Brand Name	Marketing Authorization Holder	Pharmaceutical Form	Active Ingredients (per Dose)	Dosage	Declared Effects by MAH
DEPRELLA	Organic Pharma, Warszawa	Capsules	L-tryptophan 150 mg, L-phenylalanine 150 mg, turmeric extract (*Curcuma longa*) 10:1–100 mg, saffron crocus extract 30 mg, vitamin D (cholecalciferol) 5 µg, vitamin B6 (pyridoxine hydrochloride) 1.4 mg, vitamin B9 (pteroylmonoglutamic acid) 200 µg, vitamin B12 (cyanocobalamin) 2.5 µg	1 capsule a day	Improves mood and has an antidepressant effect by using the bio-potential of a harmonious combination of ingredients that support the production of neurotransmitters and happiness hormones and the transmission of nerve impulses. The composition is enriched with the addition of B vitamins, essential for the proper functioning of the nervous system and the maintenance of mental balance.
ALINESS	MedicaLine, Karczew	Tablets	Cultivated saffron crocus extract (*Crocus sativus*) SafraSOL 30 mg, including crocin 3 mg, safranal 600 µg	1–3 tablets a day during or after a meal with water	Improves mood, helps maintain emotional balance, improves libido, helps maintain comfort before and during the menstrual cycle.
HYPERHERBA	Labofarm, Starogard Gdański	Tablets	30 mg *Hypericum perforatum* L., *herba* (St. John's wort)	1 tablet 3 times a day with water	Traditionally used to relieve temporary symptoms of mental exhaustion.
DEPREMIN	Colfarm, Mielec	Coated tablets	612 mg of extract (in the form of a dry, quantified extract) from *Hypericum perforatum* L., *herba* (St. John's wort), which corresponds to: 0.6 mg–1.8 mg of total hypericin expressed as hypericin, 36.72 mg–91.80 mg of total flavonoids per rutin, not more than 36.72 mg of hyperforin Extraction solvent: ethanol 60% (*v/v*)	1 tablet a day	Used in the short-term treatment of mild depressive disorders.
MAGNOLIAMAX	K2Pharm, s.r.o. Opava, Czech Republic	Coated tablets	350 mg of magnolia bark extract 6% (21 mg honokiol), black pepper extract—5 mg	1 tablet a day	Supports restful sleep and helps maintain a good mood. Relieves fatigue and stress.

Source: Dobrek L, Głowacka K. Depression and Its Phytopharmacotherapy—A Narrative Review. International Journal of Molecular Sciences. 2023, 24(5), 4772. https://doi.org/10.3390/ijms24054772.

- Hyperpyretic crisis, convulsions, and death may occur with MAOIs.
- Coadministration with clonidine may produce hypertensive crisis.

- Decreased effects of levodopa and guanethidine may occur with tricyclic antidepressants.
- Potentiation of pressor response may occur with direct-acting sympathomimetics.
- Increased anticoagulation effects may occur with dicumarol.
- Increased serum levels of carbamazepine occur with concomitant use of tricyclics.
- Increased risk of seizures occurs with concomitant use of maprotiline and phenothiazines.

Monoamine Oxidase Inhibitors

- Serious, potentially fatal adverse reactions may occur with concurrent use of all other antidepressants, carbamazepine, cyclobenzaprine, buspirone, sympathomimetics, tryptophan, dextromethorphan, anesthetic agents, central nervous system (CNS) depressants, and amphetamines. Avoid using within 2 weeks of each other (5 weeks after therapy with fl uoxetine).
- Hypertensive crisis may occur with amphetamines, methyldopa, levodopa, dopamine, epinephrine, norepinephrine, guanethidine, guanadrel, reserpine, vasoconstrictors, or ingestion of tyramine-containing foods.
- Hypertension or hypotension, coma, convulsions, and death may occur with opioids (avoid use of meperidine within 14 to 21 days of MAOI therapy).
- Excess CNS stimulation and hypertension may occur with methylphenidate.
- Additive hypotension may occur with antihypertensives, thiazide diuretics, or spinal anesthesia.
- Additive hypoglycemia may occur with insulins or oral hypoglycemic agents.
- Doxapram may increase pressor response.
- Serotonin syndrome may occur with concomitant use of St. John's wort.
- Hypertensive crisis may occur with ingestion of foods or other products containing high concentrations of tyramine.
- Consumption of foods or beverages with high caffeine content increases the risk of hypertension and arrhythmias.
- Bradycardia may occur with concurrent use of MAOIs and beta blockers.
- Risk of toxicity from the 5-HT-receptor agonists occurs with concurrent use of MAOIs.

Selective Serotonin Reuptake Inhibitors

- Toxic, sometimes fatal, reactions have occurred with concomitant use of MAOIs.
- Increased effects of SSRIs occur with cimetidine, l-tryptophan, lithium, linezolid, and St. John's wort.
- Serotonin syndrome may occur with concomitant use of SSRIs and metoclopramide, sibutramine, tramadol, or 5-HT-receptor agonists (triptans).

- Concomitant use of SSRIs may increase effects of hydantoins, tricyclic antidepressants, cyclosporine, benzodiazepines, beta blockers, methadone, carbamazepine, clozapine, olanzapine, pimozide, haloperidol, phenothiazines, St. John's wort, sumatriptan, sympathomimetics, tacrine, theophylline, and warfarin.
- Concomitant use of SSRIs may decrease the effects of buspirone and digoxin.
- Lithium levels may be increased or decreased by concomitant use of SSRIs.
- Decreased effects of SSRIs occur with concomitant use of carbamazepine and cyproheptadine.

Others (Heterocyclics and SNRIs)

Table 9.3. *Common Antidepressants and Their Effect on Weight*

Class	Drug	Effect on Weight	Mechanisms Involved
SSRI	Fluoxetine	-, o	5-HT +, 5-HT_{2C} -, leptin +, cortisol -
	Sertraline	-, o	5-HT +, D +
	Paroxetine	+	5-HT +, M3 -
	Citalopram	+	5-HT +, H1 -
SNRI	Venlafaxine	-	5-HT +, α1 +
	Duloxetine	o	5-HT +, α1 +
NDRI	Bupropion	--	α +, D +
Atypical	Mirtazapine	++	H1 -, α2 -, 5-HT -
	Vortioxetine	o	5-HT +/-
	Agomelatine	o	5-HT +, MT1/2 +
MAOI	Moclobemide	o	monoamines +
	Selegiline	+	monoamines +, glucose -
	Phenelzine	+	monoamines +, glucose -
TCA	Clomipramine	+	H1 -, M3 -, α1 -
	Imipramine	+	H1 -, M3 -, α1 -
	Amitriptyline	++	H1 -, M3 -, α1 -

Source: Kukucka T, Ferencova N, Visnovcova Z, Ondrejka I, Hrtanek I, Kovacova V, Macejova A, Mlyncekova Z, Tonhajzerova I. Mechanisms Involved in the Link between Depression, Antidepressant Treatment, and Associated Weight Change. International Journal of Molecular Sciences. 2024, *25(8):4511. https://doi.org/10.3390/ijms25084511.*

+/- Indicate a Stimulating or Inhibitory Effect on the Relevant Target and o Indicates a Negligible Effect on Weight. Notably, the Biphasic Effect of Certain SSRIs Facilitated 5-HT2C Downregulation. Abbreviations: SSRI—Selective Serotonin Reuptake Inhibitors, SNRI—Serotonin and Noradrenaline Reuptake Inhibitors, NDRI—Noradrenaline and Dopamine Reuptake Inhibitors, NaSSA—Noradrenergic and Specific Serotonergic Antidepressants, MAOI—Monoamine Oxidase Inhibitors, TCA—Tricyclical Antidepressants.

- Concomitant use with MAOIs results in serious, sometimes fatal, effects resembling neuroleptic malignant syndrome. Coadministration is contraindicated.
- Serotonin syndrome may occur when any of the following are used together: St. John's wort, sibutramine, trazodone, nefazodone, venlafaxine, desvenlafaxine, duloxetine, SSRIs, 5-HT-receptor agonists (triptans).
- Increased effects of haloperidol, clozapine, and desipramine may occur when used concomitantly with venlafaxine.
- Increased effects of venlafaxine may occur with cimetidine.
- Increased effects of duloxetine may occur with CYP1A2 inhibitors (e.g., fluvoxamine, quinolone antibiotics) and CYP2D6 inhibitors (e.g., fluoxetine, quinidine, paroxetine).
- Increased risk of liver injury occurs with concomitant use of alcohol and duloxetine.
- Increased risk of toxicity or adverse effects from drugs extensively metabolized by CYP2D6 (e.g., flecainide, phenothiazines, propafenone, tricyclic antidepressants, thioridazine) occurs when used concomitantly with duloxetine, desvenlafaxine, or bupropion.
- Decreased effects of bupropion and trazodone may occur with carbamazepine.
- Altered anticoagulant effect of warfarin may occur with bupropion, venlafaxine, desvenlafaxine, duloxetine, or trazodone (Table 9.3).

9.7.7.6. Side Effects

The plan of care should include monitoring for the following side effects from antidepressant medications. Nursing implications related to each side effect are designated by an asterisk (*).

May Occur With All Chemical Classes

- Dry Mouth:
  - Offer the client sugarless candy, ice, frequent sips of water.
  - Strict oral hygiene is very important.
- Sedation:
  - Request an order from the physician for the drug to be given at bedtime.
  - Request that the physician decrease the dosage or perhaps order a less-sedating drug.
  - Instruct the client not to drive or use dangerous equipment while experiencing sedation.
- Nausea:
  - Medication may be taken with food to minimize GI distress.
- Discontinuation Syndrome:
  - The risk of discontinuation syndromes varies amongst antidepressant classes. After long-term SSRI, venlafaxine, desvenlafaxine, and duloxetine therapy, abrupt withdrawal can cause headache, nausea, dizziness, and lethargy. Fluoxetine's extended half-life makes withdrawal symptoms less likely to occur. Tricyclic withdrawal abruptly can result in panic

attacks, akathisia, hypomania, cardiac arrhythmias, and gastrointestinal distress. Flulike symptoms, disorientation, hypomania, and a worsening of depressive symptoms are all part of the discontinuation syndrome linked to MAOIs. To avoid withdrawal symptoms, all antidepressant medications should be tapered gradually (Schatzberg, Cole, and DeBattista, 2007).

Most Commonly Occur With Tricyclics and Heterocyclics

- Blurred Vision:
  - Offer reassurance that this symptom should subside after a few weeks.
  - Instruct the client not to drive until vision is clear.
  - Clear small items from routine pathway to prevent falls.
- Constipation:
  - Order foods high in fiber, increase fluid intake if not contraindicated, and encourage the client to increase physical exercise, if possible.
- Urinary Retention:
  - Instruct the client to report hesitancy or inability to urinate.
  - Monitor intake and output.
  - Try various methods to stimulate urination, such as running water in the bathroom or pouring water over the perineal area.
- Orthostatic Hypotension:
  - Instruct the client to rise slowly from a lying or sitting position.
  - Monitor blood pressure (lying and standing) frequently, and document and report significant changes.
  - Avoid long hot showers or tub baths.
- Reduction of Seizure Threshold:
  - Observe clients with history of seizures closely.
  - Institute seizure precautions as specified in hospital procedure manual.
  - Bupropion (Wellbutrin) should be administered in doses of no more than 150 mg and should be given at least 4 hours apart. Bupropion has been associated with a relatively high incidence of seizure activity in anorexic and cachectic clients.
- Tachycardia' Arrhythmias:
  - Carefully monitor blood pressure and pulse rate and rhythm, and report any significant change to the physician.
- Photosensitivity:
  - Ensure that client wears sunblock lotion, protective clothing, and sunglasses while outdoors.
- Weight Gain:
  - Provide instructions for a reduced-calorie diet.
  - Encourage increased level of activity, if appropriate.

Most Commonly Occur With SSRIs and SNRIs

- Insomnia' Agitation:
  - Administer or instruct the client to take a dose early in the day.
  - Instruct client to avoid caffeinated food and drinks.
  - Teach relaxation techniques to use before bedtime.
- Headache:
  - Administer analgesics, as prescribed.
  - If relief is not achieved, physician may order another antidepressant.
- Weight Loss (may Occur Early in Therapy):
  - Ensure that client is provided with caloric intake sufficient to maintain desired weight.
  - Caution should be taken in prescribing these drugs for anorectic clients.
  - Weigh client daily or every other day, at the same time and on the same scale, if possible.
  - After prolonged use, some clients may gain weight on these drugs.
- Sexual Dysfunction:
  - Men may report abnormal ejaculation or impotence.
  - Women may experience delay or loss of orgasm.
  - If side effect becomes intolerable, a switch to another antidepressant may be necessary.
- **Serotonin Syndrome:** (may occur when two drugs that potentiate serotonergic neurotransmission are used concurrently)
  - Most frequent symptoms include changes in mental status, restlessness, myoclonus, hyperreflexia, tachycardia, labile blood pressure, diaphoresis, shivering, and tremors.
  - Discontinue the offending agent immediately.
  - The physician may prescribe medications to block serotonin receptors, relieve hyperthermia and muscle rigidity, and prevent seizures. In severe cases, artificial ventilation may be required. The histamine-1 receptor antagonist cyproheptadine is commonly used to treat the symptoms of serotonin syndrome.
  - Supportive nursing measures include monitoring vital signs, providing safety measures to prevent injury when muscle rigidity and changes in mental status are present, cooling blankets and tepid baths to assist with temperature regulation, and monitoring intake and output.
  - The condition will usually resolve on its own once the offending medication has been discontinued. However, if left untreated, the condition may progress to life-threatening complications such as seizures, coma, hypotension, ventricular arrhythmias, disseminated intravascular coagulation,

rhabdomyolysis, metabolic acidosis, and renal failure. (Prator, 2006)

Most Commonly Occur With MAOIs

- Hypertensive Crisis:
  - Hypertensive crisis occurs if the individual consumes foods containing tyramine while receiving MAOI therapy.
  - Symptoms of hypertensive crisis include severe occipital headache, palpitations, nausea/ vomiting, nuchal rigidity, fever, sweating, marked increase in blood pressure, chest pain, and coma.
  - Treatment of hypertensive crisis includes discontinuing drug immediately' monitoring vital signs' administering short-acting antihypertensive medication, as ordered by physician' using external cooling measures to control hyperpyrexia.
- Application Site Reactions: (with selegiline transdermal system [Emsam])
  - The most common reactions include rash, itching, erythema, redness, irritation, swelling, or urticarial lesions. Most reactions resolve spontaneously, requiring no treatment. However, if reaction becomes problematic, it should be reported to the physician. Topical corticosteroids have been used in treatment.

Miscellaneous Side Effects

- **Priapism:** (with trazodone)
  - Priapism is a rare side effect, but it has occurred in some men taking trazodone.
  - If the client complains of prolonged or inappropriate penile erection, withhold medication dosage and notify the physician immediately.
  - Priapism can become very problematic, requiring surgical intervention, and, if not treated successfully, can result in impotence.
- **Hepatic Failure:** (with nefazodone)
  - Cases of life-threatening hepatic failure have been reported in clients treated with nefazodone.
  - Advise clients to be alert for signs or symptoms suggestive of liver dysfunction (e.g., jaundice, anorexia, GI complaints, or malaise) and to report them to physician immediately.

Client/Family Education Related to Antidepressants

The Client Should:

- Continue to take the medication even though the symptoms have not subsided. The therapeutic effect may not be seen for as long as 4 weeks. If after this length of time no improvement is noted, the physician may prescribe a different medication.
- Use caution when driving or

operating dangerous machinery. Drowsiness and dizziness can occur. If these side effects become persistent or interfere with activities of daily living, the client should report them to the physician. Dosage adjustment may be necessary.

- Not discontinue use of the drug abruptly. To do so might produce withdrawal symptoms, such as nausea, vertigo, insomnia, headache, malaise, nightmares, and return of symptoms for which the medication was prescribed.
- Use sunblock lotion and wear protective clothing when spending time outdoors. The skin may be sensitive to sunburn.
- Report occurrence of any of the following symptoms to the physician immediately: sore throat, fever, malaise, yellowish skin, unusual bleeding, easy bruising, persistent nausea/vomiting, severe headache, rapid heart rate, difficulty urinating, anorexia/ weight loss, seizure activity, stiff or sore neck, and chest pain.
- Rise slowly from a sitting or lying position to prevent a sudden drop in blood pressure.
- Take frequent sips of water, chew sugarless gum, or suck on hard candy if dry mouth is a problem. Good oral care (frequent brushing, flossing) is very important.
- Avoid consuming the following foods or medications while taking MAOIs: aged cheese, wine (especially Chianti), beer, chocolate, colas, coffee, tea, sour cream, smoked and processed meats, beef or chicken liver, canned figs, soy sauce, overripe and fermented foods, pickled herring, raisins, caviar, yogurt, yeast products, broad beans, cold remedies, diet pills. To do so could cause a life-threatening hypertensive crisis.
- Avoid smoking while receiving tricyclic therapy. Smoking increases the metabolism of tricyclics, requiring an adjustment in dosage to achieve the therapeutic effect.
- Avoid alcohol use while taking antidepressant therapy. These drugs potentiate the effects of each other.
- Avoid use of other medications (including over-the counter medications) without the physician's approval while receiving antidepressant therapy. Many medications contain substances that, in combination with antidepressant medication, could precipitate a life-threatening hypertensive crisis.
- Notify physician immediately if inappropriate or prolonged penile erections occur while taking trazodone. If the erection persists longer than 1 hour, seek emergency department treatment. This condition is rare, but has occurred in some men who have taken trazodone. If measures are not instituted immediately, impotence can result.
- Not "double up" on medication if a dose of bupropion (Wellbutrin) is missed, unless advised to do so by the physician. Taking bupropion in divided doses will decrease the risk of seizures and other adverse effects.

- Follow the correct procedure for applying the selegiline transdermal patch:
- Apply to dry, intact skin on upper torso, upper thigh, or outer surface of upper arm.
- Apply approximately the same time each day to a new spot on the skin, after removing and discarding old patch.
- Wash hands thoroughly after applying the patch.
- Avoid exposing application site to direct heat (e.g., heating pads, electric blankets, heat lamps, hot tub, or prolonged direct sunlight).
- If patch falls off, apply new patch to a new site and resume previous schedule.

Be aware of possible risks of taking antidepressants during pregnancy. Safe use during pregnancy and lactation has not been fully established. These drugs are believed to readily cross the placental barrier' if so, the fetus could experience adverse effects of the drug. Inform the physician immediately if pregnancy occurs, is suspected, or is planned.

Be aware of the side effects of antidepressants. Refer to written materials furnished by health-care providers for safe self-administration.

Carry a card or other identification at all times describing the medications being taken.

9.8. The Suicidal Client

Since mood disorders are linked to the majority of suicides, information about suicide is provided here. "Nearly 95% of all people who commit or attempt suicide have a diagnosed mental disorder," according to a 2007 study by Sadock and Sadock. 80% are caused by depressive disorders.

9.8.1. Epidemiological Factors

The annual suicide rate in the United States is estimated to be around 30,000. According to these data, suicide ranks third among young Americans aged 15 to 24 in terms of causes of death, behind homicide and accidents. Among those aged 25 to 34, it ranks second, and among those aged 35 to 44, fourth, and among those aged 45 to 54, it ranks eighth. These statistics were provided by the National Center for Injury Prevention and Control in 2009. Many more people seriously consider suicide than actually do so, and many more attempt suicide than succeed. Today, suicide is a significant health concern in the United States.

9.9. Application of the Nursing Process with the Suicidal Client

9.9.1. Assessment

When performing a suicidal assessment, the following factors should be taken into account: the individual's demographics, presenting symptoms, medical-psychiatric diagnosis, suicidal thoughts or acts, interpersonal support network, suicidal crisis analysis, psychiatric, medical, and family history, and coping mechanisms. In his "Call to Action to Prevent Suicide," the Surgeon General discusses risk factors and protective factors. While protective factors are linked to a lower chance of suicide, risk factors are linked to a higher likelihood of suicide and suicidal behavior.

9.9.1.1. Demographics

The following demographics are assessed:

- **Age:** Suicide is highest in persons over 50. Adolescents are also at high risk.
- **Gender:** Males are at higher risk than females.
- **Ethnicity:** Whites are at higher risk than are Native Americans, who are at higher risk than African Americans.
- **Marital Status:** Single, divorced, and widowed persons are at higher risk than married persons.
- **Socioeconomic Status:** Individuals in the highest and lowest socioeconomic classes are at higher risk than those in the middle classes.
- **Occupation:** Professional health-care personnel and business executives are at highest risk. Other high-risk occupations include law enforcement, attorneys, and mechanics (Sadock & Sadock, 2007) (Tables 9.4 and 9.5).

Table 9.4. *Facts and Fables about Suicide*

FABLES	FACTS
People who talk about suicide do not commit suicide. Suicide happens without warning.	Eight out of 10 people who kill themselves have given definite clues and warnings about their suicidal intentions. Very subtle clues may be ignored or disregarded by others.
You cannot stop a suicidal person. He or she is fully intent on dying.	Most suicidal people are very ambivalent about their feelings regarding living or dying. Most are "gambling with death" and see it as a cry for someone to save them.
Once a person is suicidal, he or she is suicidal forever.	People who want to kill themselves are only suicidal for a limited time. If they are saved from feelings of self-destruction, they can go on to lead normal lives.
Improvement after severe depression means that the suicidal risk is over.	Most suicides occur within about 3 months after the beginning of "improvement," when the individual has the energy to carry out suicidal intentions.
Suicide is inherited, or "runs in families."	Suicide is not inherited. It is an individual matter and can be prevented. However, suicide by a close family member increases an individual's risk factor for suicide.
All suicidal individuals are mentally ill, and suicide is the act of a psychotic person.	Although suicidal persons are extremely unhappy, they are not necessarily psychotic. They are merely unable at that point in time to see an alternative solution to what they consider an unbearable problem.
Suicidal threats and gestures should be considered manipulative or attention-seeking behavior, and should not be taken seriously.	All suicidal behavior must be approached with the gravity of the potential act in mind. Attention should be given to the possibility that the individual is issuing a cry for help.
People usually commit suicide by taking an overdose of drugs.	Gunshot wounds are the leading cause of death among suicide victims.
If an individual has attempted suicide, he or she will not do it again.	Between 50% and 80% of all people who ultimately kill themselves have a history of a previous attempt.

Source: Adapted from Friends for Survival (2009)' The Samaritans (2009)' and USPHS (1999).

Table 9.5. *Suicide Risk Factors and Protective Factors*

RISK FACTORS	PROTECTIVE FACTORS
• Previous suicide attempt • Mental disorders—particularly mood disorders such as depression and bipolar disorder • Co-occurring mental and alcohol and substance abuse disorders • Family history of suicide • Hopelessness • Impulsive and/or aggressive tendencies • Barriers to accessing mental health treatment • Relational, social, work, or financial loss • Physical illness • Easy access to lethal methods, especially guns • Unwillingness to seek help because of stigma attached to mental and substance abuse disorders and/or suicidal thoughts • Influence of significant people—family members, celebrities, peers who have died by suicide—both through direct personal contact or inappropriate media representations • Cultural and religious beliefs—for instance, the belief that suicide is a noble resolution of a personal dilemma • Local epidemics of suicide that have a contagious influence • Isolation, a feeling of being cut off from other people	• Effective and appropriate clinical care for mental, physical, and substance abuse disorders • Easy access to a variety of clinical interventions and support for help seeking • Restricted access to highly lethal methods of suicide • Family and community support • Support from ongoing medical and mental health care relationships • Learned skills in problem solving, conflict resolution, and nonviolent handling of disputes • Cultural and religious beliefs that discourage suicide and support self-preservation instincts

Source: https://ia800602.us.archive.org/18/items/EssentialsOfPsychiatricMentalHealthNursing-Townsend/PsychBook.pdf.

- **Method:** Use of fi rearms presents a significantly higher risk than overdose of substances.
- **Religion:** Protestants are at greater risk than Catholics or Jews.
- **Family History:** Higher risk exists if the individual has a family history of suicide.

9.9.1.2. Presenting Symptoms/ Medical-Psychiatric Diagnosis

Any physical or mental health issue that the client is receiving treatment for requires the collection of assessment data. The most common disorders that precede suicide are mood disorders, specifically major depression and bipolar disorder. Addicts suffering from substance abuse disorders are also highly vulnerable. Anxiety disorders, schizophrenia, borderline and antisocial personality disorders, and other psychiatric disorders may also carry a risk of suicide (Tondo and Baldessarini, 2001). Suicidal thoughts and actions have also been sparked by other chronic and terminal medical conditions.

9.9.1.3. Suicidal Ideas or Acts

People may give away their intentions through both their words and their actions. Behavioral clues can take various forms, such as selling valuable items, organizing finances, making suicide notes, or experiencing abrupt mood swings that could signify a decision to carry out the intended action. There are two types of verbal cues: direct and indirect. Statements like "I want to die" or "I'm going to kill myself" are examples of direct statements. "This is the last time you'll see me," "I won't be around much longer for the doctor to worry about," and "I don't have anything worth living for anymore" are a few examples of indirect statements. Other evaluations involve figuring out whether the person has a plan and, if so, whether they have the resources to execute it. If the suicide will be carried out with a gun, does the person have access to a gun and ammunition? If the person plans to take pills, are they readily available and of what kind?

9.9.1.4. Interpersonal Support System

A person at high risk of suicide during an emotional crisis may not have a meaningful network of satisfying relationships. Does the person have people they can rely on for support when things get tough?

9.9.1.5. Analysis of the Suicidal Crisis

The Precipitating Stressor

Suicide may result from unfavorable life events combined with other risk factors like depression. Stressors in life that are linked to an increase in emotional disturbance include the death or divorce of a loved one, issues in significant relationships, role changes, or a serious physical illness.

Relevant History

Has the individual experienced numerous failures or rejections that would increase his or her vulnerability for a dysfunctional response to the current situation?

Life-Stage Issues

When losses and disappointments happen at times in a person's life when they are dealing with developmental issues, such as adolescence or midlife, their capacity to tolerate them is frequently weakened.

9.9.1.6. Psychiatric/Medical/Family History

The patient needs to have any prior mental health treatment for depression, alcoholism, or suicide attempts evaluated. It is important to get a medical history in order to rule out the existence of terminal, incapacitating, or chronic illnesses. Does the family have a history of depression, and has a close relative ever taken their own life?

9.9.2. Diagnosis/Outcome Identification

Nursing diagnoses for the suicidal client may include the following:

- Risk for suicide related to feelings of hopelessness and desperation;
- Hopelessness related to the absence of support systems and perception of worthlessness.

The following criteria may be used for the measurement of outcomes in the care of the suicidal client which includes:

The Client:

- Has experienced no physical harm to self;
- Sets realistic goals for self;
- Expresses some optimism and hope for the future.

9.9.3. Planning/Implementation

Nursing diagnoses are presented, along with outcome criteria, appropriate nursing interventions, and rationales for each.

9.9.3.1. Intervention with the Outpatient Suicidal Client (or Following Discharge from Inpatient Care)

Sometimes it can be found that there is little suicidal intent and no hospitalization is necessary. The client who is contemplating suicide could instead receive treatment in an outpatient environment. Guidelines for treatment of the suicidal client on an outpatient basis include the following.

- The person should not be left alone. Arrangements must be made for the client to stay with family or friends. If this is not possible, hospitalization should be reconsidered.
- Make a no-suicide agreement with the customer. Create a formal agreement in writing promising the client not to hurt themselves within a predetermined time frame. The client might write, "I will call the suicide hotline (or go to the emergency room) if I start to feel like harming myself," or "I will not harm myself in any way between now and the time of our next counseling session". A new contract is negotiated after the term of this short-term agreement has passed.
- Enlist the help of family or friends to ensure that the home environment is safe from dangerous items, such as fi rearms or stockpiled drugs. Give support persons the telephone number of counselor or emergency contact person in the event that the counselor is not available.
- Appointments may need to be scheduled daily or every other day at first until the immediate suicidal crisis has subsided.
- Establish rapport and promote a trusting relationship. It is important for the suicide counselor to become a key person in the client's support system at this time.
- Discuss the current crisis in the client's life. Use the problem-solving approach. Offer alternatives to suicide. Macnab (1993) suggests the following statements: you are incorrect in your idea that suicide is the only and the best solution to your problem. There are alternatives, and they are good. What is more, you will be alive to test them.
- Help the client identify areas of the life situation that are within his or her control and those that the client does not have the ability to control. Discuss feelings associated with these control issues. It is important for the client to feel some control over his or her life situation in order to perceive a measure of self-worth.
- The physician may prescribe antidepressants for an individual who is experiencing suicidal depression. It is wise to prescribe no more than a 3-day supply of the medication with no refills. The prescription can then be renewed at the client's next counseling session.

As the depression lifts, patients become energized and are thus able to put their suicidal plans into action. Sometimes, depressed patients, with or without treatment, suddenly appear to be at peace with themselves because they have reached a secret decision to commit suicide. Clinicians should be especially suspicious of such a dramatic clinical change, which may portend a suicidal attempt.

- Macnab (1993) suggests the following steps in crisis counseling with the suicidal client are:
    - Focus on the current crisis and how it can be alleviated.

Identify the client's appraisals of how things are and how things will be. Note how these appraisals change in changing contexts.

- Note the client's reactivity to the crisis and how this can be changed. Discuss strategies and procedures for the management of anxiety, anger, and frustration.
- Work toward restoration of the client's self-worth, status, morale, and control. Introduce alternatives to suicide.
- Rehearse cognitive reconstruction—more positive ways of thinking about the self, events, the past, the present, and the future.
- Identify experiences and actions that affirm self-worth and self-efficacy.
- Encourage movement toward the new reality, with the coping skills required to manage adaptively.
- Be available for ongoing therapeutic support and growth.

9.9.3.2. Information for Family and Friends of the Suicidal Client

The following suggestions are made for family and friends of an individual who is suicidal.

- Take any hint of suicide seriously. Anyone expressing suicidal feelings needs immediate attention.
- Do not keep secrets. If a suicidal person says, "Promise you won't tell anyone," do not make that promise. Suicidal individuals are ambivalent about dying, and suicidal behavior is a cry for help. It is that ambivalence that leads the person to confide to you the suicidal thoughts. Get help for the person and for you: find a national hotline that is available 24 hours a day.
- Be a good listener. If people express suicidal thoughts or feel depressed, hopeless, or worthless, be supportive. Let them know you are there for them and are willing to help them seek professional help.
- Many people find it awkward to put into words how another person's life is important for their own wellbeing, but it is important to stress that the person's life is important to you and to others. Emphasize in specific terms the ways in which the person's suicide would be devastating to you and to others.
- Express concern for individuals who express thoughts about committing suicide. The individual may be withdrawn and reluctant to discuss what he or she is thinking. Acknowledge the person's pain and feelings of hopelessness, and encourage the individual to talk to someone else if he or she does not feel comfortable talking with you.
- Familiarize yourself with suicide intervention sources, such as mental health centers and suicide hotlines.
- Restrict access to fi rearms or other means of self harm.

9.9.3.3. Intervention with Families and Friends of Suicide Victims

Fraser (2006) notes that a sudden and, for the most part, unexpected shattering of life occurs for many people in a post-suicide situation. The family of a suicide victim bears an additional burden in addition to the sadness and loss brought on by the death of a close relative. Their unexpected arrival in a different social environment adds to that load. Their personal grief has a public face, and they must deal with it and express their grief in a social setting with minimal frameworks for understanding their situation. They have to fight as hard as they can with the internal resources they have, which have been greatly diminished by this sad event.

Suicide of a family member can induce a whole gamut of feelings in the survivors. Macnab (1993) identifies the following symptoms, which may be evident following the suicide of a loved one are:

- A sense of guilt and responsibility.
- Anger, resentment, and rage that can never find its "object."
- A heightened sense of emotionality, helplessness, failure, and despair.
- A recurring self-searching: "If only I had done something," "If only I had not done something," "If only."
- A sense of confusion and search for an explanation: "Why did this happen?" "What does it mean?" "What could have stopped it?" "What will people think?"
- A sense of inner injury. The family feels wounded. They do not know how they will ever get over it and get on with life.
- A severe strain is placed on relationships. A sense of impatience, irritability, and anger exists between family members.
- A heightened vulnerability to illness and disease exists with this added burden of emotional stress.

Strategies for assisting survivors of suicide victims include the following:

- Encourage the clients to talk about the suicide, each responding to the others' viewpoints and reconstruction of events. Share memories.
- Be aware of any blaming or scapegoating of specific family members. Discuss how each person fits into the family situation, both before and after the suicide.
- Listen to feelings of guilt and self-persecution. Gently move the individuals toward the reality of the situation.
- Encourage the family members to discuss individual relationships with the lost loved one. Focus on both positive and negative aspects of the relationships. Gradually point out the irrationality of any idealized concepts of the deceased person. The family must be able to recognize both positive and negative aspects about the person before grief can be resolved.
- No two people grieve in the same way. It may appear that some family members are "getting over" the grief faster than others. All family members must be made to understand that if this occurs, it is not because they "care less," just that they "grieve differently." Variables that enter into this

phenomenon include individual past experiences, personal relationship with the deceased person, and individual temperament and coping abilities.

- Recognize how the suicide has caused disorganization in family coping. Reassess interpersonal relationships in the context of the event. Discuss coping strategies that have been successful in times of stress in the past and work to reestablish these within the family. Identify new adaptive coping strategies that can be incorporated.
- Identify resources that provide support: religious beliefs and spiritual counselors, close friends and relatives, support groups for survivors of suicide.

9.9.4. Evaluation

Suicidal clients are evaluated continuously as part of an ongoing process that involves goal achievement and client reassessment. Extended psychotherapy may be recommended after the immediate crisis has been resolved. The long-term goals of individual or group psychotherapy for the suicidal client would be for him or her to:

- Develop and maintain a more positive self-concept.
- Learn more effective ways to express feelings to others.
- Achieve successful interpersonal relationships.
- Feel accepted by others and achieve a sense of belonging.

A suicidal person feels worthless and hopeless. These goals serve to instill a sense of self-worth, while offering a measure of hope and a meaning for living. (APA, 2000' Karasu et al., 2006)

A Closer Look

Mental Illness

Mental illness refers to a broad range of psychological conditions that disrupt a person's thinking, feeling, mood, behavior, and daily functioning. These conditions can vary in severity and can significantly impact an individual's ability to relate to others and handle day-to-day activities. Common mental illnesses include anxiety disorders, mood disorders such as depression and bipolar disorder, psychotic disorders like schizophrenia, and personality disorders.

Anxiety disorders, the most prevalent category, involve chronic fear, worry, or anxiety that is disproportionate to the actual situation, often leading to avoidance behaviors and significant distress. Depression, characterized by prolonged periods of sadness, hopelessness, and loss of interest in activities once enjoyed, can impair physical health and social functioning. Bipolar disorder involves dramatic shifts in mood, energy, and activity levels, ranging from manic highs to depressive lows. Schizophrenia, a severe mental disorder, can cause distorted thinking, perceptions, and emotions, often manifesting as hallucinations, delusions, and disorganized behavior.

The causes of mental illness are multifactorial, involving a combination of genetic, biological, environmental, and psychological factors. Genetic predisposition plays a significant role, with individuals having a family history of mental illness being more susceptible. Neurobiological factors, such as chemical imbalances in the brain and structural brain abnormalities, also contribute to the onset of these disorders. Environmental factors, including exposure to trauma, abuse, and prolonged stress, can trigger or worsen symptoms, particularly in those with a genetic vulnerability. Psychological factors, such as personality traits and maladaptive coping mechanisms, further influence the development and progression of mental illnesses.

Diagnosis of mental illness typically involves a thorough assessment by mental health professionals, including clinical interviews, psychological evaluations, and sometimes physical exams to rule out other medical conditions. Treatment approaches are varied and often tailored to the individual's specific needs. Pharmacotherapy, involving medications like antidepressants, antipsychotics, and mood stabilizers, can help manage symptoms and improve quality of life. Psychotherapy, including cognitive-behavioral therapy (CBT), psychodynamic therapy, and other forms of counseling, aims to address the underlying psychological issues, enhance coping strategies, and provide emotional support.

Despite advances in understanding and treatment, stigma remains a significant barrier to seeking help for mental illness. Misconceptions and societal prejudices can lead to discrimination, social isolation, and reluctance to pursue treatment, exacerbating the suffering of those affected. Public education and awareness campaigns are essential to challenge stigma, promote empathy and understanding, and encourage early intervention and support.

Access to mental healthcare is another critical issue, with disparities in availability and quality of services, particularly in low-income and rural areas. Addressing these gaps requires systemic changes, including increased funding for mental health services, better integration of mental healthcare into primary healthcare systems, and the expansion of community-based support networks. Telehealth has emerged as a promising solution to improve access to mental health care, offering remote consultations and therapy sessions to those unable to attend in-person appointments.

In summary, mental illness encompasses a wide array of disorders that affect millions globally, with significant implications for individuals and society. Effective management requires a comprehensive, multi-faceted approach that includes accurate diagnosis, personalized treatment plans, and concerted efforts to reduce stigma and improve access to care. Continued research and policy initiatives are crucial to advancing our understanding and treatment of mental illness, ultimately enhancing the well-being of those affected.

Summary

- A mood disorder is a mental health condition that primarily affects your emotional state. It's a disorder in which you experience long periods of extreme happiness, extreme sadness or both. Certain mood disorders involve other persistent emotions, such as anger and irritability.
- Depression is not merely a transient feeling of sadness or a response to life's challenges' it is a complex condition that can be triggered by various factors, including genetic predisposition, biochemical imbalances, and environmental stressors.
- Mood disturbances are associated with intoxication from substances such as alcohol, amphetamines, cocaine, hallucinogens, inhalants, opioids, phencyclidine, sedatives, hypnotics, and anxiolytics.
- Depressive symptoms that occur as a consequence of a non-mood disorder or as an adverse effect of certain medications are called secondary depression.
- Bipolar disorder is a lifelong mood disorder and mental health condition that causes intense shifts in mood, energy levels, thinking patterns and behavior. There are a few types of bipolar disorder, which involve experiencing significant fluctuations in mood referred to as hypomanic/manic and depressive episodes.
- Anxiety (generalized anxiety disorder) isn't a mood disorder. It's classified as one of many anxiety disorders, including panic disorder and phobias. However, anxiety often precedes or coexists with mood disorders.
- Psychotherapy, also called talk therapy, is a term for a variety of treatment techniques that aim to help a person identify and change unhealthy emotions, thoughts and behaviors.
- Electroconvulsive therapy (ECT) is a medical procedure that involves passing a mild electric current through your brain, causing a short seizure. This procedure is proven to have strong positive effects on severe, treatment-resistant mental health conditions, including depression and bipolar disorder.

References

1. (2005). *Taber's Cyclopedic Medical Dictionary* (20th ed.). Philadelphia: FA Davis.
2. Abrams, R. (2002). *Electroconvulsive Therapy* (4th ed.). New York: Oxford University Press.
3. Administration on Aging. (2010). *A Profile of Older Americans: 2009*. Washington, DC: U.S. Department of Health and Human Services.
4. American Psychiatric Association (APA). (2000). *Diagnostic and Statistical Manual of Mental Disorders* (4th ed., Text Revision). Washington, DC: American Psychiatric Publishing.
5. Andreasen, N. C., & Black, D. W. (2006). *Introductory Textbook of Psychiatry* (4th ed.). Washington, DC: American Psychiatric Publishing.
6. Azoulay, L., Blais, L., Koren, G., LeLorier, J., & Berard, A. (2008). Isotretinoin and the risk of depression in patients with acne vulgaris: A case-crossover study. *The Journal of Clinical Psychiatry, 69*(4), 526–532.

7. Beck, A. T., Rush, A. J., Shaw, B. F., & Emery, G. (1979). *Cognitive Theory of Depression*. New York: Guilford Press.

8. Cartwright, L. (2004). Emergencies of survival: Moral spectatorship and the new vision of the child in postwar child psychoanalysis. *Journal of Visual Culture, 3*(1), 35–49.

9. Davidson, L. (2005). *Suicide and Season*. New York: American Foundation for Suicide Prevention.

10. Dubovsky, S. L., Davies, R., & Dubovsky, A. M. (2003). Mood disorders. In R. E. Hales & S. C. Yudofsky (Eds.), *Textbook of Clinical Psychiatry* (4th ed.). Washington, DC: American Psychiatric Publishing.

11. Eranti, S., Mogg, A., Pluck, G., Landau, S., Purvis, R., Brown, R. G., Howard, R., Knapp, M., Philpot, M., Rabe-Hesketh, S., Romeo, R., Rothwell, J., Edwards, D., & McLoughlin, D. M. (2007). A randomized, controlled trial with 6-month follow-up of repetitive transcranial magnetic stimulation and electroconvulsive therapy for severe depression. *American Journal of Psychiatry, 164*(1), 73–81.

12. Frackiewicz, E. J., & Shiovitz, T. M. (2001). Evaluation and management of premenstrual syndrome. *Journal of the American Pharmaceutical Association, 41*(3), 437–447.

13. Frank, L. R. (2002). Electroshock: A crime against the spirit. *Ethical Human Sciences & Services, 4*(1), 63–71.

14. Fraser, M. (2006). What about us? The legacy of suicide. Retrieved from: http://suicideandmentalhealthassociationinternational.org/whaaboutus.html (accessed on 7 September 2024).

15. Freud, S. (1957). *Mourning and Melancholia* (Vol. 14, Standard ed.). London: Hogarth Press. (Original work published 1917.)

16. Friends for Survival. (2009). Facts and fables. Retrieved from: https://friendsforsurvival.org/fables-and-facts.

17. Geddes, J. R. (2003). Efficacy and safety of electroconvulsive therapy in depressive disorders: A systematic review and meta-analysis. *The Lancet, 361*(9360), 799–808.

18. George, L. K. (1992). Social factors and depression. In K. W. Schaie, D. Blazer, & J. S. House (Eds.), *Aging, Health Behaviors, and Health Outcomes*. Hillsdale, NJ: Lawrence Erlbaum Associates.

19. Grover, S., Mattoo, S. K., & Gupta, N. (2005). Theories on mechanism of action of electroconvulsive therapy. *German Journal of Psychiatry, 8*(4), 70–84.

20. Hakko, H. (2000). *Seasonal Variation of Suicides and Homicides in Finland*. Oulu, Finland: University of Oulu.

21. Hall, J. M., & Bensing, K. (2009). Electroconvulsive therapy. *ADVANCE Newsmagazine for Nurses Online*. Retrieved from: http://nursing.advanceweb.com (accessed on 7 September 2024).

22. Harvard Medical School. (2002). Depression in children—Part I. *The Harvard Mental Health Letter*. Boston, MA: Harvard Medical School Publications Group.

23. Hudson, C. G. (2005). Socioeconomic status and mental illness: Tests of the social causation and selection hypotheses. *American Journal of Orthopsychiatry, 75*(1), 3–18.

24. Joska, J. A., & Stein, D. J. (2008). Mood disorders. In R. E. Hales, S. C. Yudofsky, & G. O. Gabbard (Eds.), *Textbook of Psychiatry* (5th ed.). Washington, DC: American Psychiatric Publishing.

25. Karasu, T. B., Gelenberg, A., Merriam, A., & Wang, P. (2006). Practice guideline for the treatment of patients with major depressive disorder (2nd ed.). *American Psychiatric Association Practice Guidelines for the Treatment of Psychiatric Disorders, Compendium 2006*. Washington, DC: American Psychiatric Publishing.

26. Kornstein, S. G. (2006). Gender and depression. *MedscapeCME*. Retrieved from: http://cme.medscape.com/viewarticle/527494 (accessed on 7 September 2024).

27. Lam, R. W., Levitt, A. J., Levitan, R. D., Enns, M. W., Morehouse, R., Michalak, E. E., & Tam, E. M. (2006). The Can-SAD Study: A randomized controlled trial of the effectiveness of light therapy and fluoxetine in patients with winter seasonal affective disorder. *The American Journal of Psychiatry, 163*(5), 805–812.

28. LaPierre, T. A. (2004). An investigation of the role of age and life stage in the moderation and mediation of the effect of marital status on depression. Paper presented at the annual meeting of the American Sociological Association, San Francisco, CA, August 14, 2004. Retrieved from: http://www.allacademic.com/meta/p109917_index.html (accessed on 7 September 2024).

29. Macnab, F. (1993). *Brief Psychotherapy: An Integrative Approach in Clinical Practice*. West Sussex, England: John Wiley & Sons.

30. Marangell, L. B., Silver, J. M., Goff, D. C., & Yudofsky, S. C. (2003). Psychopharmacology and electroconvulsive therapy. In R. E. Hales & S. C. Yudofsky (Eds.), *Textbook of Clinical Psychiatry*. Washington, DC: American Psychiatric Publishing.

31. Martinez, M., Marangell, L. B., & Martinez, J. M. (2008). Psychopharmacology. In R. E. Hales, S. C. Yudofsky, & G. O. Gabbard (Eds.), *Textbook of Psychiatry* (5th ed.). Washington, DC: American Psychiatric Publishing.

32. Mehta, A., & Sheth, S. (2006). Postpartum depression: How to recognize and treat this common condition. *Medscape Psychiatry & Mental Health, 11*(1). Retrieved from: http://www.medscape.com/viewarticle/529390 (accessed on 7 September 2024).

33. Mental Health Sanctuary. (2009). How to help a suicidal person. Retrieved from: http://www.mhsanctuary.com/suicide/sui2.htm (accessed on 7 September 2024).

34. National Center for Health Statistics (NCHS). (2009). *Health, United States, 2008*. Hyattsville, MD: NCHS.

35. National Center for Injury Prevention and Control. (2009). 20 leading causes of death, United States 2006, all races, both sexes. Retrieved from: http://www.cdc.gov/injury/wisqars/index.html (accessed on 7 September 2024).

36. National Institute of Mental Health. (2009). Antidepressant medications for children and adolescents: Information for parents and caregivers. Retrieved from: http://www.nimh.nih.gov/ (accessed on 7 September 2024).

37. Popolos, D. (2009). All about ECT. Retrieved from: http://www.schizophrenia.com/family/ect1.html (accessed on 7 September 2024).

38. Prator, B. C. (2006). Serotonin syndrome. *Journal of Neuroscience Nursing, 38*(2), 102–105.

39. Pridmore, S., Khan, U. A., Reid, P., & George, M. S. (2001). Transcranial magnetic stimulation in depression: An overview. *German Journal of Psychiatry, 4*(3), 43–50.

40. Rosenbaum, J. F., & Judy, A. E. (2004). New brain stimulation therapies for depression. *Medscape*

Psychiatry & Mental Health. Retrieved from: http://www.medscape.com/viewarticle/480897 (accessed on 7 September 2024).

41. Rupke, S. J., Blecke, D., & Renfrow, M. (2006). Cognitive therapy for depression. *American Family Physician, 73*(1), 83–86.
42. Sackeim, H. A., Prudic, J., Fuller, R., Keilp, J., Lavori, P. W., & Olfson, M. (2007). The cognitive effects of electroconvulsive therapy in community settings. *Neuropsychopharmacology, 32*(1), 244–254.
43. Sadock, B. J., & Sadock, V. A. (2007). *Synopsis of Psychiatry: Behavioral Sciences/Clinical Psychiatry* (10th ed.). Philadelphia: Lippincott Williams & Wilkins.
44. Samaritans (The). (2009). Suicide myths and misconceptions. Retrieved from: http://www.samaritansnyc.org/myths.html (accessed on 7 September 2024).
45. Schatzberg, A. F., Cole, J. O., & DeBattista, C. (2007). *Manual of Clinical Psychopharmacology* (6th ed.). Washington, DC: American Psychiatric Publishing.
46. Schimelpfening, N. (2009). A good vitamin supplement could be just what the doctor ordered. Retrieved from: http://depression.about.com/cs/diet/a/vitamin.htm (accessed on 7 September 2024).
47. Seligman, M. E. P. (1973). Fall into helplessness. *Psychology Today, 7*(1), 43–48.
48. Slattery, D. A., Hudson, A. L., & Nutt, D. J. (2004). Invited review: The evolution of antidepressant mechanisms. *Fundamental & Clinical Pharmacology, 18*(1), 1–21.
49. Substance Abuse and Mental Health Services Administration (SAMHSA). (2009). *2008 National Survey on Drug Use & Health*. Retrieved https://www.samhsa.gov/data/data-we-collect/nsduh-national-survey-drug-use-and-health.
50. Tempfer, T. C. (2006). Identifying childhood depression. Retrieved from: https://www.medscape.org/viewarticle/532598.
51. Terman, M., & Terman, J. S. (2005). Light therapy for seasonal and nonseasonal depression: Efficacy, protocol, safety, and side effects. *CNS Spectrums, 10*(8), 647–663.
52. Thase, M. E. (2007). The new "blue light" intervention for seasonal affective disorder (SAD). *Medscape Psychiatry & Mental Health*. Retrieved from: http://cme.medscape.com/viewarticle/550845 (accessed on 7 September 2024).
53. Tondo, L., & Baldessarini, R. J. (2001). Suicide: Historical, descriptive, and epidemiological considerations. Retrieved from: http://www.medscape.com/viewprogram/352 (accessed on 7 September 2024).
54. U.S. Public Health Service (USPHS). (1999). *The Surgeon General's Call to Action to Prevent Suicide*. Washington, DC: USPHS.
55. Wahlund, B., & von Rosen, D. (2003). ECT of major depressed patients in relation to biological and clinical variables: A brief overview. *Neuropsychopharmacology, 28*(Suppl 1), S21–S26.
56. Williams, D. R., Gonzalez, H. M., Neighbors, H., Nesse, R., Abelson, J. M., Sweetman, J., & Jackson, J. S. (2007). Prevalence and distribution of major depressive disorder in African Americans, Caribbean Blacks, and Non-Hispanic Whites: Results from the National Survey of American Life. *Archives of General Psychiatry, 64*(3), 305–315.

INDEX

E

F

G

N

O

P

R

S

T

Printed and bound by CPI Group (UK) Ltd, Croydon, CR0 4YY
18/09/2026
14965061-0003